Essentials in
Total Hip Arthroplasty

Essentials in
Total Hip Arthroplasty

Javad Parvizi, MD, FRCS
Department of Orthopedic Surgery
Thomas Jefferson University
The Rothman Institute
Philadelphia, Pennsylvania

Brian A. Klatt, MD
Orthopedic Surgeon
University of Pittsburgh School of Medicine
Pittsburgh, Pennsylvania

SLACK
INCORPORATED

www.Healio.com/books

ISBN: 978-1-55642-870-8

Published by: SLACK Incorporated,
6900 Grove Road
Thorofare, NJ 08086 USA
Telephone: 856-848-1000
Fax: 856-848-6091
www.Healio.com/books

Contact SLACK Incorporated for more information about other books in this field or about the availability of our books from distributors outside the United States.

Library of Congress Cataloging-in-Publication Data

Essentials in total hip arthroplasty / [edited by] Javad Parvizi, Brian Klatt.
p. ; cm.
Includes bibliographical references and index.
ISBN 978-1-55642-870-8 (alk. paper)
I. Parvizi, Javad. II. Klatt, Brian A.
[DNLM: 1. Arthroplasty, Replacement, Hip--methods. 2. Hip--surgery. 3. Hip Joint--surgery. 4. Hip Prosthesis. WE 860]

617.5'81059--dc23

2012040462

Printed in the United States of America.

Last digit is print number: 10 9 8 7 6 5 4 3 2 1

Dedication

To my lovely wife Fariba, my most loyal supporter, and my children Niosha and Cyrus, who bring joy and fun to my life.

Javad Parvizi, MD, FRCS

To my brother Tim; he inspired me to pursue a career in medicine.

Brian A. Klatt, MD

Contents

Acknowledgments

To my wife Brooke, who supports me in all my endeavors.

To my father, who read and edited the companion knee book; his insights improved this book.

To Carrie Kotlar, who believed in this project and made it a reality.

To the members of the divisions of Adult Reconstruction and Musculoskeletal Oncology at the University of Pittsburgh (Dr. Crossett, Dr. Goodman, Dr. Yates, Dr. McGough, and Dr. Weiss). Our daily interactions help me grow as a surgeon.

To the members of the Rothman Institute who put me on the path to an academic career in adult reconstruction.

Brian A. Klatt, MD

About the Editors

Javad Parvizi MD, FRCS is a Professor of Orthopedic Surgery at the Rothman Institute and Thomas Jefferson University with an interest in reconstruction of complex pelvis, hip, and knee diseases with special emphasis on joint preservation. He is a member of numerous national and international societies, such as the Hip Society, the Knee Society, and the Association of Hip and Knee Surgeons, and has served in leadership roles in a large number of national committees. He is a member of various editorial boards for orthopedic journals. He has received wide recognition for his clinical and basic science research, including the Brazilian presidential award of honor, 5 Hip Society awards, and 4 Knee Society awards, as well as numerous honors from other societies. He has authored over 350 peer-reviewed manuscripts, is the editor of 5 text books in orthopedics, and has authored over 120 chapters.

Brian A. Klatt, MD graduated from the University of Pittsburgh School of Medicine in 1997. After completing his orthopedic residency at the University of Pittsburgh, he served 4 years on active duty with the United States Air Force. The final 2 years in the military were spent working with the residency program at Wilford Hall Medical Center, and it was there that his commitment to education was solidified. After an honorable discharge from the military, Dr. Klatt completed a fellowship in adult reconstruction at the Rothman Institute, Thomas Jefferson University in Philadelphia. His decision to attend a fellowship at the Rothman Institute was a direct result of meeting Dr. Rothman at a lecture in San Antonio. Dr. Klatt has been lucky to be mentored by many of the great names in orthopedic surgery today. He is currently an Assistant Professor of Orthopedic Surgery at the University of Pittsburgh. Dr. Klatt returned to the University of Pittsburgh, where he continues to dedicate himself to the education of medical students and residents. His research interests are varied and encompass both clinical and basic science topics. He is honored to have worked with Dr. Parvizi to produce this text. This text is their second collaborative effort. Dr. Klatt hopes that it will provide a quick and easy source for residents who seek to understand the essential information required to master total hip arthroplasty.

Contributing Authors

Christopher S. Adams, PhD (Chapter 6)
Associate Professor
Philadelphia College of Osteopathic Medicine
Department of Anatomy
Philadelphia, Pennsylvania

Matt Austin, MD (Chapter 15)
Associate Professor of Orthopaedic Surgery
Thomas Jefferson University Hospital
The Rothman Institute
Philadelphia, Pennsylvania

Khalid Azzam, MD (Chapter 27)
Resident, Department of Orthopaedic Surgery
University of Nebraska Medical Center
Omaha, Nebraska

Robert L. Barrack, MD (Chapter 14)
Charles and Joanne Knight
Distinguished Professor of Orthopedic Surgery
Washington University Orthopedics
Chief of Staff for Orthopedic Surgery
Barnes-Jewish Hospital
St. Louis, Missouri

Ravi K. Bashyal, MD (Chapter 14)
NorthShore University Health System
Department of Orthopaedic Surgery
Evanston, Illinois

Benjamin Bender, MD (Chapters 11, 14, 21)
Hip and Knee Specialist
Joint Replacement Specialist
Assuta Hospital
Tel-Aviv, Israel

Hari P. Bezwada, MD (Chapter 26)
Staff Surgeon
Hip and Knee Reconstruction
Princeton Orthopaedic Associates
Princeton, New Jersey

Orhan Bican, MD (Chapter 12)
Research Fellow
The Rothman Institute
Philadelphia, Pennsylvania

James Cashman, MD (Chapters 19, 27)
Arthroplasty Fellow
The Rothman Institute
Philadelphia, Pennsylvania

Michael E. Ciminiello, MD (Chapter 19)
Attending Physician
Peconic Bay Medical Center
Riverhead, New York

Erika Davis, MD (Chapter 31)
Resident, Department of Anesthesia
Thomas Jefferson University
Philadelphia, Pennsylvania

Craig J. Della Valle, MD (Chapter 13)
Associate Professor of Orthopaedic Surgery
Rush University Medical Center
Chicago, Illinois

Joshua C. Fox, MD (Chapter 28)
Austin Bone and Joint Clinic
Austin, Texas

Mitchell K. Freedman, DO (Chapter 3)
Associate Professor in Physical Medicine
Thomas Jefferson University Hospital
Director of Physical Medicine and Rehabilitation
The Rothman Institute
Philadelphia, Pennsylvania

Kishor Gandhi, MD, MPH (Chapter 20)
Department of Anesthesiology
Division of Acute Pain Management and Regional Anesthesia
Thomas Jefferson University
Philadelphia, Pennsylvania

Elie Ghanem, MD (Chapters 15, 17)
Total Joint Replacement Fellow
Department of Orthopedics
New England Baptist Hospital
Boston, Massachusetts

Ashok Gowda, MD (Chapter 11)
New York Medical College
Orthopaedic Surgery Resident
Valhalla, New York

Eric L. Grossman, MD, FAAOS (Chapter 9)
Mount Kisco Medical Group
Northern Westchester Hospital
Co-Director of Joint Replacement
Department of Orthopedic Surgery
Mount Kisco, New York

Sanaz Hariri, MD (Chapter 22)
Fellow, Massachussets General Hospital
Harvard Medical School
Boston, Massachussets

Kristen Hines, PT (Chapter 31)
Clinical Team Leader
Rehabilitation Medicine
Thomas Jefferson University Hospital
Philadelphia, Pennsylvania

Pooya Hosseinzadeh, MD (Chapter 2)
Pediatric Orthopaedic Fellow
Shriners Hospitals for Children
Lexington, Kentucky

William J. Hozack, MD (Chapters 18, 23)
Professor of Orthopedic Surgery
Thomas Jefferson University Medical School
The Rothman Institute
Philadelphia, Pennsylvania

Ronald Huang, MD (Chapters 5, 23)
Resident
Department of Orthopaedic Surgery
Thomas Jefferson University Hospital
Philadelphia, Pennsylvania

Michael H. Huo, MD (Chapter 28)
Department of Orthopedic Surgery
University of Texas Southwestern Medical Center
Dallas, Texas

S. Mehdi Jafari, MD (Chapters 1, 23)
Assistant Professor of Orthopaedic Surgery
Tehran University of Medical Sciences
Shariati Hospital
Tehran, Iran

Thomas K. John, MD (Chapter 21)
Resident in Orthopedic Surgery
Albert Einstein Medical Center
Philadelphia, Pennsylvania

Lauren K. Kahl, MD (Chapter 12)
Harriet Lane Pediatric Residency
Johns Hopkins Hospital
Baltimore, Maryland

Steven Kurtz, PhD (Chapter 7)
Corporate Vice President and Practice Director
Biomedical Engineering
Exponent, Inc
Research Professor
School of Biomedical Science, Engineering, and Health Systems
Drexel University
Philadelphia, Pennsylvania

Lawrence P. Lai, MD, MS (Chapter 24)
Department of Orthopedic Surgery
Wake Forest University
Winston-Salem, North Carolina
Department of Physical Medicine and Rehabilitation
New Jersey Medical School
Newark, New Jersey

Eric Levicoff, MD (Chapter 16)
Clinical Instructor
University of Pittsburgh Medical Center
Department of Orthopedic Surgery
Pittsburgh, Pennsylvania

Junaid Makda, MD (Chapter 10)
Dupage Orthopedics
Bloomingdale, Illinois

Henrik Malchau, MD, PhD (Chapter 22)
Professor at Harvard Medical School
Co-Director, The Harris Orthopaedic Laboratory
Vice Chief of Orthopedics (Research)
Attending Physician, Adult Reconstructive Unit
Orthopedic Department
Massachusetts General Hospital
Boston, Massachusetts

Michael Manley, PhD (Chapter 7)
Homer Stryker Center for Orthopedic Education and Research
Mahwah, New Jersey

Richard L. McGough III, MD (Chapter 4)
Associate Professor of Orthopaedic Surgery
University of Pittsburgh
Chief, Division of Musculoskeletal Oncology
Co-Director of Sarcoma Specialty Center
University of Pittsburgh Cancer Institute
Pittsburgh, Pennsylvania

Michael A. Mont, MD (Chapter 24)
Director
Center for Joint Preservation and Reconstruction
Rubin Institute of Advanced Orthopedics
Sinai Hospital of Baltimore
Baltimore, Maryland

S.M. Javad Mortazavi, MD (Chapters 3, 5, 9)
Associated Professor of Orthopedic Surgery
Tehran University of Medical Sciences
Department of Orthopedic Surgery
Tehran, Iran

CDR M.T. Newman, MD (Chapter 26)
Vice Chairman
Department of Orthopaedic Surgery
Walter Reed National Military Medical Center
Bethesda, Maryland

Ali Oliashirazi, MD (Chapter 2)
Professor and Chair
Department of Orthopedics
Marshall University
Joan C. Edwards School of Medicine
Huntington, West Virginia

Katie O'Shea, PT, DPT, MBA (Chapter 31)
Advanced Clinician I
Rehabilitation Medicine
Thomas Jefferson University Hospital

Brett Perricelli, MD (Chapter 4)
St. Clair Memorial Hospital
South Hills Orthopaedic Surgical Associates
Bethel Park, Pennsylvania

Manny Porat, MD (Chapters 8, 16)
Resident
Department of Orthopedic Surgery
Thomas Jefferson University
Philadelphia, Pennsylvania

Luis Pulido, MD (Chapter 18)
Resident
Orthopedic Surgery
Mayo Clinic Rochester
Department of Orthopedic Surgery
Rochester, Minnesota

James J. Purtill, MD (Chapter 19)
Associate Professor
Vice Chairman
Department of Orthopedic Surgery
Thomas Jefferson University
The Rothman Institute
Philadelphia, Pennsylvania

Aaron G. Rosenberg, MD (Foreword)
Professor of Surgery
Rush Medical College
Chicago, Illinois

Adam J. Schwartz, MD (Chapter 13)
Assistant Professor
Department of Orthopaedic Surgery
Mayo Clinic
Phoenix, Arizona

Eric Schwenk, MD (Chapter 20)
Department of Anesthesiology
Division of Acute Pain Management and Regional Anesthesia
Thomas Jefferson University
Philadelphia, Pennsylvania

Thorsten M. Seyler, MD (Chapter 24)
Resident, Department of Orthopaedic Surgery
Wake Forest University School of Medicine
Winston-Salem, North Carolina

Peter F. Sharkey, MD (Chapter 9)
Professor of Orthopaedic Surgery
Thomas Jefferson University Hospital
The Rothman Institute
Philadelphia, Pennsylvania

Eric B. Smith, MD (Chapter 10)
Thomas Jefferson University
The Rothman Institute of Orthopedics
Philadelphia, Pennsylvania

Bryan D. Springer, MD (Chapter 29)
OrthoCarolina Hip and Knee Center
Charlotte, North Carolina

G. Daxton Steele, MD, PharmD (Chapter 30)
Staff Physician
Andrews Institute/BMG
Orthopaedics and Sports Medicine
Gulf Breeze, Florida

Eugene R. Viscusi, MD (Chapter 20)
Department of Anesthesiology
Division of Acute Pain Management and Regional Anesthesia
Thomas Jefferson University
Philadelphia, Pennsylvania

Kristen Vogl, PT, DPT (Chapter 31)
Clinical Team Leader
Department of Rehabilitation Medicine
Thomas Jefferson University
Philadelphia, Pennsylvania

Adolf J. Yates Jr, MD (Chapter 30)
Associate Professor
Department of Orthopaedic Surgery
University of Pittsburgh School of Medicine
Pittsburgh, Pennsylvania

Khalid M. Yousuf, MD, MS (Chapters 10, 25)
University of Oklahoma
Department of Orthopedic Surgery and Rehabilitation
Oklahoma City, Oklahoma

FOREWORD

Over the past 30 years, I have dedicated many of my efforts to teaching management of the adult hip to students of orthopedic surgery. Unfortunately, I have never found an appropriate textbook for the numerous medical students and residents approaching this field as beginners or for the more seasoned resident or young surgeon who needs review or updating. This is the text we have been waiting for. Dr. Parvizi and Dr. Klatt have provided a definitive monograph on the adult hip perfect for the student (at any level) in need of a concise, compact, yet complete source of information about hip disease and its modern treatment. While gathering important experts in the fields of osteonecrosis, complicated arthroplasty, indications for surgery, preoperative planning, outcomes, and material science, much of the text comes from clinicians at the Rothman Institute.

Richard Rothman was one of the first orthopedic clinicians to produce a comprehensive instructional monograph for both students and practitioners in the field of spine surgery. It was a landmark work and the research and educational excellence that have marked the Institute's history are exemplified by this volume. Dr. Parvizi now brings all of the talent and the industry that has produced a remarkable research career in the field of adult reconstructive orthopedics at the Rothman Institute to the task of providing a monograph on the adult hip. Perfect for medical students and residents looking for a comprehensive overview of the field while on service or the generalist looking to bring his knowledge base up to date, this volume stands alone in bringing current information to the practitioner in a concise and comprehensive manner. References are extensive but rarely outmoded or excessive; important subjects are reviewed in convenient tables and text box summaries. This text provides coverage that is comprehensive but not overwhelming.

In addition to information on biomechanics and materials as well as component design and surgical technique, there are excellent chapters on preoperative planning, indications for total hip arthroplasty, and management of complications and rehabilitation. It can be readily assimilated by the student unfamiliar with orthopedics but is best suited as a comprehensive education for the resident, or to use for review prior to board preparation.

All orthopedic surgeons interested in a comprehensive overview of the evaluation and treatment of the adult hip will benefit from this text, but those involved in education will be particularly eager to recommend this volume to their students for its comprehensive but compact exposure to the best current thought in the field.

Aaron G. Rosenberg, MD
Professor of Surgery
Rush Medical College
Chicago, Illinois

PREFACE

Performing total hip arthroplasty (THA) is a satisfying operation that can be accomplished with relative ease in the majority of patients. There are, however, patients in whom this procedure requires special attention to preoperative optimization (such as in patients with bleeding disorders or vascular disease) and may require a special set of instruments or alterations in surgical techniques (such as patients with gross deformities or Paget's disease), or the type of prosthesis may need to be altered to accommodate the anatomical aberration (such as in patients with post-traumatic arthritis).

Despite its lauded success, THA does occasionally fail, leading to a need for revision arthroplasty. Knowledge of how to prevent failures such as infection, periprosthetic fractures, and instability is critical for enhancing the success and longevity of THA. The ability to deal with these complications when they occur and perform a reconstructive procedure in patients with failed THA is also an essential part of training any reconstructive joint surgeon.

Essentials in Total Hip Arthroplasty contains relevant, practical, and important information related to disorders of the hip that a reconstruction surgeon needs to know. It is a practical manual for the practicing or training orthopedic surgeon who treats patients with disorders of the hip. This book, written by renowned experts, provides step-by-step practical guidance and relevant information for the treatment of hip problems. Brian Klatt and I decided to write this book when we became aware of the vacuum in orthopedics and the need for such a text. This book is comprehensive, reader-friendly, and useful to the practicing orthopedic surgeon. I am most grateful to all the authors who, despite their immense commitments, took on the task of writing a comprehensive, evidence-based, and illustrated text.

Last but not least, I want to thank Carrie Kotlar for her organizational skill and leadership of this project. I am also grateful to the other members of SLACK Incorporated for their support and commitment to this project.

Javad Parvizi, MD, FRCS

1

Applied Anatomy of the Hip

S. Mehdi Jafari, MD and Javad Parvizi, MD, FRCS

Operations on the hip joint through several surgical approaches are among the most common surgical procedures being performed in orthopedics. Hip arthroplasty is the most frequently performed adult reconstructive hip procedure.[1] Millions of patients with degenerative hip joint disease achieve significant improvement in their functional status and quality of life by hip replacement. In 2003, a total of 202,500 primary total hip arthroplasties (THAs) were performed nationally in the United States.[2]

Although hip arthroplasty is a relatively safe procedure with consistently good outcomes, incautious surgical dissections and reckless insertion of instruments and retractors can cause potentially limb- or life-threatening complications. Because of the increasing number of hip arthroplasties and surgeons' growing interest in using minimally invasive techniques, it is crucial for orthopedic surgeons to be thoroughly familiar with the anatomy of the hip region and the possible complications. This chapter details the clinical, surgical, and applied anatomy of the hip in arthroplasty.

Bone Anatomy

Os Coxa and Acetabulum

The acetabular surface is oriented approximately 45 degrees caudally and 15 degrees anteriorly.[3] It has predominantly a circular contour and a hemispherical depth to allow 170-degree coverage of the femoral head.[4] The labrum serves to augment the femoral head coverage, thereby increasing the depth and stability of the hip joint.

The transverse acetabular ligament (TAL) is effectively the continuation of the labrum and forms a bridge across the inferior acetabular notch. This ligament can be used as a practical landmark to identify the inferior aspect of the acetabulum and to minimize the risk of acetabular components malpositioning during primary THA (Figure 1-1) even when minimally invasive methods are being used. It defines the anteversion of the acetabular component without the need for external instrumentation and is independent of patient position.[4]

The transverse acetabular ligament may be used as a guide to acetabular reaming.[5] Maintaining a parallel orientation of the face of the reamer and subsequently the acetabular component to the TAL likely represents natural version for the patient.[5] If a gap is present between the TAL and the reamer, the acetabular component will sit too high. If the reamer is hemispherical, the inferior superficial border should sit just inside the ligament, thereby controlling for depth as well as for height.

An anterior and posterior osseous column of bone surrounds the acetabulum and functions to transmit force between the trunk and lower extremities. The thickness of the columns varies as they pass around the acetabulum. If pelvic discontinuity is suspected, a computed tomography (CT) scan should be performed.[6] Signs of pelvic discontinuity on an anteroposterior radiograph include a visible fracture line through the anterior and posterior columns, rotation of the inferior aspect of the hemipelvis relative to the superior aspect, and medial translation of the inferior aspect of the hemipelvis relative to the superior aspect.[6] The

Parvizi J, Klatt BA.
Essentials in Total Hip Arthroplasty (pp 1-11).

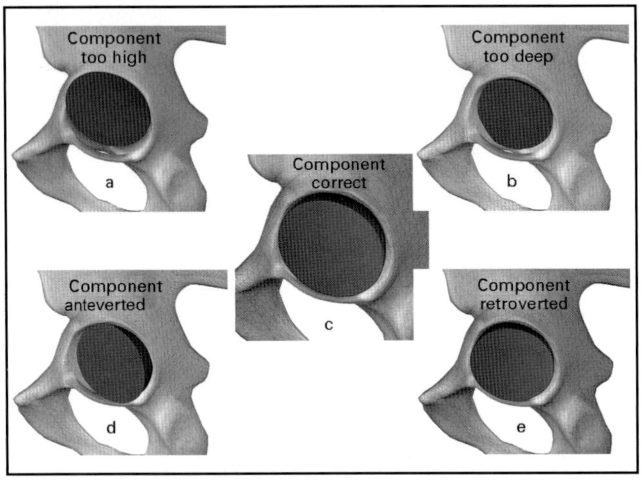

Figure 1-1. The position of the acetabular component in relation to transverse acetabular ligament: (a) high, (b) deep, (c) correct height, depth, and version, (d) correct height and depth but anteverted, and (e) correct height and depth but retroverted.

latter is seen as a break in the Kohler line. Furthermore, overreaming may remove most or all of the bone from the anterior and posterior parts of the acetabular rim, making it difficult to obtain a press-fit for cementless cups.[6] Excessive reaming of the columns may also decrease the available bone depth, limiting the screw purchase needed for peripheral and transacetabular screws to augment acetabular component fixation.[4]

Femur

The head of the femur articulates at the acetabulum and is positioned anteriorly, superiorly, and medially. The femoral neck is typically angled 125 degrees to the shaft and the center of the femoral head is at the level of the lateral aspect of the greater trochanter. The distance between the center of the femoral head and the lateral aspect of the greater trochanter can vary independent of the neck-shaft angle.[4]

The femoral neck and the metaphysis are typically positioned at 15 degrees of anteversion in relation to the posterior aspect of the femoral condyles.[7-9] Excessive anteversion limits the ability to utilize fixed stems without considerable undersizing or osteotomy. A CT scan prior to THA, although not routinely done, can evaluate the extent of anteversion. Notably, a hip in excessive anteversion is approached best through an anterolateral technique. By contrast a retroverted hip is more easily accessed through a posterolateral surgical approach.[4]

The proximal femoral metaphyseal configuration is variable and difficult to predict without CT imaging.[10-13] Generally, however, the proximal femur of younger patients tends to have a trumpet-like or champagne-fluted configuration.[14] Endosteal expansion of the isthmus with age results in a stovepipe design in more elderly patients.[14-16] The configuration of the proximal femur may affect the efficacy of cementless femoral implants with fixed proximal geometries. A cementless stem must fit the anterior-posterior and medial-lateral dimensions and also maximize contact between their porous coating and the endosteal femoral surface. The canal configuration affects the ability of the porous coating of an implant to be adequately apposed to the endosteal surface. In a femur with stovepipe configuration, adequate endosteal contact is limited and a femoral implant with a more porous surface or cemented implant may be necessary. The Dorr index attempts to characterize proximal femoral configurations by calculating a ratio of the canal diameter at the level of the lesser trochanter to the canal diameter at a point 10 cm distal.[17]

The shaft of the femoral bone is predominantly cylindrical throughout its length and is bowed anteriorly and laterally in its midportion. The extent of bowing is clinically relevant as it indicates the extent of undersizing that may be necessary for long, straight implants.[4]

Landmarks

For hip arthroplasty, several surgical landmarks exist within the bony pelvis. Even in complex revision cases with significant bone loss, these landmarks may be present, and careful identification of them is vital.

The anterior border, posterior border, and lip of the greater trochanter are used as a guide for proper skin incision. Its posterior aspect is relatively free of muscles; its anterior and lateral aspects are covered by the tensor fascia lata and the gluteus medius and minimus muscles and are much less accessible.

Specific points on the ischium, the superior pubic ramus, and superior acetabulum aid in defining a plane that allows adequate cup orientation in abduction and version.[18] Positioning of the acetabular component using these anatomical landmarks may reduce the incidence of dislocation from improper acetabular orientation. The first landmark is on the ischium and is the lowest point in the sulcus between the acetabulum and the ischeal tuberosity. Intraoperative identification of this point can be accomplished by sliding a Cobb elevator over the acetabular rim along the ischium until reaching the lowest point of the sulcus.[18] The second point is located on the lateral portion of the superior pubic ramus. The point is located at the confluence of the inferior aspect of the iliopectineal eminence and the pubic rami. This point is readily distinguishable although not an eminent osseous landmark. The point can be clearly seen or palpated at approximately 5 mm from the acetabular rim by following the ridge of the ramus toward the acetabulum.[18] The third point is the most superior aspect of the acetabulum. The orientation of the reamer and component is positioned according to the plane defined by the rim of the component passing through the first 2 landmarks and medialized to the acetabular fossa.

The anterior-superior iliac spine may aid in identification of the competent acetabular bone and guiding the placement of transacetabular screws.[4] The anterior and posterior brim may indicate if appropriate acetabular component anteversion and flexion are present.[4] The base of the fovea may serve as a guide to the extent that the acetabulum can be medially reamed.[4,11] Locating the fovea is of particular importance in the presence of a large medial osteophyte as failure to remove the osteophyte may result in a lateralized acetabular component.[4]

The transverse acetabular ligament provides a landmark to identify the inferior aspect of the acetabulum and serves as a restraint to inferior drifting of an acetabular reamer in cases where the superior acetabular bone is sclerotic.[4] It can also be used as a guide to acetabular reaming as noted above.[5]

Hip Joint Capsule

The hip joint capsule functions to restrict translation between the femur and acetabulum while allowing rotational and planar movements. The capsule is attached along the anterior and posterior margins of the acetabulum. The attachment is outside the acetabular labrum such that anterior and posterior incisions between the capsule and labrum allow retractors to be placed over the anterior and posterior columns.

Three accessory ligaments reinforce the hip joint capsule. The iliofemoral and pubofemoral reinforce the anterior portion while the ischiofemoral ligament reinforces the posterior portion. The iliofemoral and ischiofemoral ligaments are the most significant and anatomically consistent.[19] The iliofemoral ligament functions to restrict extension of the hip and provide a static restraint with full hip extension that allows erect posture to be maintained without constant muscular action.[20,21] Contracture of the iliofemoral ligament may produce a flexion/internal rotation contracture that requires release at THA. It is particularly important to correct this contracture in a posterior approach to the hip, otherwise a tendency toward hip internal rotation will result.[4] An anterolateral approach will perforce release of an internal rotation contracture.

The pubofemoral ligament becomes taut in hip extension and abduction. The ligament may need to be released to correct a hip adduction contracture during hip arthroplasty. The ischiofemoral ligament reinforces the posterior portion of the capsule and contains spiral and horizontal fibers.[4,19] The spiral fibers become taut during extension. The horizontal fibers restrict internal rotation of the hip.

In the absence of previous surgery, dislocation of the hip or injury to the hip capsule ligaments generally requires relatively high forces.[19,22] The incidence of hip dislocation following THA is approximately 3%.[23] Up to 70% of these dislocations occur 4 to 5 weeks after surgery and are most commonly the result of soft tissue laxity prior to the healing of the pseudocapsule.[24] Repair and proper tensioning of the hip capsule after THA can reduce soft tissue laxity and potentially decrease the incidence of early dislocation after surgery.

Hip Musculature

The muscles of the hip joint are unique in their large areas of origin and insertion, length, large cross section, and the extensive range of motion they permit. The hip joint may accommodate flexion 120 degrees, extension 30 degrees, abduction 45 to 50 degrees, adduction 20 to 30 degrees, internal rotation 25 degrees, and external rotation 45 degrees.[25,26] The hip musculature may be classified as flexors, extensors, abductors, adductors, external rotators, or internal rotators depending on the predominant function of the muscle.

Flexors

The primary hip flexors are the iliopsoas, rectus femoris, and sartorius. Other muscles are capable of contributing to flexion depending on the position of the hip. The tendon of the iliopsoas muscle traverses across the inferior aspect of the hip joint external to the hip capsule. The tendon serves as an important landmark for the depth to which dissection can be done during an inferior capsular resection.

The rectus femoris muscle functions to flex the hip joint and extend the knee joint. It is more effective as a hip flexor when the knee is flexed since knee flexion preloads the quadriceps muscles. When a hip flexion contracture exists or when the contracted hip has been lengthened by arthroplasty, release of the reflected head and transverse release of the rectus fascia may improve knee flexion with the hip extended.[4]

Extensors

The primary hip joint extensors are gluteus maximus and hamstring muscles. The combined strength of the hamstring muscles is less than that of the gluteus maximus muscle. The force generated by the hamstring muscles increases with hip flexion. In contrast, the gluteus maximus muscle strength is decreased as the hip flexes beyond neutral.[27]

Abductors

The gluteus medius and minimus muscles are the primary hip abductors. The gluteus medius is also active in hip flexion, internal rotation, extension, external rotation, and to provide pelvic support during one-legged stance. The gluteus minimus is also active in internal rotation and aids the gluteus medius with pelvic support and to counter hip adduction. THA may cause the gluteus minimus to tighten, resulting in an internal rotation contracture. Release of the undersurface of the muscle from caudad to cephalad may be necessary to prevent a tendency toward internal rotation that can lead to posterior hip dislocation.

The origin of the tensor fasciae lata is slightly more superficial and anterior to that of the gluteus medius. The anatomic relationship of the 2 muscles is an important element in an anterolateral approach to the hip. Incising the fascia lata posterior to the posterior margin of the tensor fasciae lata and retracting the cut fascial edge anteriorly allows separation of the 2 muscles along the intermusclar plane. Because the gluteus medius is covered and not enclosed by the fascia, it will not be retracted with the fascia. By contrast, the tensor fascia lata is enclosed by the fascia and the structures are retracted together.

Adductors

The adductor muscles of the hip include the adductor brevis, adductor longus, adductor magnus, pectineus, and gracilis. Adduction contractures are frequently found in pathologic conditions of the hip joint. An uncorrected adduction contracture may result in a dislocation diathesis. Therefore, an adductor tenotomy through a separate medial incision should be considered at the start of THA. In severe adductor contracture, release of the pubofemoral ligament and inferior capsule should be done to complete the release.

External Rotators

The external rotators of the hip include the obturator internus, the obturator externus, the superior gemellus, the inferior gemellus, the piriformis, and the quadratus femoris. Removal of the latter muscle is often necessary to adequately expose the lesser trochanter to determine the neck resection level.

Internal Rotators

Internal rotation is a secondary function of several muscles of the hip joint. The more consistent internal rotators are the anterior fibers of the gluteus medius and minimus and the tensor fascia lata muscle. Other contributing muscles include the semimembranosus, the semitendinosus, pectineus, and posterior portion of the adductor magnus muscle.

Bursa

There are numerous bursae in the hip region. The more clinically significant bursae in THA are the iliopsoas and trochanteric bursae.

Iliopsoas Bursa

The iliopsoas bursa is the largest and most constant bursa about the hip. It is present in approximately 98% of normal adults and is usually bilateral.[28,29] It is located deep to the iliopsoas tendon and functions to cushion the tendon from the structures on the anterior aspect of the hip joint capsule. Anatomic boundaries include the iliopsoas muscle anteriorly, the pectineal eminence and the joint capsule posteriorly, the iliofemoral ligament laterally, and the acetabular labrum medially.[29] The iliopsoas bursa can become inflamed and distended in many conditions, including in rare cases after THA.[30]

Trochanteric Bursa

The reported occurrence of lateral trochanteric pain (LTP) 3 or more months after THA surgery is 17% for patients who had a transtrochanteric approach and 3% for patients who had a posterior approach.[31] In general, LTP may be associated with numerous pathologies, including greater trochanteric bursitis (Figure 1-2). The diagnosis of greater trochanteric bursitis is established by a patient complaint of lateral trochanteric hip pain, palpable tenderness over the greater trochanter, and pain on resistance to active hip abduction in a side-lying position.[31] Other causes of LTP include trochanteric fracture, degenerative tendinopathy of the gluteus medius or minimus tendons, myofascial pain, overuse, femoral neck fracture, tensor fasciae femoris syndrome, abductor muscle strain, and tendinitis of the external rotators of the hip.[31,32]

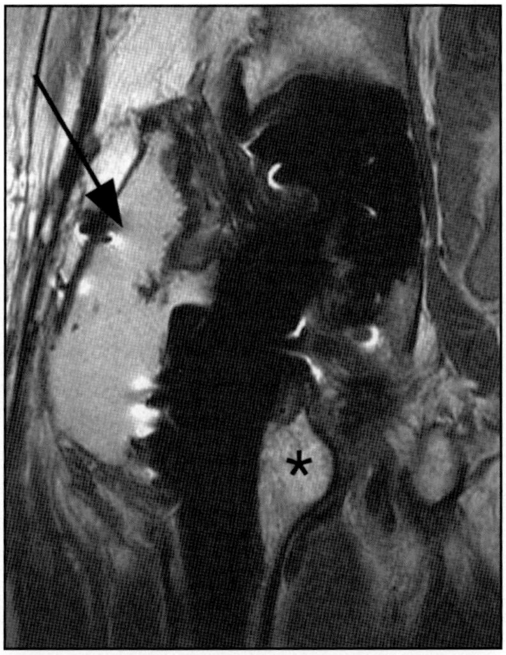

Figure 1-2. MRI demonstrating trochanteric bursitis after THA.

LTP after THA has not been studied extensively. Potential causes include all those for the nonarthroplasty population as well as infection, osteolysis, trochanteric insufficiency or nonunion, abductor insufficiency or weakness, and tensor fasciae lata insufficiency or herniation. It has been suggested that LTP may also be associated with increasing femoral offset and leg length discrepancy.[33]

Hip Vasculature

Vascular injuries are the most immediate life-threatening intraoperative or perioperative events associated with THA. Damage to the vessels may occur during the operative approach, during component insertion, or during component removal. The incidence of vascular complications may be increasing due to the prevalent use of screws in the pelvis with cementless acetabular devices, structural grafts, and antiprotrusio cages.[34] The major risk of vascular complications is associated with the use of acetabular screws.[34] The most common etiology of vascular injuries sustained during THA is thromboembolic followed by laceration, pseudoaneurysm, and arteriovenous fistula. The left side is more commonly involved than the right, and the overall mortality is 7% with a 15% incidence of major and 4% incidence of minor amputations.[35,36] Knowledge of vessel location and an understanding of the acetabular quadrant system are crucial in minimizing these potentially catastrophic complications.

The common iliac artery divides at the L5-S1 intervertebral disk level. The anterior division continues as the external iliac artery and then as the common femoral artery distal to the inguinal ligament. The posterior division becomes the internal iliac artery and will subsequently branch into an anterior and posterior division. Branches from these vessels supply the structures of the hip and lower extremities.

External Iliac Vessels

The external iliac vessels are immobile and lie close to the pelvis. Consequently, the external iliac vessels, particularly the vein, are at highest risk for injury during THA.[35] The reason for the increased susceptibility of the vein over the artery is that the vein lies within 7 mm of the anterior column of the pelvis at the level of the anterior-inferior iliac spine (AIIS) and within 4 mm at the level of the acetabular dome.[35] The external iliac artery lies within 10 mm at the AIIS and 7 mm at the acetabular dome.[35] The closer proximity to bone and thinner intima place the vein at greater risk of damage.[35]

Injury to the external iliac vessels may occur at any stage of THA. Too-medial retractor placement over the anterior column may injure the vessels.[37-39] This can be avoided by placing the retractors in a more proximal position where the iliopsoas muscle offers protection to the vessels.[37,40] Other mechanisms include excessive medial reaming, excess extra-articular cement, and cement extrusion. The latter can be limited by use of a pelvic cement restrictor or bone graft.[41]

The use of transacetabular screws for component fixation is a common mechanism for injury with resultant retroperitoneal hematoma.[42] Delayed injury may occur due to socket migration and cement spicules.[39,43-48]

Common Femoral Vessels

The common femoral artery courses directly anterior and medial to the hip capsule. At this level, only the iliopsoas tendon lies between the vessel and capsule. The common femoral vessels have been the most commonly reported extrapelvic vascular structures injured in association with THA. The femoral artery is located lateral to the femoral vein and is more likely to be injured.

Injury to the common femoral vessels typically occurs as acute-onset intraoperatively. The most commonly cited mechanism of injury has been aberrant Hohmann retractor placement during the surgical approach.[49,50] The surgeon must avoid damage by keeping close to bone and avoiding strong retraction over the lip of the acetabulum. Other mechanisms include bulk allograft placement for acetabular reconstruction, osteophyte resection, and resection of scar tissue from the anterior-inferior acetabulum.[51,52] During cemented acetabular component fixation, extrusion of excess cement anteromedially may cause intimal damage from the heat of polymerization and consequent pseudoaneurysm or thromboembolism.[37,10,53-57]

In the anterolateral approach to THA, the primary vascular complication is femoral artery and vein laceration, which are vulnerable to retractors placed too far anteriorly. The anterior retractor should be placed at the 1 o'clock position for the right hip and the 11 o'clock position for the left hip. The tip of the retractor should be placed directly on the bone and not pierce the psoas muscle, the only barrier between the acetabulum and femoral vessels. An alternative is to pass a blunt curved retractor into the pelvis at the anterior acetabulum.[35] Notably, the transverse branch of the lateral femoral circumflex artery may be encountered when splitting the vastus lateralis during this approach and must be cauterized or ligated.

The femoral vessels are also at risk during the deep dissection of the anterior THA approach because of their anterior relationship to the hip. The femoral vessels are protected if the deep dissection does not extend out of the plane of the sartorius and tensor fascia lata superficially and the gluteus medius and rectus femoris more deeply.[35] The ascending branch of the lateral femoral circumflex artery crosses the operative field at the proximal interval between the sartorius and tensor fascia lata and must be ligated or coagulated.

The course of the femoral vessels medial to the iliopectineal fascia also places them at risk with the ilioinguinal approach. Other structures at risk with this approach include the inferior epigastric vessel, bowel, bladder, and spermatic cord.[35]

Profunda Femoris Artery

The profunda femoris artery arises from the lateral side of the femoral artery approximately 3.5 cm below the inguinal ligament. Injury to the vessel or its branches is rare during THA but has been reported. Mechanisms include very medial retractor placement, extruded cement, and osteotome use.[35,37]

Superior Gluteal Vessels

The superior gluteal artery passes between the lumbosacral trunk and the first sacral nerve and courses with the superior gluteal vein and gluteal nerve. The structures leave the pelvis through the upper part of the greater sciatic foramen above the piriformis muscle. At the sciatic notch, the superior gluteal vessels are at greatest risk of injury as they lie an average of 5 mm from the bone. Injury to the superior gluteal artery in THA is rare but has been reported, such as by improper pin-retractor placement and screw fixation in the area of the sciatic notch.[35,58] Palpation of the sciatic notch prior to transacetabular screw placement will minimize this risk.

Inferior Gluteal and Internal Pudendal Vessels

The inferior gluteal and internal pudendal vessels are the terminal branches of the anterior division of the internal iliac artery. The vessels are closest to the posterior columns at the level of the ischial spine.[4] The inferior gluteal vessels lay an average of 6 mm and the pudendal vessels an average of 12 mm from the posterior column. The vessels are mobile and well-protected by a layer of fat.[59,60] Injury may occur, however, if excessively long transacetabular screws are used for component fixation. Damage to the inferior gluteal artery is the main vascular risk of the posterior approach. This vessel has many intramuscular branches, which often are cut when the gluteus maximus is split, and they must be identified and cauterized during dissection.[35]

Obturator Vessels

The obturator vessels pass through the obturator canal at the obturator foramen. At this level, the vessels lie fixed by the obturator membrane and peritoneum within 1 mm of the bony surface of the quadrilateral surface.[4,35] The vessels are protected only by the interposition of the obturator internus muscle. This places the obturator vessels at risk for damage as well by retractors or cement spicules. Notable, an aberrant obturator artery may arise from the inferior epigastric artery and pass toward the pelvic brim along the medial margin of the femoral ring.

Hip Innervation

The overall incidence of nerve injuries associated with THA is approximately 1% to 2%. High-risk groups include females, revision cases, and cases of developmental dysplasia of the hip.[61,62] Injuries to the sciatic nerve are the most common, followed by the peroneal, superior gluteal, obturator, and femoral nerves. Injury to these structures can lead to loss of function and poor outcomes. The etiology of nerve injury includes traction, contusion, hematoma, dislocation, and laceration. Nerve lengthening >4 cm generally is accepted as a risk factor for nerve injury or palsy.[63] Stretch injuries do not fare as well as direct injury.[64,65] Knowledge of nerve location and an understanding of the acetabular

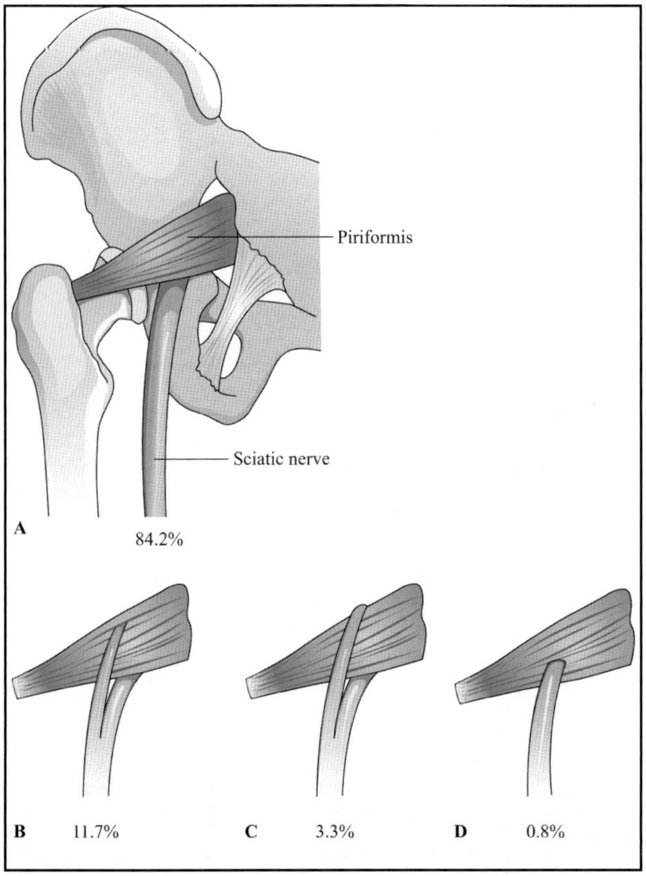

Figure 1-3. Anatomical variations of the sciatic nerve with reference to piriformis muscle.

quadrant system are crucial in minimizing these potentially catastrophic complications.

The sciatic nerve (L4-S3) arises from the sacral plexus and is the largest nerve in the body. The sciatic nerve typically divides at the superior border of the popliteal fossa into the tibial nerve and the common peroneal nerve. The common peroneal nerve has 2 relatively fixed points at the sciatic notch and the head of the fibula and it is surrounded by less connective tissue then the tibial nerve. This later feature allows the tibial nerve to sustain a larger percent of elongation before exhibiting evidence of neural compromise.[4,65]

The sciatic nerve is the most commonly injured nerve in THA. It is located anterior and medial to the piriformis muscle just proximal to where it will emerge through the greater sciatic notch. The nerve emerges as one branch in 84% of cases. In the remaining 16%, a portion of the nerve passes through the piriformis or posterior to it, placing it at greater risk (Figure 1-3).

The sciatic nerve continues vertically between 2 layers of muscle. The outer layer is formed by the gluteus maximus and the inner layer is formed by the piriformis, the superior gemellus, the obturator internus, the inferior gemellus, and the quadratus femoris. The nerve lies only 9 mm from the posterior column at the level of the acetabular dome. The nerve is more protected at the ischial spine, as the short external rotator muscles are interposed between the nerve and bone at this point is an average of 15 mm away.[66] The anatomic course of the sciatic nerve places it at risk for injury by posterior acetabular retractors and power reamers. This is even more probable as incision lengths decrease with minimal incision hip surgery.[67,68] Other mechanisms of injury are various, including entrapment by trochanteric wiring and compression over a spur of PMMA.[69-71]

Additional intraoperative risk factors for development of sciatic nerve palsy include previous trauma, particularly when there has been prior internal fixation around the acetabulum. Other cases at risk include excision of heterotopic bone in proximity to the sciatic nerve and absence of the posterior wall, particularly when there has been previous plating or bone grafting. In cases that are at risk for sciatic palsy, it is advisable to palpate and visualize the nerve, protect it with soft tissue and retractors, flex the knee, and avoid extreme positions for extended periods of time.[34,66]

In a posterior approach to the acetabulum, no internervous plane is present since the technique involves splitting the gluteus maximus in line with its fibers. The sciatic nerve is relatively protected by the short external rotators after they are detached and reflected medially. Still, the most common nerve injury during the posterior approach is contusion to the sciatic nerve.[35] Avoiding excessive traction on the nerve can minimize injury.

Femoral nerve injury is much less common than sciatic or peroneal nerve injury. The femoral nerve is the most lateral structure within the femoral triangle. It lies on the psoas muscle belly at the approximate midpoint between the anterior-superior iliac spine and pubic tubercle. It is anterior to the acetabulum and consequently is primarily at risk during capsule dissection rather than during reaming or drilling.[26] The femoral nerve may be injured in an ilioinguinal approach as well since the nerve lies under the inguinal canal on the anterior surface of the iliopsoas muscle.[35]

The superior gluteal nerve exits the sciatic notch and courses between the gluteus medius and minimum. Injury is associated with the direct lateral or anterolateral approach. It is generally well protected if the dissection does not extend beyond 5 cm above the greater trochanter.[72,73] The inferior gluteal nerve is rarely injured because it inserts into the gluteus maximus proximal and medial to the area that is split during the posterior approach to the acetabulum.[35]

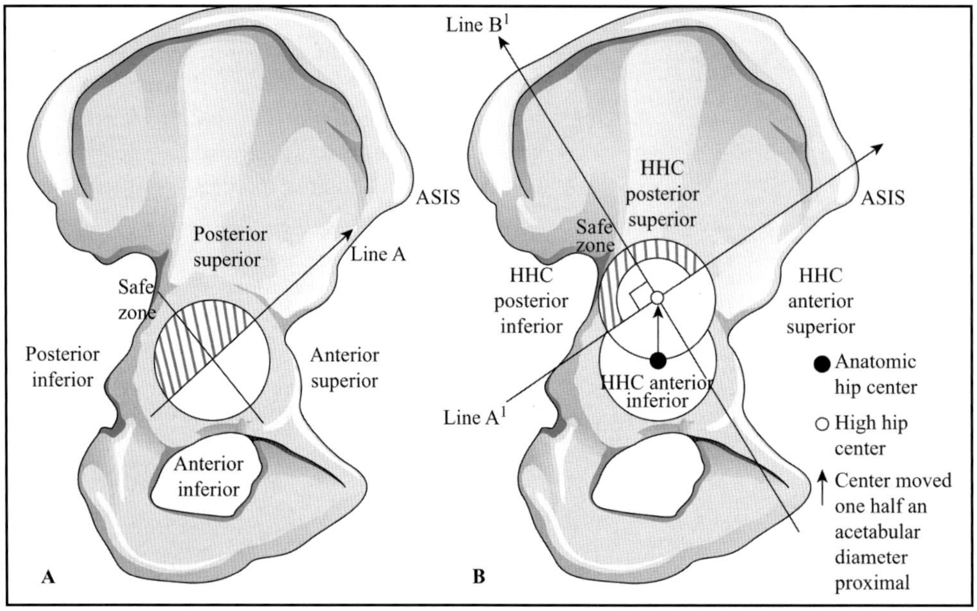

Figure 1-4. (A) Quadrants for acetabular screw placement with normal acetabular cup position. (B) Quadrants for acetabular screw placement with higher acetabular cup position.

Obturator nerve injury in THA appears to be a rare complication. Most reports of obturator neuropathy have involved violation of the medial acetabular wall and defects in the pubic ramus, drills, and cement.[74] The close proximity of the nerve to the quadrilateral surface of the acetabulum commands avoidance of the anterior-inferior acetabular area for screw placement or cement penetration.[4]

Anatomic Quadrant System

The anatomic acetabular quadrant system described by Wasielewski et al is useful for understanding acetabular anatomy and determining the location of planned acetabular screw fixation in THA to avoid neurovascular complications.[75] The system may also guide retractor placement, acetabular drilling for graft fixation, and estimation of bone depth in a specific zone. A line drawn from the anterior-superior iliac spine through the center of the acetabulum and a bisecting line at the center of the acetabulum define the 4 equal quadrants (Figure 1-4A).[75]

The anterior-superior and anterior-inferior quadrants are in close proximity to the external iliac vessels and the obturator neurovascular structures, respectively. The structures lie close to the pelvic bone with minimal protection from interposed soft tissue or muscle. In addition, the bone in the anterior quadrants is relatively sparse (Figure 1-5A). Therefore, the use of screws, anchoring holes, and cement in this area should be avoided.[75] Retraction over the anterior column should be done cautiously.

The sciatic nerve and superior gluteal structures course opposite the posterior-superior quadrant. The inferior gluteal and internal pudendal structures course opposite the posterior-inferior quadrant. By contrast to the anterior regions, however, the posterior quadrant bone depth is 25 mm or greater in the central regions.[4,75] Screws and anchoring holes may be placed relatively safely in these zones.

The high hip center (HHC) acetabular quadrant system serves a similar purpose to the anatomic system but is constructed differently. The quadrants are formed by a first line extending from the anterior-superior iliac spine through the center of the acetabulum and a second line drawn perpendicular to the first at the acetabular midpoint (Figure 1-4B). The posterior halves of the posterior-superior and posterior-inferior HHC quadrants contain the best bone stock and are relatively safe for screw placement (Figure 1-5B).

References

1. Harkess JW, Crockarell JR. Arthroplasty of the hip. In: Canale ST, Beaty JH, eds. *Campbell's Operative Orthopedics*. 11th ed. Philadelphia, PA: Mosby; 2007:314-482.

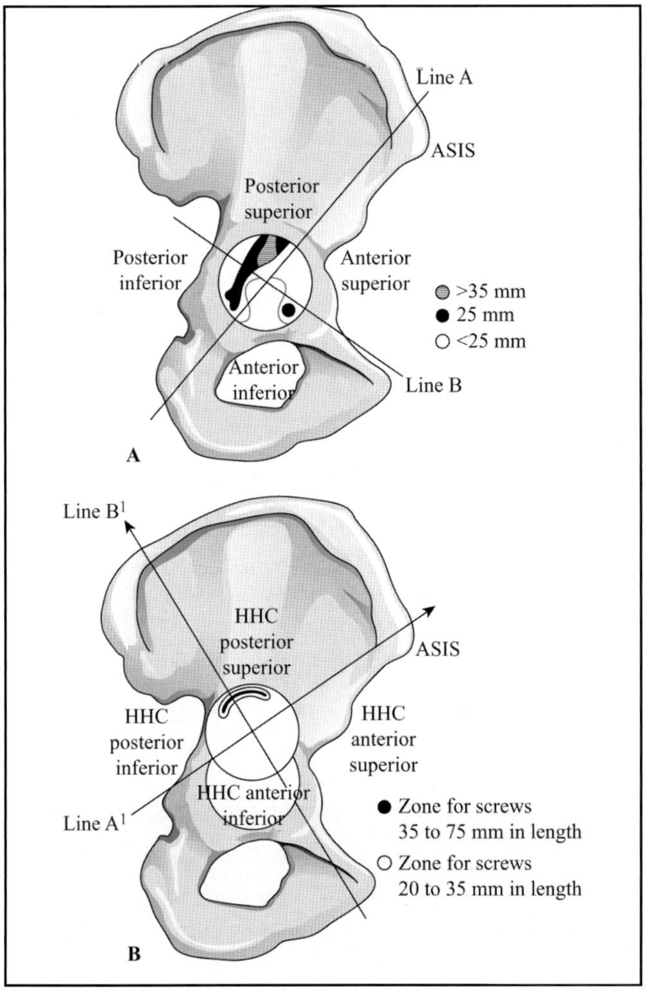

Figure 1-5. (A) Estimates of maximum screw lengths with normal acetabular cup position. (B) Estimates of maximum screw lengths with high acetabular cup position.

2. Kurtz S, Ong K, Lau E, Mowat F, Halpern M. Projections of primary and revision hip and knee arthroplasty in the United States from 2005 to 2030. *J Bone Joint Surg Am.* 2007;89(4):780-785.
3. Anda S, Svenningsen S, Dale LG, Benum P. The acetabular sector angle of the adult hip determined by computed tomography. *Acta Radiol Diagn (Stockh).* 1986;27(4):443-447.
4. Wasielewski RC. The hip. In: Callaghan JL, Rosenberg AG, Rubash HE, eds. *The Adult Hip.* 2nd ed. Philadelphia, PA: Lippincott Williams & Wilkins; 2006:51-67.
5. Archbold HA, Mockford B, Molloy D, McConway J, Ogonda L, Beverland D. The transverse acetabular ligament: an aid to orientation of the acetabular component during primary total hip replacement: a preliminary study of 1000 cases investigating postoperative stability. *J Bone Joint Surg Br.* 2006;88(7):883-886.
6. Barrack RL, Burnett SJ. Preoperative planning for revision total hip arthroplasty. *J Bone Joint Surg Am.* 2005;87(12):2800-2811.
7. Fabry G, MacEwen GD, Shands AR Jr. Torsion of the femur. A follow-up study in normal and abnormal conditions. *J Bone Joint Surg Am.* 1973;55(8):1726-1738.
8. Kingsley PC, Olmsted KL. A study to determine the angle of anteversion of the neck of the femur. *J Bone Joint Surg Am.* 1948;30A(3):745-751.
9. Reikeras O, Bjerkreim I, Kolbenstvedt A. Anteversion of the acetabulum and femoral neck in normals and in patients with osteoarthritis of the hip. *Acta Orthop Scand.* 1983;54(1):18-23.
10. Clark JM, Freeman MA, Witham D. The relationship of neck orientation to the shape of the proximal femur. *J Arthroplasty.* 1987;2(2):99-109.
11. Dai KR, An KN, Hein T. Geometric and biomechanical analysis of the femur. *Trans Orthop Res Soc.* 1986;10:99.
12. Harty M. The calcar femorale and the femoral neck. *J Bone Joint Surg Am.* 1957;39-A(3):625-630.
13. Noble PC, Alexander JW, Lindahl LJ, Yew DT, Granberry WM, Tullos HS. The anatomic basis of femoral component design. *Clin Orthop Relat Res.* 1988;(235):148-165.
14. Rubin PJ, Leyvraz PF, Aubaniac JM, Argenson JN, Esteve P, de Roguin B. The morphology of the proximal femur. A three-dimensional radiographic analysis. *J Bone Joint Surg Br.* 1992;74(1):28-32.
15. Ruff CB, Hayes WC. Subperiosteal expansion and cortical remodeling of the human femur and tibia with aging. *Science.* 1982;217(4563):945-948.
16. Smith RW Jr, Walker RR. Femoral expansion in aging women. Implications for osteoporosis and fractures. *Henry Ford Hosp Med J.* 1980;28(2-3):168-170.
17. Dorr LD, Faugere MC, Mackel AM, Gruen TA, Bognar B, Malluche HH. Structural and cellular assessment of bone quality of proximal femur. *Bone.* 1993;14(3):231-242.
18. Sotereanos NG, Miller MC, Smith B, Hube R, Sewecke JJ, Wohlrab D. Using intraoperative pelvic landmarks for acetabular component placement in total hip arthroplasty. *J Arthroplasty.* 2006;21(6):832-840.
19. Hewitt J, Guilak F, Glisson R, Vail TP. Regional material properties of the human hip joint capsule ligaments. *J Orthop Res.* 2001;19(3):359-364.
20. Fuss FK, Bacher A. New aspects of the morphology and function of the human hip joint ligaments. *Am J Anat.* 1991;192(1):1-13.
21. Jenkins DB. *Hollinshead's Functional Anatomy of the Limbs and Back.* Philadelphia, PA: Saunders; 1991.
22. Offierski CM. Traumatic dislocation of the hip in children. *J Bone Joint Surg Br.* 1981;63-B(2):194-197.
23. Hedlundh U, Ahnfelt L, Hybbinette CH, Weckstrom J, Fredin H. Surgical experience related to dislocations after total hip arthroplasty. *J Bone Joint Surg Br.* 1996;78(2):206-209.
24. Selgrath CE, Mohler CG, Collis DK, Jiranek WA. Early complications and their management. In: Callaghan JL, Rosenberg AG, Rubash HE, eds. *The Adult Hip.* 2nd ed. Philadelphia, PA: Lippincott Williams & Wilkins; 2006:1087-1108.
25. Gowitzke BA, Milner M. *Scientific Bases of Human Movement.* 3rd ed. Baltimore, MD: Williams & Wilkins; 1988.

26. Norkin CC, White DJ. *Measurement of Joint Motion: A Guide Goniometry.* 3rd ed. Philadelphia, PA: FA Davis Co; 2003.
27. Nemeth G, Ohlsen H. In vivo moment arm lengths for hip extensor muscles at different angles of hip flexion. *J Biomech.* 1985;18(2):129-140.
28. Armstrong P, Saxton H. Ilio-psoas bursa. *Br J Radiol.* 1972;45(535):493-495.
29. Dutton M. Hip Joint. *Orthopaedic: Examination, Evaluation, and Intervention.* New York, NY: McGraw-Hill; 2004:667-728.
30. Yamamoto T, Marui T, Akisue T, Yoshiya S, Hitora T, Kurosaka M. Dumbbell-shaped iliopsoas bursitis penetrating the pelvic wall: a rare complication of hip arthrodesis. A case report. *J Bone Joint Surg Am.* 2003;85-A(2):343-345.
31. Wiesman HJ Jr, Simon SR, Ewald FC, Thomas WH, Sledge CB. Total hip replacement with and without osteotomy of the greater trochanter. Clinical and biomechanical comparisons in the same patients. *J Bone Joint Surg Am.* 1978;60(2):203-210.
32. Kingzett-Taylor A, Tirman PF, Feller J, et al. Tendinosis and tears of gluteus medius and minimus muscles as a cause of hip pain: MR imaging findings. *Am J Roentgenol.* 1999;173(4):1123-1126.
33. Iorio R, Healy WL, Warren PD, Appleby D. Lateral trochanteric pain following primary total hip arthroplasty. *J Arthroplasty.* 2006;21(2):233-236.
34. Barrack RL. Neurovascular injury: avoiding catastrophe. *J Arthroplasty.* 2004;19(4 suppl 1):104-107.
35. Rue JP, Inoue N, Mont MA. Current overview of neurovascular structures in hip arthroplasty: anatomy, preoperative evaluation, approaches, and operative techniques to avoid complications. *Orthopedics.* 2004;27(1):73-81.
36. Shoenfeld NA, Stuchin SA, Pearl R, Haveson S. The management of vascular injuries associated with total hip arthroplasty. *J Vasc Surg.* 1990;11(4):549-555.
37. Nachbur B, Meyer RP, Verkkala K, Zurcher R. The mechanisms of severe arterial injury in surgery of the hip joint. *Clin Orthop Relat Res.* 1979;(141):122-133.
38. Ovrum E, Dahl HK. Vessel and nerve injuries complicating total hip arthroplasty. *Arch Orthop Trauma Surg.* 1979;95(4):267-269.
39. Todd BD, Bintcliffe IW. Injury to the external iliac artery during hip arthroplasty for old central dislocation. *J Arthroplasty.* 1990;5(suppl):S53-S55.
40. Müller ME. Total hip prostheses. *Clin Orthop Relat Res.* 1970;72:46-68.
41. Ratliff AH. Arterial injuries after total hip replacement. *J Bone Joint Surg Br.* 1985;67(4):517-518.
42. Kirkpatrick JS, Callaghan JJ, Vandemark RM, Goldner RD. The relationship of the intrapelvic vasculature to the acetabulum. Implications in screw-fixation acetabular components. *Clin Orthop Relat Res.* 1990;(258):183-190.
43. Bergqvist D, Carlsson AS, Ericsson BF. Vascular complications after total hip arthroplasty. *Acta Orthop Scand.* 1983;54(2):157-163.
44. Hennessy OF, Timmis JB, Allison DJ. Vascular complications following hip replacement. *Br J Radiol.* 1983;56(664):275-277.
45. Kettlekamp DB, Powers SR. Femoral compression neuropathy in hemorrhagic disorders. *Arch Surg.* 1969;98(3):367-368.
46. Reiley MA, Bond D, Branick RI, Wilson EH. Vascular complications following total hip arthroplasty. A review of the literature and a report of two cases. *Clin Orthop Relat Res.* 1984;(186):23-28.
47. Ryan JA, Johnson ML, Boettcher WG, Kirkpatrick JN. Mycotic aneurysm of the external iliac artery caused by migration of a total hip prosthesis. *Clin Orthop Relat Res.* 1984;(186):57-59.
48. Tazawa A, Nakamura S, Otsuka K, Nishida K, Matsushita T. Transabdominal approach for intrapelvic migration of a total hip prosthesis component. *J Orthop Sci.* 2001;6(4):362-365.
49. Aust JC, Bredenberg CE, Murray DG. Mechanisms of arterial injuries associated with total hip replacement. *Arch Surg.* 1981;116(3):345-349.
50. Mallory TH, Jaffe SL, Eberle RW. False aneurysm of the common femoral artery after total hip arthroplasty: a case report. *Clin Orthop Relat Res.* 1997;(338):105-108.
51. Bose WJ, Petty W. Femoral artery and nerve compression by bulk allograft used for acetabular reconstruction. An unreported complication. *J Arthroplasty.* 1996;11(3):348-350.
52. Fiddian NJ, Sudlow RA, Browett JP. Ruptured femoral vein. A complication of the use of gentamicin beads in an infected excision arthroplasty of the hip. *J Bone Joint Surg Br.* 1984;66(4):493-494.
53. Dorr LD, Conaty JP, Kohl R, Harvey JP Jr. False aneurysm of the femoral artery following total hip surgery. *J Bone Joint Surg Am.* 1974;56(5):1059-1062.
54. Giacchetto J, Gallagher JJ. False aneurysm of the common femoral artery secondary to migration of a threaded acetabular component. A case report and review of the literature. *Clin Orthop Relat Res.* 1988;(231):91-96.
55. Hirsch SA, Robertson H, Gorniowsky M. Arterial occlusion secondary to methylmethacrylate use. *Arch Surg.* 1976;111(2):204.
56. Neal J, Wachtel TL, Garza OT, Edwards WS. Late arterial embolization complicating total hip replacement. A case report. *J Bone Joint Surg Am.* 1979;61(3):429-430.
57. Sethuraman V, Hozack WJ, Sharkey PF, Rothman RH. Pseudoaneurysm of femoral artery after revision total hip arthroplasty with a constrained cup. *J Arthroplasty.* 2000;15(4):531-534.
58. Lozman H, Robbins H. Injury to the superior gluteal artery as a complication of total hip-replacement arthroplasty. A case report. *J Bone Joint Surg Am.* 1983;65(2):268-269.
59. Keating EM, Ritter MA, Faris PM. Structures at risk from medially placed acetabular screws. *J Bone Joint Surg Am.* 1990;72(4):509-511.
60. Wasielewski RC, Cooperstein LA, Kruger MP, Rubash HE. Acetabular anatomy and the transacetabular fixation of screws in total hip arthroplasty. *J Bone Joint Surg Am.* 1990;72(4):501-508.
61. Schmalzried TP, Amstutz HC, Dorey FJ. Nerve palsy associated with total hip replacement. Risk factors and prognosis. *J Bone Joint Surg Am.* 1991;73(7):1074-1080.

62. Schmalzried TP, Noordin S, Amstutz HC. Update on nerve palsy associated with total hip replacement. *Clin Orthop Relat Res.* 1997;(344):188-206.

63. Johanson NA, Pellicci PM, Tsairis P, Salvati EA. Nerve injury in total hip arthroplasty. *Clin Orthop Relat Res.* 1983;(179):214-222.

64. Ahlgren SA, Elmqvist D, Ljung P. Nerve lesions after total hip replacement. *Acta Orthop Scand.* 1984;55(2):152-155.

65. Edwards BN, Tullos HS, Noble PC. Contributory factors and etiology of sciatic nerve palsy in total hip arthroplasty. *Clin Orthop Relat Res.* 1987;(218):136-141.

66. Barrack RL, Butler RA. Avoidance and management of neurovascular injuries in total hip arthroplasty. *Instr Course Lect.* 2003;52:267-274.

67. Belsky MR. What's new in orthopaedic surgery. *J Am Coll Surg.* 2003;197(6):985-989.

68. Wenz JF, Gurkan I, Jibodh SR. Mini-incision total hip arthroplasty: a comparative assessment of perioperative outcomes. *Orthopedics.* 2002;25(10):1031-1043.

69. Gudmundsson GH, Pilgaard S. Prevention of sciatic nerve entrapment in trochanteric wiring following total hip arthroplasty. *Clin Orthop Relat Res.* 1985;(196):215-216.

70. Edwards MS, Barbaro NM, Asher SW, Murray WR. Delayed sciatic palsy after total hip replacement: case report. *Neurosurgery.* 1981;9(1):61-63.

71. Casagrande PA, Danahy PR. Delayed sciatic-nerve entrapment following the use of self-curing acrylic. A case report. *J Bone Joint Surg Am.* 1971;53(1):167-169.

72. Jacobs LG, Buxton RA. The course of the superior gluteal nerve in the lateral approach to the hip. *J Bone Joint Surg Am.* 1989;71(8):1239-1243.

73. Ramesh M, O'Byrne JM, McCarthy N, Jarvis A, Mahalingham K, Cashman WF. Damage to the superior gluteal nerve after the Hardinge approach to the hip. *J Bone Joint Surg Br.* 1996;78(6):903-906.

74. Eftekhar NS, Kiernan HA Jr, Stinchfield FE. Systemic and local complications following low-friction arthroplasty of the hip joint. A study of 800 consecutive operations. *Arch Surg.* 1976;111(2):150-155.

75. Wasielewski RC, Crossett LS, Rubash HE. Neural and vascular injury in total hip arthroplasty. *Orthop Clin North Am.* 1992;23(2):219-235.

2

Hip Biomechanics

Pooya Hosseinzadeh, MD and Ali Oliashirazi, MD

The hip is likely the most heavily studied joint from a biomechanical perspective. Understanding hip biomechanics is important in evaluating and treating patients with hip pathology, planning hip reconstruction, and improving implant designs. For example, decreasing joint reaction forces and improving implant designs could decrease the risk of implant failure in total hip arthroplasty (THA). The most investigated areas in hip biomechanics include range of motion, kinematics, and joint reactive forces during standing and daily routine activities. Various methods are used for these studies. Kinematic studies are usually performed in the setting with gait analysis. Joint reaction forces could be measured with both in vivo and in vitro methods. In this chapter forces at the hip joint, their implications in clinical settings, and gait and functional adaptations in hip pathologies will be discussed.

Forces at the Hip Joint

Determining the resultant force at the hip joint at different positions is fundamental in investigating the behavior and mechanism of failure of total hip replacements (THR). Forces have been studied in both in vivo and in vitro analysis.

In Vivo Measurement

No in vivo contact stress measurements in native hips are reported yet, as there is no device available to measure these forces. However, with the use of special strain-gauged hip prostheses, in vivo measurement of forces at the hip joint is possible. These in vivo measurement studies are usually limited to a small number of patients due to their complexity. Failure of the equipment in some studies limited the study to a short postoperative period, when the results could be affected by acute postoperative phase as the patients were ambulating with assistive devices during this period. These studies are not ideal, but the results are worth studying. What we have learned from these studies is described in the remainder of this section.

During normal gait, peak hip joint forces vary between 1.8 to 4.3 body weight. In stance phase, the orientation of the force in frontal plane is medial and inferior, but in sagittal plane the force is oriented posteriorly in the first half of the stance and anteriorly in the second half.[1,2]

During daily activities, the hip joint is also loaded with some out-of-plane forces. These forces can cause torsional moments around the femoral axis. These forces are affected by anteversion angle, type of the activity, and speed. For example, stair climbing induces significant out-of-plane loads and torsional moments.[1,2]

Contact pressure between the femoral head and acetabulum has been measured during daily routine activities. During gait, the maximum pressure occurs between heel strike and midstance at the superior-anterior part of the femoral head. Rising from a chair increases this pressure significantly.[3,4]

Parvizi J, Klatt BA.
Essentials in Total Hip Arthroplasty (pp 13-17).

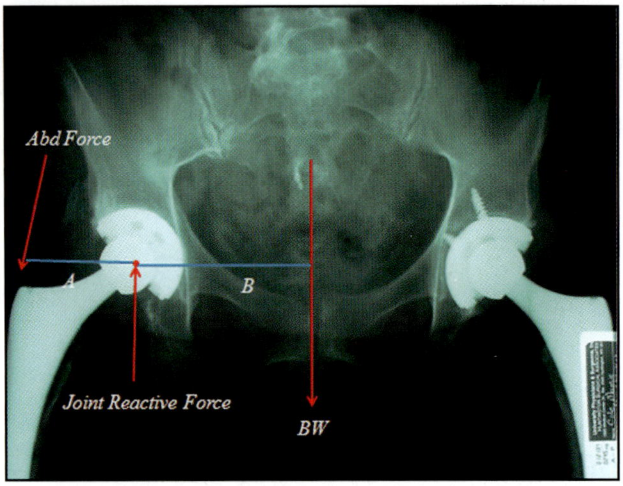

Figure 2-1. Moments caused by body weight (BW) and abductors acting on the hip joint (abductor force x A = BW x B).

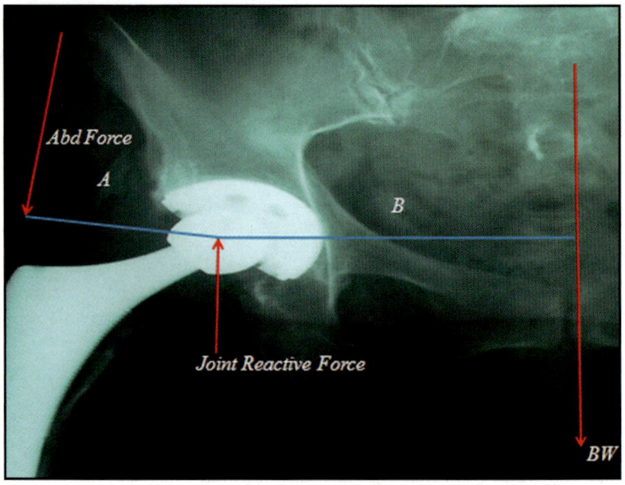

Figure 2-2. Increased moment arm of abductors (A) as seen in varus hip, increased offset and neck length of component, medialization of acetabulum, and lateral transfer of greater trochanter results in decreased joint reaction force.

In Vitro Measurement

Most of the current information regarding biomechanics of the hip joint is based on analytical studies. A common simple form describes 2-dimensional analysis of a one-legged stance (Figure 2-1). In this model, the active forces around the hip joint include body weight, abductor muscle force, and hip joint reaction force. Body weight and abductor forces produce moments around the center of the femoral head. Joint reaction force does not produce moment since it is applied directly to the femoral head similar to the reaction force at the hinge in a seesaw. According to Newton's first law of mechanics, for the hip to be in equilibrium, the moments produced by body weight and abductors should be in opposite directions and equal in magnitude. The body weight is applied from the center of gravity (in front of the second sacral vertebrae). It acts in vertical direction and is assumed to be five-sixths of the total body weight as to account for the weight of the supporting extremity. The abductor muscle force is oriented 30 degrees from the vertical axis. The lever arm for body weight can be measured from radiographic studies. The lever arm of the abductor muscles is usually one-half of the body weight. On the other hand, in this simple one-legged stance model, the sum of forces acting on the hip joint should be 0. Force triangle is used to calculate the joint reaction force based on the parallelogram law. The 3 forces acting on the hip joint should make a closed triangle. Based on this method, hip joint reaction force of 2.75 BW has been calculated[5] (Figure 2-2).

Analytical approaches can be used to estimate joint reaction forces during dynamic activities. Complex 3-dimensional models are used to estimate the joint reaction forces in dynamic settings. Newton's second law of motion is the basis of these studies. It states that if the resultant force on an object is not 0, the object will have acceleration in the direction of the force and proportional to the magnitude of the force. Intersegmental hip forces can be calculated by measuring external forces and locating the position of joint centers during activities. In these methods, extremity motions are measured by various opto-electronic methods and a force plate is used to measure the foot ground reaction force. Forces and moments around the hip joint are used to estimate the internal joint forces using a method similar to the 2-dimensional analysis described earlier. The moment generated by internal joint forces should be equal and in the opposite direction of the measured external joint moment. Using the above-mentioned techniques, the hip joint peak forces during walking have been calculated and are reported to be 4.5 to 5 BW during slow walking and increase to 7.6 BW during fast walking.[6]

In vivo data are only available for patients with hip replacement. Hip joint reaction forces estimated by analytical methods are usually higher compared to in vivo studies done in patients after THR. This might be caused by anatomic simplifications and normal function assumption in analytic studies. In fact, patients with arthritis and after THR have an altered gait that could also explain a part of the differences in joint reaction forces between analytical and in vivo studies. Kinematics and kinetics of a patient with hip replacement was incorporated in an analytical study and a straight line muscle model was modified.[7] These modifications reduced the contact forces to 2.5 to 3.5 BW

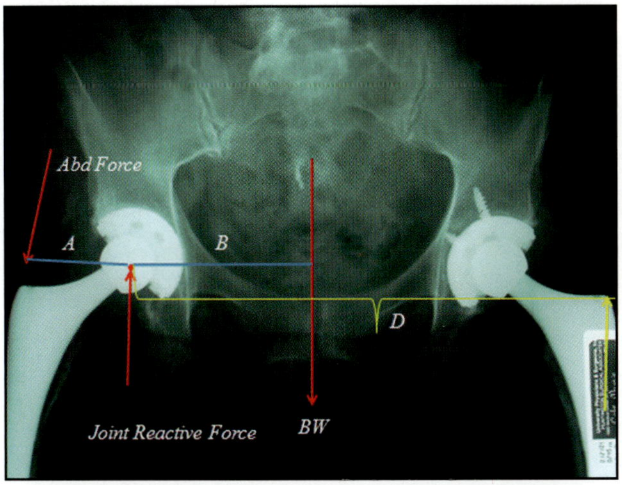

Figure 2-3. Holding a cane in the opposite hand decreases abductor and joint reaction forces by increasing abductor moment arm (D).

during the gait cycle, which are still higher than the in vivo measurements of 1.8 to 3.2 BW. Limitation of the in vivo studies to early postoperative period could also explain some of the differences in the force estimates.

Finite elemental analyses have rapidly evolved in the engineering sophistication and clinical relevance and a significant portion of the information on hip biomechanics is based on these studies. These studies usually investigate the stress distribution on hip prostheses. Recently these studies are performed to investigate the impact of implant design and surgical positioning on dislocation potential and to estimate the wear of prosthesis-bearing surfaces. In this method, the articular surface and the prosthesis are divided into very small units and force and stress on each unit is measured and contact stress and forces on the articular surface is calculated by a computational model. Detailed description of this method is beyond the scope of this chapter.

Determining contact area and pressure of the hip joint is of great interest in the context of joint degenerative disease, reconstructive osteotomies, treatment of intra-articular fractures, and failure of hip replacement. Measurement areas are constantly evolving in this area. Sheet array sensors like Tekscan (Tekscan, South Boston, MA) that are widely used in knee and shoulder studies have been unsuccessful in hip studies due to the fact that they wrinkle, forcing them to conform to the geometry of the hip joint.

The Impact of Walking Aids

It has been shown in both in vitro and in vivo studies that using a cane in the opposite hand decreases the hip joint reactive forces. The moment produced by the body weight should be equal and opposite to the moment produced by hip abductors and the cane. The cane has a much larger moment arm compared to the hip abductors and subsequently reduces the joint reactive forces significantly. Joint reactive forces can be reduced to almost 50% when 15% of body weight is applied to the cane.[8] Kinematic studies and analytical models in preoperative THR patients has shown that those who used a cane had joint reaction force of just 65% of those who did not use a cane.[9] Joint forces in postoperative THR patients have been measured using in vivo methods and showed that ambulation with crutches deceases the joint reaction forces to 2.6 to 2.8 BW (Figure 2-3).[10]

The Impact of Rotational Moments About the Axis of Implant

Implant stability in hip replacement is affected by out-of-plane forces especially in uncemented stems.[11-14] This fact is often overlooked because the hip mechanical forces are most commonly depicted in the frontal plane (coronal plane). Most fractures propagate from the anterolateral cortex and result from a combination of forces acting longitudinally and posteriorly.[12] It has also been shown that posteriorly directed forces that happen during hip flexion can cause retroversion of the stem and may have a significant part in the loosening of femoral stems.[15] Loose stems are often found in a retroverted position. It is crucial that a stem achieve immediate torsional stability for effective ingrowth to occur. Otherwise, the stem will move with these forces and ingrowth will fail.

The Impact of Joint Geometry

Various diseases and surgical procedures can alter the position of the femoral head or the greater trochanter, and these changes alter the forces at the hip. Most importantly, changes to the geometry of the joint can affect strength and moments generated by abductor muscles. This can have a significant impact on the biomechanics of the joint. Alteration of the neck length, neck angle, or location of the hip center can change hip biomechanics. When performing THA, surgeons attempt to reconstruct the neck and hip center with attention to these biomechanical considerations.

Neck Length and Neck Angle

Typically, the center of the femoral head is at the level of the greater trochanter. Decreasing head-neck angle (varus

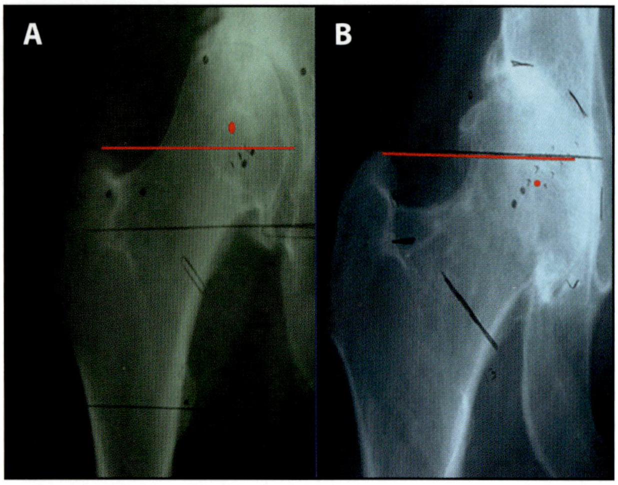

Figure 2-4. Relationship of center of femoral head to greater trochanter in valgus (A) and varus hips (B).

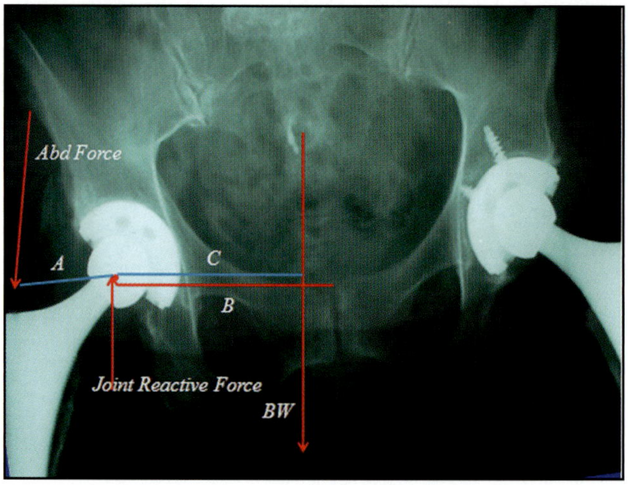

Figure 2-5. Shifting the body toward the affected side (weak abductors) compensates for weak abductors by decreasing moment arm of body weight. (B) Moment arm before shift, (C) moment arm after shift.

position neck angle) puts the center of the femoral head below the top of the greater trochanter. This increases the mechanical advantage of hip abductors by increasing their moment arm. Therefore, joint reaction forces are decreased in this position.[16] Increasing the neck length and moving the greater trochanteric position more lateral have the same impact on hip abductors. On the other hand, varus position increases moment arm for forces transmitted to proximal femur and therefore increases the bending moments in proximal femur and component, which over time can lead to loosening (Figure 2-4).

Valgus position (increased neck angle) and decreased neck length decrease the bending moments in the proximal femur by decreasing the moment arm. On the other hand, this position decreases the moment arm of abductors.[17]

Neck length and neck angle can be modified by choice and position of the femoral implant in THA. Preoperative planning as discussed in the templating chapter is crucial to recreating the desired length and offset of the femoral neck.

Hip Center

Movement of the hip center medially, inferiorly, and anteriorly decreases the hip joint reaction forces.[17] This position increases the moment arm for abductors and decreases the external moment by bringing the hip center closer to the line of action of foot-floor reaction force.[16,18] Hip center location can be altered in certain pathologic conditions like osteoarthritis. In this condition, the femoral head displaces posteriorly, superiorly, and laterally. It has been shown by analytical models that the highest joint reaction forces and moments occur with a femoral head located superior, lateral, and posterior to its original location.[16] This position decreases the mechanical advantage of hip abductors, flexors, adductors, and extensors by reducing muscle lengths and moment arms. This is one reason why the high hip center position is discouraged for the acetabular component in hip dysplasia.

Analytical and experimental results on the effects of joint geometry on hip joint forces are consistent with clinical studies. Higher loosening rates have been reported in implants placed superior or lateral compared to anatomic position.[19,20] Decreased femoral offsets and abductor moment arm have been associated with higher volumetric polyethylene wear.[17]

In THA surgery, the position of the acetabular component is planned by the surgeon preoperatively to create desired hip function.

Gait Adaptations

Individuals with hip joint pathology change their daily activities and how they are performed in adaptation to pain, instability, and decreased muscle strength. For example, some extent of Trendelenberg gait is common in patients with hip pathology due to weak abductors.[17] In these patients, gait is adapted to decrease the demand on theses muscles. Shifting the body toward the affected side partially compensates for weak abductors by decreasing the moment arm of the body weight acting on the hip joint (Figure 2-5).

Decreased step lengths and cadences both result in slow walking speeds in candidates for THR.[21] Decreased swing time and step length on the affected side are caused by painful motion of the hip and loss of hip extension during stance phase, respectively.[22,21]

Decreased hip flexion-extension is common in THR candidates.[21,23-25] This limited motion is compensated partially by increasing pelvic anterior-posterior tilt. After THR, hip pain is significantly decreased and hip function is restored to a great extent. Gait velocities, hip motion, and step length increase after THR. Hip sagittal motion increases and Trendelenberg gait improves after THR.[17]

Summary

Forces acting on the hip joint can be measured with analytical and in vivo measures. Both of these methods have shown that the hip joint is subject to substantial amounts of force during activities of daily living. In vivo studies with transducers are the only way of accurately measuring the reaction forces on the hip joint, but these studies are invasive and cannot be used to evaluate the effect of changes in anatomy of the joint or implant design on the joint reactive forces. Analytical studies are noninvasive and can be performed on a large number of patients but they only approximate the forces.

The effect of external and internal forces on the hip joint and the stability of the implant depend on both the magnitude and direction of the force. It is important for the surgeon to understand how forces act around the hip. With this knowledge, a surgeon can understand cane use, implant design, implant placement, and gait abnormalities.

References

1. Bergmann G, Graichen F, Rohlmann A. Hip joint loading during walking and running measured in two patients. *J Biomechanics.* 1993;26(8):969-990.
2. Bergmann G, Graichen F, Rohlmann A. Is staircase walking a risk for fixation of hip implants? *J Biomechanics.* 1995;28(5):535-553.
3. Hodge WA, Carlson KL, Fijan SM, et al. Contact pressures from an instrumented hip endoprosthesis. *J Bone Joint Surg.* 1989;71A(9):1378-1385.
4. Kerbs DE, Elbaum L, Riley PO, Hodge WA. Exercise and gait effects on in vivo hip contact pressures. *Phys Ther.* 1991;9:301-309.
5. Frankle VH, Nordin M. *Basic Biomechanics of the Skeletal System.* Philadelphia, PA: Lea and Febiger; 1980:303-309.
6. Paul JP. Approaches to design: force actions transmitted by joints in the human body. *Proc R Soc Lond B Biol Sci.* 1976;192:163-172.
7. Brand RA, Pederson DR, Davy DT, Kotzar GM, Heiple KG, Goldberg VM. Comparison of hip force calculation and measurements in the same patient. *J Arthroplasty.* 1994;9(1):45-51.
8. Cochran GVB. *A Primer of Orthopedic Biomechanics.* New York, NY: Churchill Livingstone; 1982;240-250.
9. Brand RA, Crowninshield RD. The effect of cane use on hip contact stress force. *Clin Orthop.* 1980;147:181-184.
10. Davy DT, Kotzar GM, Brown RH, et al. Telemetric force measurement across the hip after total hip arthroplasty. *J Bone Joint Surg.* 1988; 70A(1):45-50.
11. Berzins A, Summer DR, Andriacchi TP. Stem curvature and load angle influence the initial relative bone-implant motion of cementless femoral stems. *J Orthop Res.* 1993;11(5):758-769.
12. Galante JO. Current concepts review: causes of the fractures of the femoral component in total hip replacement. *J Bone Joint Surg.* 1980;62(A):670-673.
13. Hampton SJ, Andriacchi TP, Galante JO. Three dimensional stress analysis of the femoral stem of a total hip prosthesis. *J Biomechanics.* 1980;13:443-448.
14. Philips TW, Nguyen LT, Munro SD. Loosening of cementless femoral stems: a biomechanical analysis of immediate fixation with loading vertical, femur horizontal. *J Biomechanics.* 1991;24(1):37-48.
15. Charnely J. *Low Friction Arthroplasty of the Hip: Theory and Practice.* New York, NY: Springer-Verlag; 1979:186-289.
16. Johnston RC, Brand RA, Crowninsheild RD. Reconstruction of the hip. *J Bone Joint Surg.* 1979;61A(5):639-652.
17. Hurwitz DE, Andriacchi TP. Biomechanics of the hip. In: Callahan J, Rubash H, Rosenberg A, eds. *The Adult Hip.* Philadelphia, PA: Lippincott Williams & Wilkins; 1998:75-89.
18. Delp SL, Maloney W. Effects of hip center location on the moment generating capacity of muscles. *J Biomechanics.* 1993;26(4,5):485-499.
19. Box G, Noble PC. The position of joint center and the functional outcome of total hip replacement. *Trans ORS.* 1993;18:525.
20. Yoder SA, Brand RA, Pederson DR, O'Gorman TW. Total hip acetabular component position affects component loosening rates. *Clin Orthop Relat Res.* 1988;228:79-87.
21. Murray MP, Gore DR, Clarkson BH. Walking patterns of patients with unilateral hip pain due to osteoarthritis and avascular necrosis. *J Bone Joint Surg.* 1971;53A(2):259-274.
22. Berman AT, Quinn RH, Zarro VJ. Quantitative gait analysis in unilateral and bilateral total hip replacement. *Arch Phys Med Rehabil.* 1991;72:190-193.
23. Hulet C, Hurwitz DE, Andriacchi TP, Galante JO, Rosenberg AG. Gait adaptations in patients with hip osteoarthritis. *Gait & Posture.* 1996;4(2):188.
24. Hurwitz DE, Chertack CC, Andriacchi TP. How gait changes in preoperative and postoperative patients with total hip replacement. Proceeding of the Second North American Congress on Biomechanics. 1992;313-314.
25. Wadsworth JB, Smidt GL, Johnson RC. Gait characteristics of subjects with hip disease. *Phys Ther.* 1972;52(8):829-839.

3

Approach to the Patient With Hip and Groin Pain

S.M. Javad Mortazavi, MD and Mitchell K. Freedman, DO

Hip pain and symptoms related to hip abnormalities are extremely common in adults. Approximately 14.3% of adults aged 60 years or older reported substantial hip pain on most days of the previous 6 weeks.[1] Osteoarthritis is the most common form of arthritis and one of the leading causes of chronic disability in the elderly.[2] The incidence rate of symptomatic, radiographic hip osteoarthritis is 88 per 1,000,000 person-years (95% CI, 75 to 101).[3] The prevalence of hip osteoarthritis has been reported to be 3% for women and 3.2% for men aged 55 to 74 years according to the National Health and Nutrition Survey (NHANES-I)[3] and 15.1% for women and 14.1% for men over 55 years according to the Rotterdam study.[4] Approximately 2.5% of all sports-related injuries relate to the hip.[5]

The complex anatomy of the hip joint and surrounding anatomic structures and potential pain generators offers challenges to diagnosing and appropriately treating a painful hip. The hip joint consists of the femoral head articulating with the acetabulum. The acetabulum is deepened by the labrum, a fibrocartilaginous structure, around its border. The joint is enclosed by a strong fibrous capsule. The other important structures around the hip are muscles and their tendons (abductors, adductors, extensors, flexors, and hamstrings) and bursae (greater trochanteric, iliopectineal, and ischiogluteal). Major vessels and nerves cross the hip joint on their way from the intra-abdominal region to the periphery of the legs. The pain may also arise from the muscular and osseous elements of the pelvis, the lumbar disc and facet joints, the sacroiliac joint, the abdominal wall, and the neurologic and visceral structures in the retroperitoneal space.

A systematic approach is necessary to distinguish intra-articular versus extra-articular lesions that can cause pain in the area of the hip (Table 3-1). This includes a thorough history and physical examination in combination with appropriate laboratory and imaging investigations. While this will identify the majority of clinically important pathologic entities, it may be difficult to establish the exact cause of pain in some cases. Furthermore, the reasons for pain may be multifactorial, especially in the presence of degenerative changes in both the hip and the lumbar spine.[6]

History

Pain secondary to hip joint pathology classically presents in the groin, thigh (anterior more than lateral or posterior thigh), and buttock. On rare occasions it can radiate to the knee or foot.[7] It is generally more achy than sharp, although the semantics of the descriptors vary greatly with the individual patient. The pain intensifies with weight bearing and certain movements. It is better with sitting or laying. Patients often complain of an accompanying limp. Lateral hip pain may present secondary to trochanteric bursitis, a tight tensor fascia lata, or hip abductor tendonitis. Buttock pain can result from ischial bursitis or piriformis syndrome, which may result in local buttock pain or radiating pain into the lower extremity. Medial groin pain may be secondary to adductor tendonitis, inflammation of the pubic symphysis, or pelvic fractures.

Patients with intra-articular hip pathology may also have concurrent complaints from the lumbosacral spine.[6] A

Parvizi J, Klatt BA.
Essentials in Total Hip Arthroplasty (pp 19-27).

Table 3-1

Differential Diagnosis of Hip Pain

Intra-Articular Etiologies

- Trauma
  - Fractures
  - Labral tears
- Inflammation
  - Seronegative arthropathies
    - Ankylosing spondylosis
    - Reiter
    - Inflammatory bowel disease
    - Psoriatic
  - Rheumatoid arthritis
  - Systemic lupus erythematosis
- Infection
  - Septic arthritis
  - Osteomyelitis
  - Tuberculosis
  - Brucellosis
  - Bursitis
  - Lyme disease
- Avascular necrosis
  - Idiopathic
  - Secondary
    - Alcoholism
    - Corticosteroid
    - Sickle cell anemia
- Transient osteoporosis (transient bone marrow edema syndrome)
- Childhood disorders
  - Developmental dysplasia of the hip
  - Legg-Calvé-Perthes disease
  - Slipped capital femoral epiphysis
- Femoral acetabular impingement
- Degenerative osteoarthritis
- Metabolic
  - Osteomalacia
  - Gout
  - Pseudogout
  - Paget's disease
  - Hemochromatosis
  - Hematologic
  - Hemophilia
- Neurologic
  - Charcot joint

Extra-Articular Etiologies

- Bursitis
- Tendonitis
  - Adductor
  - Iliopsoas
  - Piriformis
  - Tensor fascia lata
- Spine and pelvis
  - Fracture
  - Metastasis
  - Prolapsed intervertebral disc
  - Spondylolisthesis
  - Proximal radiculopathy
  - Sacroiliac joint
  - Facet joint dysfunction
- Visceral
  - Inguinal hernia
  - Testicular pathology
  - Urolithiasis
  - Intrapelvic pathology
  - Intravaginal pathology
- Vascular
  - Aneurysm
  - Arterial insufficency
- Neurologic
  - Mononeuropathies
    - Ilioinguinal
    - Iliohypogasteric
    - Femoral
    - Meralgia paresthetica

specific history pertinent to those structures must be performed as well, depending on the nature of the complaints. Lumbar spondylosis, spondylolisthesis, stenosis, and disc herniations can result in radiating pain to the buttock, groin, and further down the leg. Lumbar stenosis generally causes pain to radiate into the extremity with ambulation and is better with rest. Pain secondary to intervertebral disc herniations or internal disc derangements is frequently worse with sitting and is better with walking brief distances. Sacroiliac joint dysfunction can result in local pain near the sacroiliac joint as well as in groin pain and can occasionally radiate down below the knee.[8] Lumbar radiculopathy results in pain into the proximal, middle, and distal anterior thigh with injuries to the L1, L2, and L3 nerve roots, respectively. L4 radiculopathy can radiate into the anterior and or posterior thigh to the medial shin while L5 radiates posteriorly to the dorsum of the foot and S1 radiates posteriorly to the plantar aspect of the foot. Paresthesias are present with neurologic problems as opposed to joint disorders. Thus, the presence of paresthesias in the aforementioned distributions must raise suspicion of a neurologic disorder. Injuries to nerves in the retroperitoneum (resulting in femoral and obturator nerve lesions) can result in pain into the anterior thigh with accompanying weakness in the proximal lower extremity. Lateral thigh pain or paresthesias may point toward meralgia paresthetica (lateral femoral cutaneous nerve syndrome).

The instigating features resulting in the pain syndrome should be thoroughly scrutinized. Sudden onset of hip pain usually indicates trauma as the major cause. Trauma can result in a labral tear or other intra-articular injuries, while overstretch or overuse injuries may lead to extra-articular injuries like a strain, tendonitis, or bursitis. Pain secondary to a herniation of the intervertebral disc may be noted shortly after lifting a heavy object or even an innocuous event, such as a cough or sneeze. Hip pain secondary to inflammation or infection can have a sudden or gradual onset. A degenerative process such as hip osteoarthritis usually has a gradual onset of pain. However, there may be periods of acute exacerbations of the symptoms in patients with hip osteoarthritis related to an increase in activity, certain movements, or changes in the weather. Pain due to spinal stenosis or zygapophyseal joint dysfunction has also a gradual onset over a period of time.[9,10] The pain secondary to stress fracture and insufficiency fractures of the hip, femur, and pelvis is generally vague and nonspecific but may be severe and interfere with weight bearing. Osteoporosis and osteomalacia should be considered as the major risk factor to these types of fractures. Intermittent pain, especially unilateral pain radiating from the groin down the anterior thigh, usually indicates an intra-articular problem, including ischemic necrosis of the involved hip.[8]

Chronic inflammatory back pain, enthesopathy, and tender sacroiliac joint are common presentations of seronegative spondyloarthropathies. Nocturnal back pain that is relieved by varying degrees of activity may indicate ankylosing spondylitis.[11] Morning stiffness, or stiffness that appears after a long period of inactivity, that resolves within approximately 15 min is typical of osteoarthritis, while stiffness that lasts at least 1 hr is reminiscent of rheumatic disease.

Unexplained weight loss, fever, and night sweats indicate the possibility of a systemic inflammatory process. Nocturnal pain, weight loss, history of malignancy, and age over 65 raise concerns about a potential underlying malignancy.[12] Genitourinary and gastrointestinal symptoms may indicate that pathology is located in one of these areas instead of the hip. Inguinal or abdominal hernias must be a consideration with groin or suprapubic pain. Aortic and femoral artery aneurysms must be evaluated with groin or thigh pain. Vascular insufficiency must be considered with radiating pain into the extremity that is worse with ambulation. A careful search for these symptoms is indicated for patients with history of disease in these systems, as well as for patients who do not have findings consistent with musculoskeletal disease.[13]

Physical Examination

A stepwise approach to the physical examination is essential to ensure that important findings are not missed. Inspection of gait, pelvic symmetry, and curvature of back and leg length is very important. An antalgic gait may indicate a functional abnormality in the foot, ankle, knee, hip, pelvis, or lower back. A compensated Trendelenburg gait occurs when there is listing of the trunk over the affected side during weight bearing; this is a result of severe weakness of the ipsilateral hip abductors or pain secondary to hip osteoarthritis. Lesser degrees of weakness of the gluteus medius muscle leads to an uncompensated Trendelenburg gait in which the pelvis on the contralateral side dips with weight bearing, causing protrusion of the stationary affected hip. In a stiff hip gait, the patient walks by rotating the pelvis and swinging the legs in a circular fashion, so these patients show excessive motion in the spine and ipsilateral knee.[14] A labral tear in the hip may result in complaints of instability when the patient is standing with the hip in external rotation. Pelvic obliquity may be assessed using calibrated blocks and determined as to whether it is fixed or not.[15] The lumbar spine should be evaluated for hyperlordosis, which may indicate compensation for a fixed flexion deformity of the hip or a spondylolisthesis.

Lumbar flexion and extension should be evaluated while the patient is standing. The pattern of pain and the movement that provokes the pain should be noted for diagnostic purposes as well as to establish the therapeutic exercise program if therapy is indicated. Palpation of the sacroiliac joint, lower lumbar musculature, piriformis muscle, and trochanteric bursa can be evaluated in a standing or prone position. Asymmetries in the muscle bulk of the buttock, thigh, and calf should be noted.

The hip joint should be evaluated for specific areas of tenderness. In a supine position, the anterior hip capsule is palpated just inferior to the inguinal ligament over the femoral triangle. This area should be assessed both in supine and standing position for lymphadenopathy, inguinal, or femoral hernia and the presence of a femoral pulse or aneurysm. The popliteal, dorsalis pedis, and posterior tibial pulses should be evaluated. Leg length discrepancy should be evaluated in a supine position by measuring the distance from the umbilicus and anterior superior iliac spine to the medial malleoli to see if the problem is a leg length asymmetry or secondary to a scoliosis.

Hip range of motion should be evaluated in a supine position. Limited and painful range of motion in the hip joint points toward intra-articular joint pathology. Limited internal rotation of the hip is often one of the most sensitive findings for hip osteoarthritis. A painful click may suggest the presence of a labral tear, but sounds are nonspecific. Tenderness over the hip adductors can be seen with tendonitis of the adductor tendons. If there is tendonitis, then resistance to active hip adduction and passively stretching the hip adductors will replicate the pain. Similarly, with tendonitis of the hip abductors or hip flexors, the examiner palpates the site and passively stretches the tendon followed by having the patient perform an active contraction of the muscle and tendon in question. Pain secondary to trochanteric bursitis can often be reproduced with active contraction of the hip abductors or passive stretch of the hip abductors in addition to palpation over the bursa.

The Thomas flexion test involves flexing one of the hips in a supine position. If the contralateral hip flexes, there is a hip flexion contracture. Ober's test evaluates the tensor fascia lata and the patient is in a lateral recumbent position. The hip that is next to the table is flexed to eliminate lumbar lordosis while the hip that is away from the table is abducted and extended so that the thigh aligns with the body. If the hip is released then the leg will maintain an abducted position secondary to tightness of the iliotibial band. The muscle should be palpated as it is stretched and one side should be compared to the other side.[16] The straight leg rest should be checked in a supine position. Pain that radiates below the knee to the calf or foot between 30 and 70 degrees of hip flexion is compatible with radicular pain. Pain that radiates to the knee can be a result of radicular pain or secondary to hamstring tightness. The reverse straight leg test (femoral nerve stretch test) involves placing the patient into a prone position while the knee is flexed and the hip is extended. With upper lumbar or femoral nerve pathology, the pain radiates into the anterior thigh.[16]

Gaenslen's and Patrick's tests are 2 tests that have been used to help with diagnosis of sacroiliac joint dysfunction. Gaenslen's test involves having the patient in a supine position with his or her hip flexed while his or her hands are around the ipsilateral flexed knee. The contralateral hip is extended off of the table. The examiner is on the side of the extended hip. Pain is produced in the area of the sacroiliac joint. Patrick's test involves having the patient in a supine position and rotating the hip into flexion, abduction, and external rotation (FABER). Both tests can produce pain in patients with spine, hip, and sacroiliac dysfunction and are not specific.

The Pace test and the Freiberg tests are utilized to diagnose sacroiliac joint dysfunction. The Pace test provokes ipsilateral hip pain with resistance to active abduction and external rotation of the hip. The Freiberg test reproduces ipsilateral buttock pain with passive hip abduction and internal rotation. Patients with femoral acetabular impingement (FAI) will have pain with adduction and internal rotation of the hip at 90 degrees of hip flexion.

Knee and ankle examination should be performed. Patients with hip pathology can have pain referred to the knee. Furthermore, ambulation is a result of the entire lower extremity chain. Alteration in structures distal to the hip can also change forces through the hip and predispose patients to hip pain with ambulation.

Neurologic testing should be performed. Strength in the hip flexors may be compromised in L1, L2, and L3 radiculopathy. Quadriceps and hip adductors may be weak with L2-L4 radiculopathy. Retroperitoneal lesions can result in weakness of the hip flexors, hip adductors, and knee extensors. Femoral and obturator nerve lesions result in weakness of the knee extensors and hip adductors, respectively. L4 lesions can cause weakness into the knee extensors and ankle dorsiflexors (quadriceps and tibialis anterior). L5 lesions result in weakness of the ankle and toe dorsiflexors as well as the hip abductors while the S1 radiculopathy causes weakness in the ankle and toe plantar flexors and the hip extensors. Sciatic nerve lesions cause weakness in the dorsi and plantar flexors but spare the hip abductors and extensors unless there is a very proximal lumbosacral lesion that injures the superior and/or inferior gluteal nerves.

While an abnormal patellar reflex suggests involvement of the L2, L3, or L4 nerve root, an abnormal ankle jerk reflex suggests S1 nerve root involvement. A medial hamstring reflex is diminished with L5 nerve root involvement. Upper motor neuron findings such as a Babinski sign, hyperreflexia, or clonus should be evaluated as well.

Sensory examination of both the dermatomal and peripheral nerve pattern must be performed. The L1, L2, and L3 nerve roots innervate the anterior middle and distal anterior thigh, respectively. L4 innervates the medial shin while L5 is evaluated by checking the dorsal aspect of the foot and S1 innervates the area just below the lateral malleolus. The lateral femoral cutaneous nerve innervates the lateral upper thigh while the femoral nerve innervates the anterior thigh. A sciatic nerve lesion can result in hypesthesia of the entire foot. Proprioception should be checked in the great toe and the ankle.

Imaging Studies

Once the pain has been attributed to the hip joint, a differential diagnosis has to be considered to determine the most suitable imaging and laboratory studies to determine the etiology of the pain.[17] Standard radiographs remain the basis for the evaluation of the adult hip. The standard views include an anteroposterior view of the pelvis and commonly a cross-table lateral view of the symptomatic hip. Cross-table lateral (groin lateral) views better display the anterosuperior portion of the femoral neck than the frog-leg view. This is an important consideration regarding femoroacetabular impingement.[18] On the other hand, a subcortical lucent line, which is a sign of avascular necrosis (AVN) of the femoral head, is better viewed on frog-leg lateral. The signs of AVN are scattered areas of lucencies and sclerosis and femoral head collapse. In addition, in patients with suspected fracture of the hip, the cross-table lateral view should be ordered instead of the frog-leg lateral view. The plain radiographs should be scrutinized for any signs of malalignment, such as broken Shenton's line. The mineralization may diminish in osteoporosis, osteomalacia, inflammatory arthritides, and AVN. The joint line should be investigated since a narrowed joint space is 1 of the 4 radiological signs of osteoarthritis, which may be secondary to dysplasia.[19,20] The other radiographic signs of osteoarthritis are sclerosis of the joint line, osteophyte formation, and subchondral cyst. Radiographs of the hip fail to show early degenerative changes in the joint. One recent study showed arthroscopic evidence of osteoarthritis in 32% of patients with normal radiographs.[21] Findings typical of hip dysplasia include distortions of the femoral head, deviations of center-edge angle, and acetabular roof obliquity.[22] Although the plain radiography is not a standard measure for soft tissue evaluation, some clues such as lateral subluxation of the femoral head, absence of vacuum effect, and demineralization of subchondral bone refer to a problem in the joint space. Calcification within the soft tissue indicates abnormality in muscle, capsule, or bursae. The finding of calcification is nonspecific and could be observed in various conditions like rheumatoid arthritis, systemic lupus erythematous, and heterotopic ossification. Detection of a neoplastic lesion involving bone solely based on radiography requires at least 50% of tissue erosion.

Sonography is a useful tool for detection of muscle and tendon injuries and the presence of bursitis, hernia, and joint effusion. In addition, it allows dynamic evaluation of patients with snapping hip.[17,23] It also can optimally guide joint aspirations and therapeutic injections.[24]

Bone scan localizes an osseous lesion when there are wide spread pain complaints and the history and physical examination do not determine the etiology of the pain. It is now limited to evaluating disorders that are likely to involve multiple skeletal locations such as metastatic tumors and Paget's disease, or when there is ongoing suspicion of a stress fracture when other studies, such as magnetic resonance imaging (MRI), computed tomography (CT) scan, or plain x-ray are negative.

The main indication for performing CT scan in patients with hip pain is trauma. CT scan not only demonstrates fractures of the femoral neck that have not been detected on standard radiographs, but is also important for grading and surgical planning of complex fractures of the pelvis, acetabulum, and proximal femur.

Fractures, infection, tumors, and avascular necrosis should be ruled out early because they require immediate treatment to prevent damage to the joint. CT allows detection of calcifications and their localization. The 3-dimensional CT is very helpful in the assessment of acetabular and femoral version and dysplasia.[18,25]

MRI is the imaging study of choice in patients with hip pain whose radiographs are negative or inconclusive. However, different imaging protocols of the hip region are appropriate depending on the suspected diagnosis. In addition, the decision should be made as to whether to image the affected hip or both hips. In patients with suspected osteonecrosis or metastasis, bilateral imaging seems to be more appropriate. In most other situations, single hip imaging provides better spatial and contrast resolution due to the small field of view and use of a dedicated surface coil.[17] For patients with acute hip pain, MRI is the most sensitive and specific imaging technique for detecting and staging hip fractures, osteochondral injuries, soft tissue injuries, and inflammation.[26,27] Patients with contraindications to MRI (pacemakers, metallic implants, etc) may need to get a bone scan or CT scan in suspected fractures or metastasis where plain x-rays are unrevealing. Congenital deformities, degenerative osteoarthritis, stress fractures, and osteoarthritis are well characterized by MRI. MRI arthrography is both sensitive and specific for detecting labral tears, loose bodies in the joint space, chondral injuries, synovial chondromatosis, and ligamentum teres sprains.[19,28]

MRI of the lumbar spine and pelvis may be valuable studies to help to distinguish spine versus hip pathology. However, one must not forget that the presence of discogenic changes in the lumbar spine can be seen in asymptomatic patients.[29] Similarly, the presence of degenerative changes in the hip joint does not mean that the hip is the cause of the symptoms. One must compare these studies to the history and physical. Electromyography and nerve conduction velocity studies can be useful studies to look for objective evidence of lower motor nerve lesions. Lumbar discography is the gold standard for the diagnosis of internal disc disruption but false positive and false negative responses may occur.[30] The diagnostic injection is the gold standard for diagnosing sacroiliac joint dysfunction[31] and zygapophyseal joint pain.[32] At least 2 blocks are performed, and in excess of 75% pain relief is expected, as the false positive rate for one block is 38% in zygapophyseal joint blocks.[33] Fluoroscopically guided hip injections have also been used to delineate hip from spine pathology[34] and prognosticate on the outcome of hip arthroplasty.[35] Hip arthroscopy has been suggested as diagnostic and therapeutic mode for the diagnosis of labral tears and damage to the ligamentum teres. High rates of negative studies have been reported, however, and have limited the use of arthroscopy as an initial diagnostic procedure.[19,36,37]

Laboratory Investigation

Laboratory investigation should be tailored to the problems of the patient. Analysis of the blood helps in determining the presence of infection or inflammation as the cause of pain. Elevated white cell count may indicate infection, and anemia and thrombocytosis suggest chronic inflammation associated with RA.[8] Elevated blood urea nitrogen (BUN) and serum creatinine levels suggest renal disease that may be associated with chronic renal failure. Elevated liver enzymes may be compatible with a diagnosis of alcoholism, which could cause avascular necrosis of the femoral head. Erythrocyte sedimentation rate, C-reactive protein, serum Ig levels, and other acute-phase reactants are typically elevated in patients with inflammatory or infectious disease. Certain tests, such as rheumatoid factor, antinuclear antibodies, and HLA B-27, may be helpful in the diagnosis of systemic inflammatory disease. Synovial fluid analysis for cell count and differential, culture and gram stain, and crystal analysis provide precious information to differentiate different forms of arthritis, infections, gout, and pseudogout.

Differential Diagnosis of Intra-Articular Causes of Hip Pain

Osteoarthritis is one of the most common causes of hip pain in adults.[38,39] It usually occurs in the elderly, but it can occur at any age. Rheumatoid arthritis, ankylosing spondylitis, and other seronegative arthropathies can also involve the hip joint. In patients receiving corticosteroids for the treatment of inflammatory arthritis, the risk of avascular necrosis of the femoral head increases.[38] The hip is a common site for occult fracture. Stress fractures may result from abnormal stress on normal bone (fatigue fracture) or from the normal stress on abnormal bone. These fractures may not stop the patient from bearing weight and usually are not visible on the initial radiograph, so repeated radiographs and bone scan or MRI may be needed in doubtful cases.[17] The pelvis is a common site of involvement in Paget's disease and it may be presented as hip pain. In addition, these patients may have an associated osteoarthritis of the hip. Pain that originates in an arthritic Paget joint may be attributed to the occurrence of microfractures or to increased vascularity of the bone.[40]

Avascular necrosis of the femoral head is a pathological process that is associated with numerous conditions and therapeutic interventions including trauma, corticosteroid administration, alcohol use, sickle cell hemoglobinopathies, systemic lupus erythematous, Gaucher's disease, chronic renal failure, and pregnancy.[41] Clinical outcome is related to the percentage of involved weight bearing femoral area in relation to the acetabular roof.[42] The process most often is progressive, resulting in joint destruction and osteoarthritis within 3 to 5 years if left untreated.

Transient osteoporosis of the hip, now known as transient bone marrow edema syndrome, is typically seen in overweight middle-aged men and in women during the third trimester of pregnancy. It may be part of a continuum of bone marrow abnormalities including stress-related edema-like changes, subchondral fractures, and osteonecrosis.[17,43] On MRI images, extensive bone marrow edema in the femoral head and neck, possibly associated with joint effusion, is seen.[17] The absence of additional circumscribed, subchondral changes has a 100% positive predictive value for the transient nature of disease. In the presence of such changes, the probability for irreversible disease is increasing depending on the size of the lesion.[44]

Infectious arthritis of the hip is not common in adults but it can present as an acute septic arthritis or insidious septic arthritis in immune-compromised patients. As the hip joint capsule is strong and the joint space is small, any acute infection can lead to an increase in intra-articular pressure, which in turn can cause disturbances in critical blood supply to the femoral head.[38] In addition, the possibility of brucellosis and tuberculosis should always be kept in mind. The rate of osteoarticular infection in HIV-positive patients with tuberculosis has been reported as high as 60%.[45]

Torn acetabular labrum is a known cause of hip pain. The patient with a labral tear may complain of instability. Most labral abnormalities are associated with hip deformities including developmental dysplasia and femoroacetabular impingement. They are often considered a part of a spectrum of morphological changes resulting in labral tears, cartilage delamination, and early osteoarthritis.[46-48]

Crystalline arthropathies such as gout and pseudogout can produce extreme pain in the hip joint and often go undetected if the disease is limited to the hip joint. The patient may present with normal serum uric acid level and a joint effusion detected by ultrasound or MRI.[49]

Pigmented villonodular synovitis is a benign proliferative disorder of the synovial membrane but tends to locally destroy the joint. The hip joint is the second most commonly involved location after the knee joint.[50] It is usually seen in young adults who present with progressive pain and stiffness of the involved joint. In patients with advanced pigmented villonodular synovitis (PVNS) of the hip, juxta-articular erosions and osteoarthritis usually are seen on standard radiographs.[51] MRI is the modality of choice for assessment of PVNS.[52] Synovial chondromatosis is a metaplastic condition that results in production of numerous loose bodies. After the knee, the hip is the most common site of involvement.[53] Patients usually present in the second to fifth decades of life with nonspecific clinical symptoms that typically include dull, aching joint pain; catching; locking sensation; or mild limitation of motion.[54] The initial radiographic picture is often negative with the characteristic juxta-articular radiopacities not seen until much later in the disease process.[54] Since the clinical presentations are often insidious, there are usually delays in accurate diagnosis and initiation of the treatment.[54,55]

Both benign and malignant bone tumors may involve the proximal femur. Osteoid osteoma, osteoblastoma, chondroblastoma, chondrosarcoma, multiple myeloma, and metastasis should be considered depending on the patient's age and associated symptoms.[56] Standard radiographs remain the first-step imaging modality in suspected patients. MRI is very helpful in determining the extent of the tumor. CT scan may not only demonstrate cortical destruction and periosteal reaction, but may also show the subtle soft-tissue calcification not seen on standard radiographs.[17]

References

1. Christmas C, Crespo CJ, Franckowiak SC, Bathon JM, Bartlett SJ, Andersen RE. How common is hip pain among older adults? Results from the Third National Health and Nutrition Examination Survey. *J Fam Pract.* 2002;51(4):345-348.
2. Lawrence R, Helmick CG, Arnett FC, et al. Estimates of the prevalence of arthritis and selected musculoskeletal disorders in the United States. *Arthritis Rheum.* 1998;41(5):778-799.
3. Oliveria SA, Felson DT, Reed JI, Cirillo PA, Walker AM. Incident of symptomatic hand, hip and knee osteoarthritis among patients in a health maintenance organization. *Arthritis Rheum.* 1995;38(8):1134-1141.
4. Odding E, Valkenburg HA, Algra D, Vandenouweland FA, Grobbee DE, Hofman A. Associations of radiological osteoarthritis of the hip and knee with locomotor disability in the Rotterdam study. *Ann Rheum Dis.* 1998;57(4):203-208.
5. Anderson K, Strickland SM, and Warren R. Hip and groin injuries in athletes. *Am J Sports Med.* 2001;29(4):521-533.
6. McNamara MJ, Barrett KG, Christie MJ, Spengler DM. Lumbar spinal stenosis and lower extremity arthroplasty. *J Arthroplasty.* 1993;8(3):273-277.
7. Lesher JM, Dreyfuss P, Hager N, Kaplan M, Furman M. Hip joint pain referral patterns: a descriptive study. *Pain Med.* 2008;9(1):22-25.
8. Troum OM, Crues JV III. The young adult with hip pain: diagnosis and medical treatment, circa 2004. *Clin Orthop Relat Res.* 2004;(418):9-17.
9. Mazanec D, Podichetty V, Hsia A. Lumbar canal stenosis: start with nonsurgical therapy. *Cleve Clin J Med.* 2002;69(11):909-917.
10. Schwarzer A, Aprill CN, Derby R, Fortin J, Kine G, Bogduk N. Clinical features of patients with pain stemming from the lumbar zygapophyseal joints. *Spine.* 1994;19(10):1132-1137.
11. Khan MA. Update on spondyloarthropathies. *Ann Intern Med.* 2002;136:896-907.
12. Deyo RA, Diehl AK. Cancer as a cause of back pain: frequency, clinical presentation, and diagnostic strategies. *J Gen Intern Med.* 1988;3(3):230-238.

13. Adkins SB III, Figler RA. Hip pain in athletes. *Am Fam Physician.* 2000; 61(7):2109-2118.

14. Karol LA, Halliday SE, Gourineni P. Gait and function after intra-articular arthrodesis of the hip in adolescents. *J Bone Joint Surg Am.* 2000;82(4):561-569.

15. Gross MT, Burns CB, Chapman SW, et al. Reliability and validity of rigid lift and pelvic leveling device method in assessing functional leg length inequality. *J Orthop Sports Phys Ther.* 1998;27(4):285-294.

16. Malanga GA, Nadler S. *Musculoskeletal Physical Examination: an Evidence-Based Approach.* Philadelphia, PA: Elsevier Mosby; 2006:xiii, 353.

17. Mengiardi B, Pfirrmann CW, Hodler J. Hip pain in adults: MR imaging appearance of common causes. *Eur Radiol.* 2007;17(7):1746-1762.

18. Peters CL, Erickson J. The etiology and treatment of hip pain in the young adult. *J Bone Joint Surg Am.* 2006;88(suppl 4):20-26.

19. Hickman JM, Peters CL. Hip pain in the young adult: diagnosis and treatment of disorders of the acetabular labrum and acetabular dysplasia. *Am J Orthop.* 2001;30(6):459-467.

20. Takatori Y, Ninomiya S, Nakamura S, et al. Long-term results of rotational acetabular ostomy in patients with slight narrowing of the joint space on preoperative radiographic findings. *J Orthop Sci.* 2001;6(2):137-140.

21. Santori N, Villar RN. Arthroscopic findings in the initial stages of hip osteoarthritis. *Orthopedics.* 1999;4:405-409.

22. Murphy SB, Kijewski PK, Millis MB, Harless A. Acetabular dysplasia in the adolescent and young adult. *Clin Orthop Relat Res.* 1990;261:214-223.

23. Miller TT. Abnormalities in and around the hip: MR imaging versus sonography. *Magn Reson Imaging Clin N Am.* 2005;13(4):799-809.

24. Sofka CM, Saboeiro G, Adler RS. Ultrasound-guided adult hip injections. *J Vasc Interv Radiol.* 2005;16(8):1121-1123.

25. Parvizi J, Campfield A, Clohisy JC, Rothman RH, Mont MA. Management of arthritis of the hip in the young adult. *J Bone Joint Surg Br.* 2006;88(10):1279-1285.

26. Yamamoto T, Takabatake K, Iwamoto Y. Subchondral insufficiency fracture of the femoral head resulting in rapid destruction of the hip joint: a sequential radiographic study. *Am J Roentgenol.* 2002;178:435-437.

27. Hong SH, Kim SM, Ahn JM, Chung HW, Shin MJ, Kang HS. Tuberculous versus pyogenic arthritis: MR imaging evaluation. *Radiology.* 2001;218:848-853.

28. Petersilge CA. MR arthrography for evaluation of the acetabular labrum. *Skeletal Radiol.* 2001;30:423-430.

29. Boden SD, Davis DO, Dina TS, Patronas NJ, Wiesel SW. Abnormal magnetic-resonance scans of the lumbar spine in asymptomatic subjects. A prospective investigation. *J Bone Joint Surg Am.* 1990;72(3):403-408.

30. Carragee EJ, Lincoln T, Parmar VS, Alamin T. A gold standard evaluation of the "discogenic pain" diagnosis as determined by provocative discography. *Spine.* 2006;31(18):2115-2123.

31. Dreyfuss P, Michaelsen M, Pauza K, McLarty J, Bogduk N. The value of medical history and physical examination in diagnosing sacroiliac joint pain. *Spine.* 1996;21(22):2594-2602.

32. Dreyer SJ, Dreyfuss PH. Low back pain and the zygapophysial (facet) joints. *Arch Phys Med Rehabil.* 1996;77(3):290-300.

33. Schwarzer AC, Aprill CN, Derby R, Fortin J, Kine G, Bogduk N. The relative contributions of the disc and zygapophyseal joint in chronic low back pain. *Spine.* 1994;19(7):801-806.

34. Pateder DB, Hungerford MW. Use of fluoroscopically guided intra-articular hip injection in differentiating the pain source in concomitant hip and lumbar spine arthritis. *Am J Orthop.* 2007;36(11):591-593.

35. Odoom JE, Allen GM, Wilson DJ. Response to local anaesthetic injection as a predictor of successful hip surgery. *Clin Radiol.* 1999;54(7):430-433.

36. Berend KR, Vail TP. Hip arthroscopy in the adolescent and pediatric athlete. *Clin Sports Med.* 2001;20(4):763-778.

37. O'Leary J, Berend AK, Vail TP. The relationship between diagnosis and outcome in arthroscopy of the hip. *Arthroscopy.* 2001;17(2):181-188.

38. Zacher J, Gursche A. Regional musculoskeletal conditions: 'hip' pain. *Best Pract Res Clin Rheumatol.* 2003;17(1):71-85.

39. Hamer AJ. Pain in the hip and knee. *BMJ.* 2004;328(7447):1067-1069.

40. Hadjipavlou AG, Gaitanis IN, Kontakis GM. Paget's disease of the bone and its management. *J Bone Joint Surg Br.* 2002;84(2):160-169.

41. Assouline-Dayan Y, Chang C, Greenspan A, Shoenfeld Y, Gershwin ME. Pathogenesis and natural history of osteonecrosis. *Semin Arthritis Rheum.* 2002;32(2):94-124.

42. Lafforgue P, Dahan E, Chagnaud C, Schiano A, Kasbarian M, Acquaviva PC. Early-stage avascular necrosis of the femoral head: MR imaging for prognosis in 31 cases with at least 2 years of follow-up. *Radiology.* 1993;187(1):199-204.

43. Guerra JJ, Steinberg ME. Distinguishing transient osteoporosis from avascular necrosis of the hip. *J Bone Joint Surg Am.* 1995;77(4):616-624.

44. Vande Berg BC, Malghem JJ, Lecouvet FE, Jamart J, Maldague BE. Idiopathic bone marrow edema lesions of the femoral head: predictive value of MR imaging findings. *Radiology.* 1999;212(2):527-535.

45. Tuli SM. General principles of osteoarticular tuberculosis. *Clin Orthop Relat Res.* 2002;(398):11-19.

46. McCarthy JC, Noble PC, Schuck MR, Wright J, Lee J. The Otto E. Aufranc Award: the role of labral lesions to development of early degenerative hip disease. *Clin Orthop Relat Res.* 2001;(393):25-37.

47. Ganz R, Parvizi J, Beck M, Leunig M, Nötzli H, Siebenrock KA. Femoroacetabular impingement: a cause for osteoarthritis of the hip. *Clin Orthop Relat Res.* 2003(417):112-120.

48. Leunig M, Podeszwa D, Beck M, Werlen S, Ganz R. Magnetic resonance arthrography of labral disorders in hips with dysplasia and impingement. *Clin Orthop Relat Res.* 2004;(418):74-80.

49. McCarthy JC. Hip arthroscopy: when it is and when it is not indicated. *Instr Course Lect.* 2004;53:615-621.

50. Cotten A, Flipo RM, Chastanet P, Desvigne-Noulet MC, Duquesnoy B, Delcambre B. Pigmented villonodular synovitis of the hip: review of radiographic features in 58 patients. *Skeletal Radiol.* 1995;24(1):1-6.

51. Llauger J, Palmer J, Rosón N, Bagué S, Camins A, Cremades R. Nonseptic monoarthritis: imaging features with clinical and histopathologic correlation. *Radiographics.* 2000;20:S263-278.

52. Bancroft LW, Peterson JJ, Kransdorf MJ. MR imaging of tumors and tumor-like lesions of the hip. *Magn Reson Imaging Clin N Am.* 2005;13(4):757-774.

53. Ogilvie-Harris DJ, Saleh K. Generalized synovial chondromatosis of the knee: a comparison of removal of the loose bodies alone with arthroscopic synovectomy. *Arthroscopy.* 1994;10(2):166-170.

54. Schoeniger R, Naudie DD, Siebenrock KA, Trousdale RT, Ganz R. Modified complete synovectomy prevents recurrence in synovial chondromatosis of the hip. *Clin Orthop Relat Res.* 2006;451:195-200.

55. Lim SJ, Chung HW, Choi YL, Moon YW, Seo JG, Park YS. Operative treatment of primary synovial osteochondromatosis of the hip. *J Bone Joint Surg Am.* 2006;88(11):2456-2464.

56. Beltran J, Opsha O. MR imaging of the hip: osseous lesions. *Magn Reson Imaging Clin N Am.* 2005;13(4):665-676, vi.

4

Preoperative Evaluation of Patients for Total Hip Arthroplasty

Brett Perricelli, MD and Richard L. McGough III, MD

The evaluation of patients for total hip arthroplasty (THA) involves obtaining the correct diagnosis, assessing physical function and limitations, and evaluating medical comorbidities. It begins with an initial consultation that involves a history and physical examination. Hip disease must be accurately diagnosed and differentiated from spine, buttock, and knee pathology. Comorbidities, prior surgeries, the reasons for previous failed surgery, and infection risk must be identified and addressed. An accurate determination of the patient's functional status will address rehabilitation needs and allow for the correct expectations following surgery.

History

An in-depth analysis of hip pain and the differential was conducted in Chapter 3. It will be assumed for the purpose of this chapter that the proper diagnosis has been reached, and one is planning for hip replacement surgery.

Previous Treatment

Documenting the use of conservative measures in the treatment of hip arthritis is important. Some patients may have had some type of treatment prior to presentation. This treatment may have been either patient directed or physician prescribed. Patients need to be questioned about previous pharmacologic, physical, and occupational therapy. Not uncommonly will patients present with a several month or year history of nonsteroidal anti-inflammatory use, narcotic use, chiropractic care, and/or personal training. Primary care physicians may have ordered physical therapy, ambulatory assist devices, and therapeutic or diagnostic hip injections.

Patients with longstanding hip pathology may have already had surgical intervention. This may include an osteotomy, arthroscopy, or prior arthroplasty procedure. In a revision setting, the original diagnosis should be obtained as well as the operative report to verify the approach, fixation, and implants utilized. The evaluation of the painful arthroplasty needs to include an evaluation of infection, lysis, loosing, and dislocation.

Rating Scales

It is prudent to use standardized forms as an evaluation tool. Completing these before surgery is crucial so that the surgeon has an understanding of the preoperative disability present in the patient population. Rating scales have been designed to capture the essential elements of pain, stiffness, and physical disability in patients with osteoarthritis of the major joints. The Harris hip score is scored by the examiner and emphasizes range of motion, pain, and function. The Western Ontario McMaster Universities Osteoarthritis Index (WOMAC) is scored by the patient. It is used for both knee and hip pathology and it also assesses pain stiffness and function. A more general outcome score is the SF-36 Health Status Survey, which evaluates the patient's physical and emotional health and is completed by the patient. The process of completion of any of these surveys will give both the clinician and the patient further insight to the diagnosis, expectations, and goals of treatment.

Parvizi J, Klatt BA.
Essentials in Total Hip Arthroplasty (pp 29-37).

Past Medical History

The importance of past medical history and general health level cannot be overemphasized. As the majority of arthroplasty patients are over the age of 50, many if not most have medical comorbidities, some of which will be quite serious. The orthopedist should be aware of any concurrent illness, pertinent history, medications, allergies, previous surgeries, and previous anesthetics. Many medical comorbidities, such as diabetes, rheumatoid arthritis, poor nutrition, obesity, and the use of corticosteroids, are well known to increase the risk of infection or lead to poor prognosis.[1-4] Subpopulations of arthroplasty patients, most notably those who have undergone solid organ or bone marrow transplantation, as well as those suffering from avascular necrosis due to chronic corticosteroid use may be substantially immunocompromised. While this may not preclude hip arthroplasty, immunosuppression certainly alters the expected infection rate and should be included in the risk-benefit discussion.

Infection

Due to the gravity of infectious complications, a history of prior or recurrent infections should be specifically elicited. A history of joint infection, genitourinary infection, diverticular disease, nonhealing ulcers, and dentition must be pursued and corrected prior to any arthroplasty procedure.[3,5] Dental clearance is a topic of some controversy but it is the practice of many to require a dental evaluation prior to THA.

Diabetes Mellitus

There is excellent evidence that surgical site infection can be decreased by close control of perioperative glucose levels in diabetics.[6] When controlling for age, sex, and procedure, diabetes mellitus increases the risk of developing a late prosthetic infection after THA.[5,7] Diabetics, especially those patients who are insulin dependent, need to have excellent glucose control both pre- and postoperatively.

Anticoagulation and Venous Thromboembolism

Anticoagulant use is common among arthroplasty candidates. While aspirin is the most widely used and best studied antiplatelet agent, the use of clopidogrel (Plavix [Bristol-Myers Squibb, New York, NY]) has increased substantially in recent years. Heavy marketing to physicians and direct-to-consumer advertising have now made it the second best-selling drug in the world after Lipitor (atorvastatin calcium) (Pfizer, New York, NY).[8] Approximately 5.9% of people over the age of 65 suffer from atrial fibrillation, many treated with warfarin.[9] Anticoagulants should be stopped in the appropriate manner so the effects are mitigated or reversed.

Venous thromboembolism (VTE) is one of the most frequent and serious complications after total hip arthroplasty, total knee arthroplasty, and hip fracture surgery.[10] In the absence of thromboprophylaxis, approximately 50% of individuals after hip arthroplasty and hip fracture will go on to develop a deep venous thrombosis (DVT).[11] After even a single first episode of DVT, there is a 30% cumulative risk of recurrent DVT at 8 years.[12] It is important to document VTE history and plan for prophylaxis and prevention.

Anesthesia History

In patients that have a history of anesthetic problems, preoperative planning and anesthesia consultation can increase patient safety and save time. This consultation can also substantially reduce anxiety for the patient and the anesthesia team. Examples of historical factors that can complicate the delivery of anesthesia include narcotic use, malignant hyperthermia, prior lumbar surgery, spinal deformity, obstructive sleep apnea, and other airway disorders.

Patients who have used narcotics for an extended period of time will develop tolerance to the medications. Controlling the pain in these patients will require higher doses of narcotics, and if this fact is recognized early, it makes the pain control smoother. Malignant hyperthermia needs to be discovered in the patient's history or the family history.

THA is often done under spinal anesthesia, and many patients have misconceptions about what this involves. If the surgeon prepares the patient for anesthesia with a brief mention of his or her preferences, this can ease the discussion with anesthesia. Patients with severe lumbar stenosis, prior lumbar surgery, and spinal scoliosis may not be able to undergo spinal anesthesia.

A history of difficult intubation or prior anesthetic complication should be elicited and reported to the anesthesia providers preoperatively. A fiber-optic intubation may be needed if the airway is difficult and having the equipment in the OR requires planning.

More detail on anesthesia options can be found in Chapter 20.

Medications

A detailed medication and drug history is required. This includes over-the-counter medications, nutritional products, inhalers, and prescription medications. The use of herbal remedies and its effects on surgery can present detrimental effects.[13-16] Doses and schedule should be documented for all medications, especially narcotics. Resumption of rheumatoid medications can also be explained at this time. Many of the newer agents used to treat rheumatologic diseases have an immune modulating effect, and they have to be held to improve wound healing and to lower infection risks. An excellent guide to perioperative medication management in patients with rheumatoid arthritis is provided in the *Journal of the American Academy of Orthopaedic Surgeons.*

Social History and Family History

A full social history including social support systems, level of physical activity, alcohol use, occupation, and a smoking history should be obtained. This will allow the clinician and team to plan for a smooth postoperative stay and rehabilitation. Family history of anesthetic problems and VTE should also be noted.

One of the most frequently missed social history items surrounds the patient's domicile and cohabitants. In planning for postoperative care, a lot must be known regarding the patient's physical space. The home layout, number of stairs to enter or exit, and availability of bathrooms can change discharge planning substantially, and can make transfer to a rehabilitation or skilled nursing facility necessary. Likewise, the availability of caregivers strongly affects the initial rehabilitation efforts. Does the patient live alone? Do family members or friends who are willing to assume a caregiving role live in close proximity? Who would the patient call if "stuck" on a sofa, toilet, or floor? Does the patient's spouse have substantial physical disabilities that would negate his or her abilities to function as an active caregiver? All of these issues require exploration to assure a safe, functional rehabilitation.

Physical Examination

The physical exam begins with inspection as soon as the clinician observes the patient, either going into the exam room or with clinician entry into the exam room. What type of posture does the patient have when he or she walks into the room? Is the patient independent or is he or she using an assistive device or a wheelchair? Can the patient easily transfer from a chair to the examination table? These factors will determine discharge location and ability to rehabilitate.

Inspection

Inspection begins after the patient is gowned and disrobed. Surgical and traumatic scars are noted along with any muscular atrophy of the trunk, buttocks, or spine. Surgical scars over the hip are taken into consideration when planning the surgical incision. The spine should be examined for range of motion, abnormal curves, deformity, and irregular hair distribution. Spinal scars and deformity can alert the surgeon to a patient who may need general anesthesia and to a patient who might have spine-related weakness in the limb. Attention is then focused on the pelvis, usually with the examiner behind the patient. Bony landmarks can be palpated for tenderness. These landmarks include the posterior-superior iliac spine, anterior-superior iliac spine, greater trochanter, and ischial tuberosity. At this time, pelvic obliquity can be determined with the examiner's hands on the iliac crests. Apparent obliquity must be differentiated from fixed obliquity, which can be secondary to lumbar spine disease. This is most commonly done with blocks placed under the short limb. While the patient is still standing, a Trendelenburg test is performed by asking the patient to stand on the involved leg. The Trendelenburg sign is a signal of gluteus medius weakness or relative inhibition. In a positive sign, the pelvis will drop on the uninvolved side and the pelvis will be unlevel.[17] In a more subtle positive test, the patient will shift the upper torso over the standing leg, indicating more subtle abductor weakness with preserved balance. A patient with a functional gluteus medius will be able to maintain a level pelvis from the preserved gluteus medius strength. If the patient has a weakness of the abductors preoperatively, then this will likely persist into the postoperative period.

Gait is then observed and evaluated. An abnormality exists in approximately 15% of people older than 64 years and this increases to 40% by age 85.[18] A coxalgic gait of a painful hip is characterized by the shifting of the thorax toward the painful side during the single-limb stance phase on the affected hip. This maneuver results in a decreased joint reactive force on the painful hip. In a coxalgic gait, the stance phase is decreased on the affected side, with increasing time spent on swing phase (Figure 4-1). Coxalgic gait should be corrected by the THA. A Trendelenburg gait is similar to the coxalgic gait; however, it involves tilt of the pelvis. The abductor dysfunction of the affected side is noted with the drop of the pelvis of the contralateral side. This differs from the aforementioned coxalgic gait in which the pelvis remains level and the upper torso shifts toward the painful hip during the single-limb stance. Stance and swing phases remain symmetric in a Trendelenburg gait (see Figure 4-1).[17]

Palpation

The patient is then asked to lie down upon the exam table, again with notice to agility, speed, and assistance

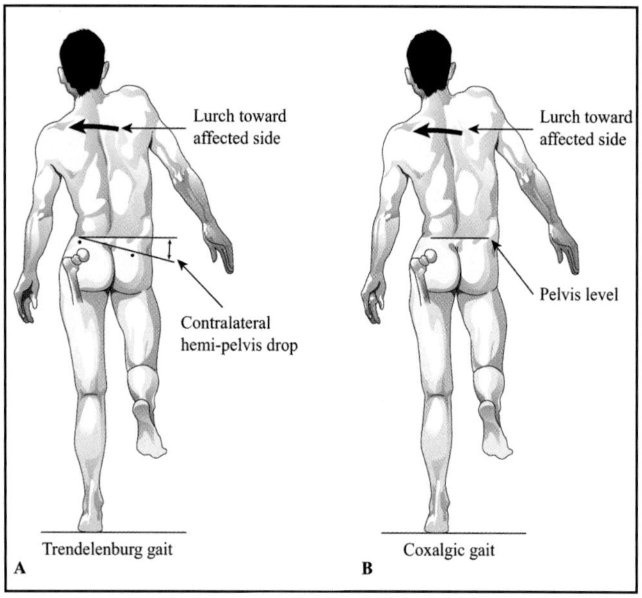

Figure 4-1. Trendelenburg gait. The Trendelenburg gait is very similar in appearance to a coxalgic gait, with one main distinguishing feature: the tilt of the pelvis. In the Trendelenburg gait (A), the contralateral hemipelvis drops during the single-limb stance phase on the affected side because of severve abductor insufficiency. In the coxalgic gait (B), the pelvis remains level.

needed. Palpation of the pubic symphysis, lymph nodes, greater trochanter, and pulse should be performed. Active and passive hip motion are then observed and recorded. Hip flexion/extension in neutral, internal, and external rotation is measured. Hip flexion should be done with the patient supine and knee flexed to eliminate hamstring tightness. Extension is best measured prone: normal is between 0 to 15 to 30 degrees, and frequently decreases with increasing age. Hip abduction and adduction should be measured with the patient supine and a level pelvis as judged by the bilateral anterior superior iliac spines.

Special Tests

The Thomas test can be used to assess for a hip flexion contracture. Hip flexion contracture may require release of the anterior capsule for correction. With the patient supine on the exam table, both knees and hips are flexed to the patient's chest. This maneuver stabilizes the pelvis and flattens the spine, which eliminates any lumbar lordosis. The hip to be examined is then extended to neutral. Fixed hip flexion is then easily measured. Ely's test is then used to evaluate a tight rectus femoris. The patient is positioned prone and passive knee flexion is applied. A contracted rectus femoris will yield hip flexion on the affected side; normally the hip would remain flat on the exam table.

Ober's test evaluates the iliotibial (IT) band and contraction.[19] The patient is positioned lateral with the affected side up. The examiner assists the patient with hip abduction with the hip and knee flexed to 90 degrees. The leg is then released from abduction to neutral. An IT band contracture will prevent the leg from falling back into adduction. A normal IT band will fall into neutral.

Hamstring tightness is also evaluated by measuring the popliteal angle. While the patient is supine, the hip and knee are flexed to 90 degrees. The knee is then passively extended. Full extension is a 0-degree popliteal angle.

Differentiation of intra-articular pain from posterior sacroiliac (SI) pain can be evaluated with Patrick's test (FABER or figure 4 test). The hip in question is flexed, abducted, and externally rotated. The foot is then placed on the contralateral anterior thigh/knee. An external rotation force is then applied to the ipsilateral knee. The test result is considered to be positive if the patient reports reproduction of hip pain in this position. Pain posterior may be indicative of SI pathology and groin pain is most likely from intra-articular pathology.[20]

Apprehension tests may then be performed indicative of labral pathology. Specifically the hip is flexed, adducted, and internally rotated. Pain during this maneuver may be indicative of anterior labral pathology.

Neurocirculatory Examination

Neurocirculatory examination is then addressed. It is crucial to document preoperative function so that any deficiencies postoperatively are recognized. This exam includes muscle testing, sensation, and vascular examination. Functional groups of flexors, extensors, adductors, abductors, and rotators are tested. Strength is judged on the 5-point scale as established by the National Foundation of Infantile Paralysis, Inc, Committee on After-Effects, and adopted by the American and British Academies of Orthopaedic Surgeons (Table 4-1).[21]

Vascular examination of the femoral, popliteal, dorsalis pedis, and posterior tibialis pulses are then performed and recorded. The Ankle-Brachial Index should be obtained if no palpable pulse is present.

Assessment of Leg Length

Planning for correction of leg length inequality is part of the preoperative planning. Leg length is assessed while the patient is supine—this involves 2 measurements. True leg length is determined by the distance from the anterior-superior iliac spine to the medial malleolus and reflects the

Table 4-1

MANUAL MUSCLE TESTING SCALE FROM 0 TO 5

GRADE	FINDINGS
0	No muscle contraction visible or palpated.
1	Examiner can see or palpate a contraction when the patient attempts to contract the muscle.
2	The patient can actively move the muscle in the plane of gravity.
3	The patient can move the muscle against gravity, but cannot move against any resistance from the examiner.
4	The patient can move the muscle against some resistance from the examiner, but cannot overcome full resistance
5	The patient can overcome full resistance of the examiner. This is full/normal muscular strength.

actual length of the extremity. Apparent leg length takes into account contractures about the hip as well as lumbar spine pathology that may result in pelvic obliquity. Apparent leg length is measured from the umbilicus, or a fixed point in the center of the body, to the medial malleolus. It is possible for the true leg length measurement to identify the involved hip as shorter than the contralateral normal hip while the apparent leg length suggests the involved extremity is longer secondary to either a hip abduction contracture on the involved side or a fixed pelvic obliquity from lumbar spine disease.

Both of these conditions result in elevation of the unaffected hemipelvis and give the appearance of shortening of the unaffected leg. Pelvic obliquity, possibly from lumbar spine pathology, results in an apparent leg length discrepancy. The surgeon must realize this preoperatively and inform these patients that a hip operation cannot equalize apparent leg length discrepancy. Attempting to do so could lead to significant lengthening or shortening of the true leg length, both of which are associated with potential problems. Shortening of the true leg length can lead to hip instability. Lengthening of the lower extremity beyond the true leg length can be associated with nerve injury or obvious cosmetic and functional problems.[22,23]

Hip pathology can produce an apparent leg length discrepancy through the development of either an adduction or abduction contracture; both may lead to pelvic obliquity. An abduction contracture results in an obliquity with the involved hemipelvis being lower than the uninvolved side and yields an apparently long leg. An adduction contracture does just the opposite, pelvic obliquity with the involved hemipelvis being higher than the uninvolved side and giving the appearance of a short leg. Patients with hip adduction contracture and osteoarthritis of the hip will appear to have a very short leg because the 2 factors are additive. The hip arthroplasty will alleviate the pelvic obliquity related to an adduction contracture and over time the pelvis will once again balance.

RADIOGRAPHIC EVALUATION

The next step in the process involves analysis of radiographs. The radiographs should be used to confirm the clinical history and exam. In addition, the use of preoperative templating to identify the level of the osteotomy cut, neck length, and femoral offset is important in re-establishing hip biomechanics and minimizing leg length discrepancy. Chapter 3 provides an in-depth review of imaging studies used in the evaluation of hip pain.

Rheumatoid arthritis (RA) typically lacks osteophyte formation unless it is longstanding and the patient has developed secondary osteoarthritis. RA commonly presents with periarticular osteoporosis and global joint space narrowing. Patients with RA should also have routine cervical spine films performed to evaluate for instability prior to surgery.[24] With regard to other possible diagnoses, one must keep in mind that a metastatic lesion must destroy 30% to 50% of bone and reach a size of 1 cm to be seen on plain radiographs.[25] Hip and thigh pain with negative radiographs often necessitates a further work-up.

Cases that involve complex acetabular pathology should be evaluated with Judet's view and any patient with a history of a pelvic fracture should have inlet and outlet views obtained. A patient with a lower extremity deformity or history of growth arrest should have long leg cassette views and/or scanograms for leg length discrepancy.

Computed Tomography, Radioscintigraphy, Magnetic Resonance Imaging, and Arthrography

Under certain circumstances, computed tomography (CT) scanning may help with preoperative evaluation. CT has traditionally been utilized and considered superior to magnetic resonance imaging (MRI) for bony assessment and congruity. CT is useful for acetabular or femoral anteversion determination, as well as determination of the size and shape of both the femoral neck and the acetabulum. In patients with a history of traumatic dislocation, CT is also useful for evaluating loose bodies. In the revision with bone loss from osteolysis or other causes, the CT can give an accurate idea of the remaining bone available for cup support.

A bone scan may be useful to identify osteoblastic activity in the lumbosacral spine, SI joint, or the hip joint. It may also be useful in the revision setting if one is worried about aseptic loosening. Bone scan has largely been replaced by MRI as the most sensitive tool for diagnosing occult hip fractures and avascular necrosis (AVN).

MRI has historically been used for soft tissue evaluation but it can also be useful in some bony conditions. MRI is superior to all other modalities in the early detection of stress fractures and AVN. MRI combined with arthrography appears to increase the utility in the diagnosis of labral tears and intra-articular pathology. When trying to detect a labral lesion, the sensitivity for MR arthrography was 95% and the accuracy of MR arthrography was 88% when correlated with surgical findings.[26]

Hip arthrography and intra-articular injection can be a useful adjunct as both therapy and a diagnostic tool to help delineate hip from spine or pelvis pathology. A response to an intra-articular injection of anesthetic has been reported to be up to 90% accurate for detecting the presence of intra-articular abnormality.[27] Rarely, a hip aspiration should be performed if inflammatory joint disease or infection are suspected.

LOGISTICS

Preoperative Clinic Visit

PREOPERATIVE CLEARANCE

Many tasks need to be completed on the preoperative visit after a decision for surgery is made. The purpose of preoperative evaluation is not to "give medical clearance" but rather to evaluate the patient's current medical status. Preoperative evaluation has been shown to reduce the number of canceled surgical procedures and increase physician satisfaction.[28]

The extent of a preoperative evaluation is patient specific. It will depend upon the patient's medical condition, the proposed surgical procedure, and the anesthetic choice. An octogenarian with unstable angina and diabetes will have different needs than a younger patient with no medical problems or medications. As a basic rule of thumb, if the patient has a significant medical history, a recent unstable condition, or is on a medication that may need to be modified due to surgery, consultation among the patient primary care provider and anesthesia staff is appropriate. Examples of medications that may require perioperative modifications include insulin, corticosteroids, oral hypoglycemics, anticoagulants, and chronic narcotic use.

Laboratory Evaluation

Much controversy exists with regard to routine preoperative screening. It has been shown in other disciplines of surgery that routine testing is not useful or cost-effective.[29-31] Despite this controversy, preoperative studies are the norm at many institutions and are frequently required prior to surgery. Preoperative laboratory testing should be based on age, gender, concomitant medical disease, and type of operation to be performed.[29-31]

A complete blood count with differential is done to check red cell levels, platelet counts, and the total white blood cell count. It is not uncommon to have a patient present with anemia on routine screening, and the reason for this is both complex and frequently multifactorial. Persistent iron deficiency anemia or anemia of another type should undergo a hematologic work-up. A basic metabolic panel is used for evaluation of electrolyte imbalance and renal failure, specifically for those on dialysis, as well as those taking diuretic medications or digitalis. A urinalysis (UA) is done for infectious screening; it can also be utilized to verify glucose levels and red blood cell levels. These may lead to a diagnosis of diabetes or genitourinary tumor. Either of these should be worked up prior to arthroplasty intervention.

An electrocardiogram (EKG) is used for cardiac evaluation, often revealing new and old ischemic changes, arrhythmias, or prior pulmonary emboli. EKG findings may identify patients at risk of postoperative ischemia or dysrhythmia.[32]

Chest radiography was traditionally done for evaluation of chest lesions; now it is a useful screen for cardiac, pulmonary, and volume status. Recently, it has been recommended that clinical findings instead of age cutoffs direct preoperative testing.[33] Any patient with a history of malignancy, tuberculosis (TB), pulmonary infection, sleep apnea, and congenital heart disease of suspected intrathoracic conditions should have a chest radiograph performed.

Less well defined is the need for a cardiology specific medical evaluation. In 2002, the American College of Cardiology and the American Heart Association established

Table 4-2

Clinical Predictors of Increased Perioperative Cardiovascular Risk

Major Clinical Predictors
Unstable coronary syndrome
Decompensated congestive heart failure
Significant arrhythmias
Severe valvular disease
Intermediate Clinical Predictors
Mild angina pectoris
History of myocardial infarction, diabetes mellitus, or chronic renal failure with serum creatinine greater than 2 mg/dL

a framework for considering cardiac risk of noncardiac surgery in a variety of patients and surgical situations.[34,35] These guidelines have been further modified to include when a cardiology referral is indicated.[36] The noncardiologist physician, whether an anesthesiologist, a generalist, or an orthopedic surgeon, should assess 1) the presence or absence of major or intermediate clinical predictors, 2) the patient's functional status, and 3) the risk of surgery, as well as obtain information about previous cardiac intervention and testing (Table 4-2). Figure 4-2 is a basic protocol of which patients need to have a cardiac consultation prior to operative intervention.

Information

Patients have better outcomes when they are informed and empowered. The preoperative clinic visit is the ideal place for information to be distributed. Examples of patient information topics can be found in Table 4-3. Basic information about arthroplasty, anesthetic blocks, drains, and postoperative therapy should be distributed.

Operating Room Needs

Implant selection and special operating room equipment (somatosensory evoked potentials, instruments, etc) should be noted or ordered during the pre-operative visit (discussed in other chapters).

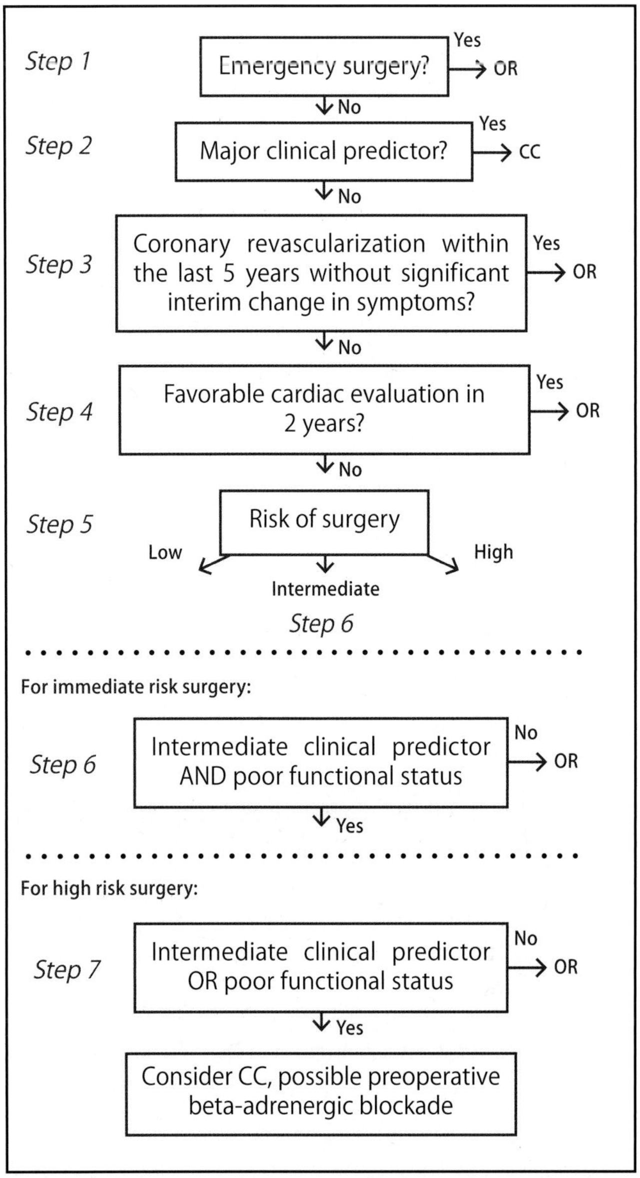

Figure 4-2. Modification of the ACC-AHA guidelines to highlight indications for cardiology consultation. OR, operating room; CC, cardiology consultation. The clinical predictors, high-risk and intermediate-risk surgery, and poor functional status are defined in the text. CC may be indicated (1) for patients with a major clinical predictor, (2) for patients undergoing an intermediate-risk surgery who have poor functional status and an intermediate clinical predictor, and (3) for patients undergoing a high-risk surgery who have poor functional status or an intermediate clinical predictor.

References

1. Cierny G III, DiPasquale D. Periprosthetic total joint infections: staging, treatment, and outcomes. *Clin Orthop Relat Res.* 2002;(403):23-28.

Table 4-3

PATIENT INFORMATION TOPICS

- Venous thromboembolic events and prevention
- Preoperative antimicrobial skin preparation
- What the patient should bring (sleep apnea device, dentures, glasses, etc)
- Directions to the hospital, parking, family visitation hours
- Anesthesia information (general, spinal, blocks, and patient-controlled analgesia)
- Medication to stop prior to surgery
- Sequential compression devices
- Foley catheter
- Surgical drains
- Cardiac monitors
- Who the patient will meet in the hospital (surgeons, internists, nurses, physical therapists, social work, case management)
- Incisional care
- Braces and immobilizers
- Home care, visiting nurses and setting it up
- Postoperative rehabilitation guidelines and timetables

2. Peersman G, Laskin R, Davis J, Peterson M. Infection in total knee replacement: a retrospective review of 6489 total knee replacements. *Clin Orthop Relat Res.* 2001;(392):15-23.
3. Wilson MG, Kelley K, Thornhill TS. Infection as a complication of total knee-replacement arthroplasty. Risk factors and treatment in sixty-seven cases. *J Bone Joint Surg Am.* 1990;72(6):878-883.
4. Winiarsky R, Barth P, Lotke P. Total knee arthroplasty in morbidly obese patients. *J Bone Joint Surg Am.* 1998;80(12):1770-1774.
5. Wymenga AB, van Horn JR, Theeuwes A, Muytjens HL, Slooff TJ. Perioperative factors associated with septic arthritis after arthroplasty. Prospective multicenter study of 362 knee and 2,651 hip operations. *Acta Orthop Scand.* 1992;63(6):665-671.
6. Zerr KJ, Furnary AP, Grunkemeier GL, Bookin S, Kanhere V, Starr A. Glucose control lowers the risk of wound infection in diabetics after open heart operations. *Ann Thorac Surg.* 1997;63(2):356-361.
7. Lai K, Bohm ER, Burnell C, Hedden DR. Presence of medical comorbidities in patients with infected primary hip or knee arthroplasties. *J Arthroplasty.* 2007;22(5):651-656.
8. The Independent Drug Information Service. Anti-platelet therapy. URL: http://www.rxfacts.org/professionals/antiplatelet.php. Accessed August 2011.
9. Feinberg WM, Blackshear JL, Laupacis A, Kronmal R, Hart RG. Prevalence, age distribution, and gender of patients with atrial fibrillation. Analysis and implications. *Arch Intern Med.* 1995;155(5):469-473.
10. Geerts WH, Pineo GF, Heit JA, et al. Prevention of venous thromboembolism: the Seventh ACCP Conference on Antithrombotic and Thrombolytic Therapy. *Chest.* 2004;126(3 suppl):338S-400S.
11. Gallus AS. Applying risk assessment models in orthopaedic surgery: overview of our clinical experience. *Blood Coagul Fibrinolysis.* 1999;10(suppl 2):S53-61.
12. Prandoni P, Villalta S, Bagatella P, et al. The clinical course of deep-vein thrombosis. Prospective long-term follow-up of 528 symptomatic patients. *Haematologica.* 1997;82(4):423-428.
13. Petry JJ. Surgically significant nutritional supplements. *Plast Reconstr Surg.* 1996;97(1):233-240.
14. Petry JJ. Garlic and postoperative bleeding. *Plast Reconstr Surg.* 1995;96(2):483-484.
15. Burnham BE. Garlic as a possible risk for postoperative bleeding. *Plast Reconstr Surg.* 1995;95(1):213.
16. Cheema P, El-Mefty O, Jazieh AR. Intraoperative haemorrhage associated with the use of extract of Saw Palmetto herb: a case report and review of literature. *J Intern Med.* 2001;250(2):167-169.
17. Trendelenburg F. Uber den gang bei angeborener huftgelenksluxation. *Dtsch Med Wchenschr.* 1895(21):21-24.
18. Sudarsky L. Geriatrics: gait disorders in the elderly. *N Engl J Med.* 1990;322(20):1441-1446.
19. Ober F. The role of the iliotibial band and fascia lata as a factor in the causation of low-back disabilities and sciatica. *J Bone and Joint Surgery.* 1936;18:105-110.
20. Slipman CW, Sterenfeld EB, Chou LH, Herzog R, Vresilovic E. The predictive value of provocative sacroiliac joint stress maneuvers in the diagnosis of sacroiliac joint syndrome. *Arch Phys Med Rehabil.* 1998;79(3):288-292.
21. Hoppenfeld S. *Orthopaedic Neurology: A Diagnostic Guide to Neurologic Levels.* Philadelphia, PA: JB Lippincott Company; 1977.
22. Maloney WJ, Keeney JA. Leg length discrepancy after total hip arthroplasty. *J Arthroplasty.* 2004;19(4 suppl 1):108-110.
23. Ireland J, Kessel L. Hip adduction/abduction deformity and apparent leg-length inequality. *Clin Orthop Relat Res.* 1980(153):156-157.
24. Kwek TK, Lew TW, Thoo FL. The role of preoperative cervical spine x-rays in rheumatoid arthritis. *Anaesth Intensive Care.* 1998;26(6):636-641.
25. Stephen D. Management of metastatic osseous lesions of the lower extremity. *Techniques in Orthopaedics.* 2004;19(1):15-24.
26. Czerny C, Kramer J, Neuhold A, Urban M, Tschauner C, Hofmann S. [Magnetic resonance imaging and magnetic resonance arthrography of the acetabular labrum: comparison with surgical findings]. *Rofo.* 2001;173:702-707.

27. Byrd JW, Jones KS. Diagnostic accuracy of clinical assessment, magnetic resonance imaging, magnetic resonance arthrography, and intra-articular injection in hip arthroscopy patients. *Am J Sports Med.* 2004;32(7):1668-1674.
28. Marcus D, Magallanes M. The perioperative medicine service: an innovative practice at Kaiser Bellflower Medical Center. *Perm J.* 2002;6(3):13-16.
29. Velanovich V. Preoperative laboratory screening based on age, gender, and concomitant medical diseases. *Surgery.* 1994;115(1):56-61.
30. Velanovich V. The value of routine preoperative laboratory testing in predicting postoperative complications: a multivariate analysis. *Surgery.* 1991;109(3 pt 1):236-243.
31. Kaplan EB, Sheiner LB, Boeckmann AJ, et al. The usefulness of preoperative laboratory screening. *JAMA.* 1985;253(24):3576-3581.
32. Velanovich V. Preoperative screening electrocardiography: predictive value for postoperative cardiac complications. *South Med J.* 1994;87(4):431-434.
33. Lim EH, Liu EH. The usefulness of routine preoperative chest x-rays and ECGs: a prospective audit. *Singapore Med J.* 2003;44(7):340-343.
34. Eagle KA, Berger PB, Calkins H, et al. ACC/AHA guideline update for perioperative cardiovascular evaluation for noncardiac surgery--executive summary. A report of the American College of Cardiology/American Heart Association Task Force on practice guidelines (committee to update the 1996 guidelines on perioperative cardiovascular evaluation for noncardiac surgery). *Anesth Analg.* 2002;94(5):1052-1064.
35. Fleisher LA, Beckman JA, Brown KA, et al. ACC/AHA 2006 guideline update on perioperative cardiovascular evaluation for noncardiac surgery: focused update on perioperative beta-blocker therapy: a report of the American College of Cardiology/American Heart Association Task Force on practice guidelines (writing committee to update the 2002 Guidelines on Perioperative Cardiovascular Evaluation for Noncardiac Surgery): developed in collaboration with the American Society of Echocardiography, American Society of Nuclear Cardiology, Heart Rhythm Society, Society of Cardiovascular Anesthesiologists, Society for Cardiovascular Angiography and Interventions, and Society for Vascular Medicine and Biology. *Anesth Analg.* 2006;113(22):2662-2674.
36. Park KW. Preoperative cardiology consultation. *Anesthesiology.* 2003;98(3):754-762.

Suggested Reading

Howe CR, Gardner GC, Kadel NJ. Perioperative medication management for the patient with rheumatoid arthritis. *J Am Acad Orthop Surg.* 2006;14(9):544-551.

5

Osteoarthritis of the Hip
Epidemiology, Pathogenesis, and Pathology

Ronald Huang, MD and S.M. Javad Mortazavi, MD

Osteoarthritis (OA) is the most common form of arthritis and one of the leading causes of disability, especially in the elderly.[1] In addition to the toll it takes on quality of life, OA also has a tremendous economic impact. Nearly 27 million Americans are affected by OA.[2] In a recent study by Pop et al, it was found that 10% of all patients in rehabilitation, rheumatology, and orthopedic departments or receiving care at physiotherapy centers were composed of patients suffering from degenerative joint disease of the hip or knee.[3] Direct and indirect costs of these patients have been shown to be greater when associated with poorer general quality of life and increased severity of the OA.[4,5] A recent report by the Centers for Disease Control and Prevention states that OA costs in 2003 were up to $128 billion per year, with $81 billion associated with direct medical expenditures and $47 million associated with lost wages.[6]

Progression of hip OA to disability is the leading cause for total hip arthroplasty (THA). However, most hip OA cases do not require THA, and for these patients, the most important treatment is nonoperative management of symptoms and preservation of the native hip joint. Thus, it is important to understand the pathophysiology and pathogenesis of OA in order to attenuate disease progression and maintain mobility in the hip joint.

The classification of hip OA is usually primary (idiopathic) and secondary hip OA. Primary hip OA develops spontaneously with no previous injury or deformity, except for some evidence of genetic predisposition for primary hip OA.[7] Other risk factors that have been studied, such as occupational and physical activity and body mass index, show an inconsistent correlation with development of primary hip OA.[8,9] Primary hip OA primarily affects individuals over 50 and under 70 years of age.

Secondary hip OA develops following localized trauma to the hip such as fracture or a hip abnormality such as Legg-Calvé-Perthes disease, developmental hip dysplasia, slipped capital femoral epiphysis, or Paget's disease.[10] Patients with traumatic hip dislocation or subluxation have a 16% chance of developing hip OA, and those who experience acetabular fracture have an 88% chance of developing hip OA.[11] Secondary hip OA is mostly seen in individuals aged 20 to 50; thus, any young individual presenting with hip OA must be evaluated to determine the biomechanics of the OA in order to attempt to attenuate progression of the disease.

Epidemiology

Incidence and Prevalence

The prevalence of hip OA has been reported to be 16% for men and 6% for women, both between the ages of 65 and 74 years among a population in England.[12,13] It has also been reported at 3% for women and 3.2% for men between 55 and 74 years according to the National Health and Nutrition Survey (NHANES-I)[14] and 15.1% for women and 14.1% for men older than 55 years, according to the Rotterdam study.[15] The increased incidence and prevalence of OA with age is probably due to decreased

Parvizi J, Klatt BA.
Essentials in Total Hip Arthroplasty (pp 39-45).

ability of chondrocytes to respond to growth factors and to repair cartilage, leading to thinning of the articular cartilage. With the growing elderly population throughout the world, we can expect to see increasing number of hip OA cases in coming years, and thus, an increase in the demand of total hip replacements, since the most common diagnosis leading to hip THA is OA. It is reported that over 238,000 patients underwent total hip arthroplasty in 2005, resulting in over 9.2 billion dollars spent directly on hospitalization costs alone.[16]

Overall, there is a higher prevalence of general OA in women than men. However, under the age of 50, OA is more prevalent in men; over 50, OA in most joints is more prevalent in women, and the sex difference increases with age.[17] This fits with the theory that after women undergo menopause, they have hormone deficiencies that make them more susceptible to develop OA. Nonetheless, hip OA has been shown to be more prevalent in men across the whole age spectrum.[17]

PATHOGENESIS

Development of OA consists of 2 arms: joint vulnerability and joint loading. A vulnerable joint whose protectors are dysfunctional can develop OA with minimal levels of loading, perhaps even levels encountered during every day activities. On the other hand, in a young joint with competent protectors, a major acute injury or long-term overloading is necessary to precipitate disease. Joint capsule and ligaments, synovial fluid, muscle and tendons, sensory afferents, and underlying bone are the major joint protectors. Joint capsule and ligaments serve as joint protectors by providing a limit to excursion, thereby fixing the range of joint motion. Rupture of ligaments is a well-known cause of the early development of OA.[18] Muscles and tendons that bridge the joint are key joint protectors. Their cocontractions at the appropriate time in joint movement provide the appropriate power and acceleration for the limb to accomplish its tasks. As a consequence, these muscles and tendons can assume the right tension at appropriate points in joint excursion to act as optimal joint protectors, anticipating joint loading. Focal stress across the joint is minimized by muscle contraction that decelerates the joint before impact and assures that when joint impact arrives, it is distributed broadly across the joint surface. The ligaments, along with overlying skin and tendons, contain mechanoreceptor sensory afferent nerves. These mechanoreceptors fire at different frequencies throughout a joint's range of motion, providing feedback by way of the spinal cord to muscles and tendons. Charcot arthropathy, which is a severe and rapidly progressive OA, develops when minor joint injury occurs in the presence of posterior column peripheral neuropathy.[19] The bone underneath the cartilage may also provide a shock-absorbing function, as it may give way subtly to an oncoming impulse load. Synovial fluid reduces friction between articulating cartilage surfaces, thereby serving as a major protector against friction-induced cartilage wear. This lubrication function depends on the molecule *lubricin*, a mucinous glycoprotein secreted by synovial fibroblasts whose concentration diminishes after joint injury and in the face of synovial inflammation.[20] Both the smooth frictionless surface and the compressive stiffness of cartilage serve as protective mechanisms preventing joint injury. The compressible stiffness of cartilage compared to bone provides the joint with impact-absorbing capacity.

Risk factors for OA can be understood in terms of their effect either on joint vulnerability or on loading.

Systemic Risk Factors

Systemic risk factors such as increasing age, female gender, genetic predisposition, high bone density, estrogen deficiency, and vitamin C and D deficiency do not themselves cause OA, but contribute to the susceptibility of the joint to developing OA.

AGE

Age is the most potent risk factor for OA. It is uncommon in younger individuals under the age of 50, but very common in the elderly over age 50.[14] Although increasing age does not directly cause OA, it is clear that incidence and prevalence of the disease increases significantly as age increases. Aging increases joint vulnerability through several mechanisms affecting joint protectors. Cartilage thins with age and thinner cartilage experiences higher shear stress at basal layers and is at greater risk of cartilage damage.[21] In addition, muscles are weaker, ligaments are less competent, and sensory response is slower in elderly people.

GENDER

Older women are at high risk of OA in all joints, a risk that emerges as women reach their sixth decade. While hormone loss with menopause may contribute to this risk, there is little understanding of the vulnerability of older women's joints to OA.

GENETICS

OA is a highly heritable disease, but its heritability varies by joint. Possibly over 50% of the hand and hip OA in the community is attributable to inheritance (ie, to disease present in other members of the family).[22] Genetic factors have been shown to play a major role in influencing development of hip OA.[23] In twin studies, heritability of hip OA was shown to be 58% in female twins.[24] However, male twins showed a much weaker genetic association than females. A recent study suggests that the mode of inheritance is through a major Mendelian gene with a residual multifactorial component. This study also demonstrated stronger heritability in females than males.[25]

The exact mechanism through which genetic defects influence OA is not known. However, many genes have been identified that may play a role in development of OA. The majority of these are involved in synthesis of matrix proteins, such as the gene COL2A1 on chromosome 12 that is responsible for synthesis of type II procollagen, the precursor for type II collagen, a major component of articular cartilage. Other genes associated with hip OA have been linked to loci on chromosomes 2, 4, 6, and 16.[26,27]

Global Considerations

There have been many studies done across different ethnicities and nationalities, providing a better picture of the etiology of OA. In Asian populations, prevalence of hip OA is much lower than in White populations; accordingly, the rate of hip arthroplasty in the United States is lower in Asians than in Whites.[28] Statistics on patients who underwent total hip replacement for primary OA in San Francisco and Hawaii demonstrated a virtual absence of the condition in Asians and low rates in the Black and Hispanic populations.[29] In a study by Nevitt et al, it is reported that the Chinese have a far lesser prevalence of symptomatic and radiographic hip OA than Whites from the United States.[30]

Hormonal Factors

The critical role of estrogens in bone homeostasis is well known; however, there is some evidence of a role for estrogens in the development of OA. Low levels of estrogens in postmenopausal women have been associated with an increased risk of OA in some studies. Nevertheless, the effect of estrogen replacement therapy in protection against the development of OA is controversial. Some studies have shown that estrogen supplementation decreases cartilage thickness by inhibiting proliferation and maturation of chondrocytes,[31,32] while estrogen replacement therapy has also been correlated with a reduction of risk of hip and knee OA.[33-35]

Nutritional Factors

Nutritional factors such as vitamins also play a role in OA. Vitamin C has many functions within cartilage, including protection against reactive oxygen species and serving as a cofactor for type II collagen synthesis. In a study based in Framingham, low vitamin C intake was associated with progression of OA but did not affect incidence of the disease. Vitamin D was also determined, with the same population, to be necessary in bone turnover, which may play an important role in OA.[36]

Bone Density

The role of bone in serving as a shock absorber for impact load is not well understood, but persons with increased bone density might be at a higher risk of OA,[37,38] suggesting that the resistance of bone to impact during joint use may play a role in disease development. Women with osteoporosis (low bone density) have a lower-than-expected prevalence of OA[39] according to some studies; however, there are other studies that show the opposite result or no association between bone density and OA.[40-42]

Local Risk Factors

Along with the systematic risk factors, the local risk factors are another set of factors that influence development of OA, either by changing the joint vulnerability or loading.

Major Joint Injury

OA is associated with major joint injuries such as ruptured ligaments, articular fractures, avascular necrosis, and joint dislocations. This damage alters the way that the joint distributes stress along its surface, thus increasing the risk of OA. As mentioned previously, the risk of developing OA with these factors increases when compounded with increasing age. Additionally, increased contact stress on the joint caused by incongruities on the articular surface may lead to early development of disease.[43] Another source of anatomic abnormality is malalignment across the joint. Malalignment causes this effect by decreasing contact area during loading, increasing stress on a focal area or cartilage, which then breaks down. There is evidence that malalignment in the knee not only causes cartilage loss but leads to underlying bone damage, producing bone marrow lesions seen on MRI.[44,45]

Developmental Abnormalities

Three uncommon major developmental abnormalities have been identified that occur in early life and later lead to hip OA during adulthood: developmental hip dysplasia, Legg-Calvé-Perthes disease, and slipped femoral capital epiphysis.[46]

Obesity

Obesity is very common in the United States today; over 34 million people are obese, including 13 million who are morbidly obese as defined by body mass index (BMI). Obesity's effect on the development and progression of disease is mediated mostly through the increased loading in weight-bearing joints that occurs in overweight persons.[47] However, a modest association of obesity with an increased risk of hand OA suggests that there may be a systemic metabolic factor circulating in obese persons that also affects disease risk.[48]

A linear relationship has been identified with weight and risk of knee OA; with each increase of 2 BMI units, there is a 36% increase in risk.[49] Accordingly, each reduction of 2 units of BMI lowers the risk of developing symptomatic OA by 50%.[48] Weight reduction in obese patients should be attempted in order to reduce risk of OA and to improve their general health. Not only is obesity a risk factor for OA in weight-bearing joints, but obese persons have more severe symptoms of the disease.[50,51]

Occupation

Repetitive use of a joint, particularly repetitively overstressing the joint, leads to OA. In jobs such as farming, workers perform repetitive activities such as bending, lifting, moving heavy objects, and walking on rough ground, which puts them at high risk for hip OA.[52] Jobs that require squatting also may lead to increased risk of hip OA. The Framingham study data suggest that farming activities stated above account for 15% to 30% of cases of hip OA in males.[53]

Physical Activity

Similar to occupational activities, repetitive overuse of a joint leads to increased risk of OA. Studies have shown that elite runners have increased risk of knee and hip OA, but had inconclusive results about recreational runners.[54] Additionally, it was shown that people who squat and lift heavy weights are at increased risk for developing hip OA.[55] Sports injuries are another significant risk factor for OA; high intensity impact, ligament damage, and other sports injuries should be treated promptly with a goal of preserving joint-surface integrity.[37]

Pathology

Although it is not certain whether the cartilage or bone undergoes change first,[56] it is well established that OA eventually progresses to affect all aspects of the synovial joint, including the articular cartilage, subchondral bone, synovial tissue, ligaments, joint capsule, and muscles that act across the joint.[37] The characteristic changes of articular cartilage include fibrillations and loss of the articular cartilage, thickening and remodeling of the subchondral bone, and full thickness loss of joint space.

During early OA, fibrillation and irregularities develop in the superficial zone of the articular cartilage and extend into the transitional zone.[57] This degradation is generally agreed to be due to an increased synthesis and activation of extracellular proteinases, mainly matrix metalloproteinases. The main proteinases that degrade cartilage matrix are the collagenase MMP13[58] and the aggrecanase ADAMTS5 or ADAMTS4.[59,60] At first, the chondrocytes attempt to make up for the loss by increasing production of collagen and proteoglycans. However, the chondrocytes demonstrate changes in gene expression and the collagen and proteoglycans that they produce are smaller than normal, causing decreased stiffness and loss of the normal tight weave of matrix proteins.[56] This leads to an increase in water content in the matrix and swelling and softening of the cartilage. Repetitive mechanical forces on this weakened cartilage accelerate the degenerative process.[52] As the disease progresses, matrix repair mechanisms are overwhelmed by the degradative enzymes and the matrix continues to be degraded, with the possibility of the bone being exposed. Without a large amount of intact aggrecan, the joint loses its ability to bear weight.[59]

Increased osteogenesis is also significant in OA, but the timing of this process in relation to changes in cartilage is still unclear.[61-63] New bone is deposited on trabeculae,[64] and osteophytes are produced around the joint. It is suggested that osteophyte formation is a result of growth in an attempt to repair osteoarthritic lesions rather than a result of degradation of the bone.[65] Transforming growth factor (TGF-β) has been implicated in many studies to play a key role in osteophyte formation and protection against cartilage destruction.[66-68] It may work to increase osteophyte formation by activating macrophages that produce cytokines, growth factors, and bone morphogenic proteins that stimulate chondrogenesis and osteogenesis.[69] TGF-β also stimulates chondrocytes to produce extracellular matrix components and counteracts catabolic cytokines.[66] A study by Scharstuhl et al demonstrates that inhibition of TGF-β leads to loss of proteoglycans and cartilage loss, probably due to up-regulation of MMPs.[67] Therefore, TGF-β can be identified as a significant factor that protects against destruction of existing cartilage and also stimulates osteophyte formation. In particular, TGF-β3 has been identified to play a role in early osteophyte development.[68] These fibrous, cartilaginous, osseous prominences often develop along the degenerating joint surfaces[37] and around the femoral head-neck junction, providing stability to the osteoarthritic joint,[70] but also limiting the range of motion. They are mainly seen on the mediodorsal surface of the femur from the rim of the femoral neck to the fovea capitis (medial epiarticular osteophytes), and also along the periphery of the articular cartilage (marginal osteophytes).[71,72] The radiographic presence of osteophytes is considered an important factor that differentiates between hip pain due to OA and hip pain due to other causes.[73]

If there is excessive load on the affected joint, microfractures can occur, which are healed by callus formation and remodeled. The remodeled trabeculae are stiffer than normal bone, leading to a lessened shock-absorbing quality of the subchondral bone.[64] The exact role of subchondral bone in the genesis of OA is not clear because the changes caused by remodeling precede the degradation of articular cartilage, but may not actually cause cartilage degeneration.[74]

Although OA is not an inflammatory disease, the synovial membrane becomes inflamed due to shards of articular cartilage separated from the matrix during degradation.[75] The synoviocytes and macrophages of the inflamed membrane produce metalloproteinases, cytokines, and growth factors, causing a cascade by influencing chondrocytes to produce even more metalloproteinases and aggrecanases, causing further matrix degradation.[76] Additionally, the interleukin-1 produced by the macrophages stimulates production of prostaglandin E2 by synoviocytes, which may be the cause of pain in the joint.

Summary

OA of the hip is highly prevalent and takes a toll on the quality of life of many patients. An important part of treating these patients is understanding the pathogenesis and pathology of this debilitating process.

References

1. Lawrence RC, Helmick CG, Arnett FC, et al. Estimates of the prevalence of arthritis and selected musculoskeletal disorders in the United States. *Arthritis Rheum.* 1998;41(5):778-799.
2. Lawrence RC, Felson DT, Helmick CG, et al. Estimates of the prevalence of arthritis and other rheumatic conditions in the United States. Part II. *Arthritis Rheum.* 2008;58(1):26-35.
3. Pop T, Szczygielska D, Druzbicki M. Epidemiology and cost of conservative treatment of patients with degenerative joint disease of the hip and knee. *Ortop Traumatol Rehabil.* 2007;9(4):405-412.
4. Gupta S, Hawker GA, Laporte A, Croxford R, Coyte PC. The economic burden of disabling hip and knee osteoarthritis (OA) from the perspective of individuals living with this condition. *Rheumatology (Oxford).* 2005;44(12):1531-1537.
5. Rabenda V, Manette C, Lemmens R, Mariani AM, Struvay N, Reginster JY. Direct and indirect costs attributable to osteoarthritis in active subjects. *J Rheumatol.* 2006;33(6):1152-1158.
6. MMWR. National and State Medical Expenditures and Lost Earnings Attributable to Arthritis and Other Rheumatic Conditions. United States, 2003; 2007.
7. Mustafa Z, Chapman K, Irven C, et al. Linkage analysis of candidate genes as susceptibility loci for osteoarthritis-suggestive linkage of COL9A1 to female hip osteoarthritis. *Rheumatology (Oxford).* 2000;39(3):299-306.
8. Chitnavis J, Sinsheimer JS, Suchard MA, Clipsham K, Carr AJ. End-stage coxarthrosis and gonarthrosis. Aetiology, clinical patterns and radiological features of idiopathic osteoarthritis. *Rheumatology (Oxford).* 2000;39(6):612-619.
9. Cvijetic S, Dekanic-Ozegovic D, Campbell L, Cooper C, Potocki K. Occupational physical demands and hip osteoarthritis. *Arh Hig Rada Toksikol.* 1999;50(4):371-379.
10. Woodward JL. Section f: hip and thigh. In: *Frontera: Essentials of Physical Medicine and Rehabilitation on MD Consult*; 2002.
11. Rodriguez-Merchan EC. Coxarthrosis after traumatic hip dislocation in the adult. *Clin Orthop Relat Res.* 2000;(377):92-98.
12. Kellgren JH. Osteoarthrosis in patients and populations. *BMJ.* 1961;2(5243):1-6.
13. Lawrence JS, Bremner JM, Bier F. Osteo-arthrosis. Prevalence in the population and relationship between symptoms and x-ray changes. *Ann Rheum Dis.* 1966;25(1):1-24.
14. Oliveria SA, Felson DT, Reed JI, Cirillo PA, Walker AM. Incidence of symptomatic hand, hip, and knee osteoarthritis among patients in a health maintenance organization. *Arthritis Rheum.* 1995;38(8):1134-1141.
15. Odding E, Valkenburg HA, Algra D, Vandenouweland FA, Grobbee DE, Hofman A. Associations of radiological osteoarthritis of the hip and knee with locomotor disability in the Rotterdam Study. *Ann Rheum Dis.* 1998;57(4):203-208.
16. American Academy of Orthopaedic Surgeons. Facts on Hip Replacements. URL: http://www.aaos.org/research/stats/Hip_Facts.pdf. Accessed August 2011.
17. van Saase JL, van Romunde LK, Cats A, Vandenbroucke JP, Valkenburg HA. Epidemiology of osteoarthritis: Zoetermeer survey. Comparison of radiological osteoarthritis in a Dutch population with that in 10 other populations. *Ann Rheum Dis.* 1989;48(4):271-280.
18. Fleming BC, Hulstyn MJ, Oksendahl HL, Fadale PD. Ligament injury, reconstruction and osteoarthritis. *Curr Opin Orthop.* 2005;16(5):354-362.
19. Slowman-Kovacs SD, Braunstein EM, Brandt KD. Rapidly progressive Charcot arthropathy following minor joint trauma in patients with diabetic neuropathy. *Arthritis Rheum.* 1990;33(3):412-417.
20. Jay GD, Torres JR, Rhee DK, et al. Association between friction and wear in diarthrodial joints lacking lubricin. *Arthritis Rheum.* 2007;56(11):3662-3669.
21. Wang Y, Wei HW, Yu TC, Cheng CK. Parametric analysis of the stress distribution on the articular cartilage and subchondral bone. *Biomed Mater Eng.* 2007;17(4):241-247.

22. Spector TD, MacGregor AJ. Risk factors for osteoarthritis: genetics. *Osteoarthritis Cartilage.* 2004;12(suppl A):S39-44.
23. Lanyon P, Muir K, Doherty S, Doherty M. Assessment of a genetic contribution to osteoarthritis of the hip: sibling study. *BMJ.* 2000;321(7270):1179-1183.
24. Spector TD, Cicuttini F, Baker J, Loughlin J, Hart D. Genetic influences on osteoarthritis in women: a twin study. *BMJ.* 1996;312(7036):940-943.
25. Kaprio J, Kujala UM, Peltonen L, Koskenvuo M. Genetic liability to osteoarthritis may be greater in women than men. *BMJ.* 1996;313(7051):232.
26. Loughlin J, Mustafa Z, Irven C, et al. Stratification analysis of an osteoarthritis genome screen-suggestive linkage to chromosomes 4, 6, and 16. *Am J Hum Genet.* 1999;65(6):1795-1798.
27. Loughlin J, Mustafa Z, Smith A, et al. Linkage analysis of chromosome 2q in osteoarthritis. *Rheumatology (Oxford).* 2000;39(4):377-381.
28. Hoaglund FT, Oishi CS, Gialamas GG. Extreme variations in racial rates of total hip arthroplasty for primary coxarthrosis: a population-based study in San Francisco. *Ann Rheum Dis.* 1995;54(2):107-110.
29. Hoaglund FT, Steinbach LS. Primary osteoarthritis of the hip: etiology and epidemiology. *J Am Acad Orthop Surg.* 2001;9(5):320-327.
30. Nevitt MC, Xu L, Zhang Y, et al. Very low prevalence of hip osteoarthritis among Chinese elderly in Beijing, China, compared with whites in the United States: the Beijing osteoarthritis study. *Arthritis Rheum.* 2002;46(7):1773-1779.
31. Talwar RM, Wong BS, Svoboda K, Harper RP. Effects of estrogen on chondrocyte proliferation and collagen synthesis in skeletally mature articular cartilage. *J Oral Maxillofac Surg.* 2006;64(4):600-609.
32. Richette P, Corvol M, Bardin T. Estrogens, cartilage, and osteoarthritis. *Joint Bone Spine.* 2003;70(4):257-262.
33. Spector TD, Nandra D, Hart DJ, Doyle DV. Is hormone replacement therapy protective for hand and knee osteoarthritis in women? The Chingford Study. *Ann Rheum Dis.* 1997;56(7):432-434.
34. Hannan MT, Felson DT, Anderson JJ, Naimark A, Kannel WB. Estrogen use and radiographic osteoarthritis of the knee in women. The Framingham Osteoarthritis Study. *Arthritis Rheum.* 1990;33(4):525-532.
35. Lee YJ, Lee EB, Kwon YE, et al. Effect of estrogen on the expression of matrix metalloproteinase (MMP)-1, MMP-3, and MMP-13 and tissue inhibitor of metalloproternase-1 in osteoarthritis chondrocytes. *Rheumatol Int.* 2003;23(6):282-288.
36. Lane NE, Gore LR, Cummings SR, et al. Serum vitamin D levels and incident changes of radiographic hip osteoarthritis: a longitudinal study. Study of Osteoporotic Fractures Research Group. *Arthritis Rheum.* 1999;42(5):854-860.
37. Garstang SV, Stitik TP. Osteoarthritis: epidemiology, risk factors, and pathophysiology. *Am J Phys Med Rehabil.* 2006;85(11 suppl):S2-11; quiz S12-14.
38. Nevitt MC, Lane NE, Scott JC, et al. Radiographic osteoarthritis of the hip and bone mineral density. The Study of Osteoporotic Fractures Research Group. *Arthritis Rheum.* 1995;38(7):907-916.
39. Hart DJ, Mootoosamy I, Doyle DV, Spector TD. The relationship between osteoarthritis and osteoporosis in the general population: the Chingford Study. *Ann Rheum Dis.* 1994;53(3):158-162.
40. Arokoski JP, Arokoski MH, Jurvelin JS, Helminen HJ, Niemitukia LH, Kroger H. Increased bone mineral content and bone size in the femoral neck of men with hip osteoarthritis. *Ann Rheum Dis.* 2002;61(2):145-150.
41. Sandini L, Arokoski JP, Jurvelin JS, Kroger H. Increased bone mineral content but not bone mineral density in the hip in surgically treated knee and hip osteoarthritis. *J Rheumatol.* 2005;32(10):1951-1957.
42. Haara MM, Arokoski JP, Kroger H, et al. Association of radiological hand osteoarthritis with bone mineral mass: a population study. *Rheumatology (Oxford).* 2005;44(12):1549-1554.
43. Buckwalter JA, Brown TD. Joint injury, repair, and remodeling: roles in post-traumatic osteoarthritis. *Clin Orthop Relat Res.* 2004(423):7-16.
44. Hunter DJ, Zhang Y, Niu J, et al. Structural factors associated with malalignment in knee osteoarthritis: the Boston osteoarthritis knee study. *J Rheumatol.* 2005;32(11):2192-2199.
45. Felson DT, McLaughlin S, Goggins J, et al. Bone marrow edema and its relation to progression of knee osteoarthritis. *Ann Intern Med.* 2003;139(5 pt 1):330-336.
46. Felson DT. Risk factors for osteoarthritis: understanding joint vulnerability. *Clin Orthop Relat Res.* 2004(427 suppl):S16-21.
47. Felson DT. Does excess weight cause osteoarthritis and, if so, why? *Ann Rheum Dis.* 1996;55(9):668-670.
48. Haara MM, Heliovaara M, Kroger H, et al. Osteoarthritis in the carpometacarpal joint of the thumb. Prevalence and associations with disability and mortality. *J Bone Joint Surg Am.* 2004;86-A(7):1452-1457.
49. Hart DJ, Spector TD. The relationship of obesity, fat distribution and osteoarthritis in women in the general population: the Chingford Study. *J Rheumatol.* 1993;20(2):331-335.
50. Jinks C, Jordan K, Croft P. Disabling knee pain--another consequence of obesity: results from a prospective cohort study. *BMC Public Health.* 2006;6:258.
51. Nunez M, Nunez E, del Val JL, et al. Health-related quality of life in patients with osteoarthritis after total knee replacement: factors influencing outcomes at 36 months of follow-up. *Osteoarthritis Cartilage.* 2007;15(9):1001-1007.
52. Croft P, Coggon D, Cruddas M, Cooper C. Osteoarthritis of the hip: an occupational disease in farmers. *BMJ.* 1992;304(6837):1269-1272.
53. Felson DT, Hannan MT, Naimark A, et al. Occupational physical demands, knee bending, and knee osteoarthritis: results from the Framingham Study. *J Rheumatol.* 1991;18(10):1587-1592.

54. Spector TD, Harris PA, Hart DJ, et al. Risk of osteoarthritis associated with long-term weight-bearing sports: a radiologic survey of the hips and knees in female ex-athletes and population controls. *Arthritis Rheum.* 1996;39(6):988-995.

55. Kujala UM, Kettunen J, Paananen H, et al. Knee osteoarthritis in former runners, soccer players, weight lifters, and shooters. Arthritis Rheum. 1995;38(4):539-546.

56. Huber M, Trattnig S, Lintner F. Anatomy, biochemistry, and physiology of articular cartilage. *Invest Radiol.* 2000;35(10):573-580.

57. Guilak F, Fermor B, Keefe FJ, et al. The role of biomechanics and inflammation in cartilage injury and repair. *Clin Orthop Relat Res.* 2004(423):17-26.

58. Knauper V, Lopez-Otin C, Smith B, Knight G, Murphy G. Biochemical characterization of human collagenase-3. *J Biol Chem.* 1996;271(3):1544-1550.

59. Fosang AJ, Little CB. Drug Insight: aggrecanases as therapeutic targets for osteoarthritis. *Nat Clin Pract Rheumatol.* 2008;4(8):420-427.

60. Hardingham T. Extracellular matrix and pathogenic mechanisms in osteoarthritis. *Curr Rheumatol Rep.* 2008;10(1):30-36.

61. Burr DB, Schaffler MB. The involvement of subchondral mineralized tissues in osteoarthrosis: quantitative microscopic evidence. *Microsc Res Tech.* 1997;37(4):343-357.

62. Jeffery AK. Osteogenesis in the osteoarthritic femoral head. A study using radioactive 32 P and tetracycline bone markers. *J Bone Joint Surg Br.* 1973;55(2):262-272.

63. Matsui H, Shimizu M, Tsuji H. Cartilage and subchondral bone interaction in osteoarthrosis of human knee joint: a histological and histomorphometric study. *Microsc Res Tech.* 1997;37(4):333-342.

64. Lajeunesse D, Reboul P. Subchondral bone in osteoarthritis: a biologic link with articular cartilage leading to abnormal remodeling. *Curr Opin Rheumatol.* 2003;15(5):628-633.

65. Neuman P, Hulth A, Linden B, Johnell O, Dahlberg L. The role of osteophytic growth in hip osteoarthritis. *Int Orthop.* 2003;27(5):262-266.

66. Blaney Davidson EN, Vitters EL, van der Kraan PM, van den Berg WB. Expression of transforming growth factor-beta (TGFbeta) and the TGFbeta signalling molecule SMAD-2P in spontaneous and instability-induced osteoarthritis: role in cartilage degradation, chondrogenesis and osteophyte formation. *Ann Rheum Dis.* 2006;65(11):1414-1421.

67. Scharstuhl A, Glansbeek HL, van Beuningen HM, Vitters EL, van der Kraan PM, van den Berg WB. Inhibition of endogenous TGF-beta during experimental osteoarthritis prevents osteophyte formation and impairs cartilage repair. *J Immunol.* 2002;169(1):507-514.

68. Uchino M, Izumi T, Tominaga T, et al. Growth factor expression in the osteophytes of the human femoral head in osteoarthritis. *Clin Orthop Relat Res.* 2000(377):119-125.

69. van Lent PL, Blom AB, van der Kraan P, et al. Crucial role of synovial lining macrophages in the promotion of transforming growth factor beta-mediated osteophyte formation. *Arthritis Rheum.* 2004;50(1):103-111.

70. Jordan GR, Loveridge N, Bell KL, et al. Increased femoral neck cancellous bone and connectivity in coxarthrosis (hip osteoarthritis). *Bone.* 2003;32(1):86-95.

71. Harrison MH, Schajowicz F, Trueta J. Osteoarthritis of the hip: a study of the nature and evolution of the disease. *J Bone Joint Surg Br.* 1953;35-B(4):598-626.

72. Jeffery AK. Osteophytes and the osteoarthritic femoral head. *J Bone Joint Surg Br.* 1975;57(3):314-324.

73. Altman R, Alarcon G, Appelrouth D, et al. The American College of Rheumatology criteria for the classification and reporting of osteoarthritis of the hip. *Arthritis Rheum.* 1991;34(5):505-514.

74. Li B, Aspden RM. Mechanical and material properties of the subchondral bone plate from the femoral head of patients with osteoarthritis or osteoporosis. *Ann Rheum Dis.* 1997;56(4):247-254.

75. Myers SL, Flusser D, Brandt KD, Heck DA. Prevalence of cartilage shards in synovium and their association with synovitis in patients with early and endstage osteoarthritis. *J Rheumatol.* 1992;19(8):1247-1251.

76. Bondeson J, Wainwright SD, Lauder S, Amos N, Hughes CE. The role of synovial macrophages and macrophage-produced cytokines in driving aggrecanases, matrix metalloproteinases, and other destructive and inflammatory responses in osteoarthritis. *Arthritis Res Ther.* 2006;8(6):R187.

6

Biomaterials

Christopher S. Adams, PhD

The process of development of highly specialized hip implants has seen only a few changes in material choices since Sir John Charnley opened the era of modern hip replacement in the early 1960s. The past 50 years has seen hip implants largely assembled from 5 basic materials: titanium alloys, cobalt chromium alloys, alumina and zirconia ceramics, and ultra-high molecular weight polyethylene (UHMWPE). The characteristics of these materials will be discussed in this section.

The 3 primary components of the hip implant are assembled from different materials. The stem, which forms a strong interface with the femur, is frequently manufactured from a titanium or cobalt chromium alloy. The articulating ball, replacing the head of the femur, is manufactured from titanium alloy, cobalt chromium alloy, or an alumina or zirconia ceramic. Finally, the cup, which replaces the acetabulum and is osseointegrated into the skeleton of the pelvis, is frequently assembled in 2 parts, with a ceramic or UHMWPE articulating lining and a titanium alloy or cobalt chromium alloy making up the base.

Hip implants, like other skeletal implants, have been designed with a number of criteria in mind. There are 2 criteria that primarily determine the applicability of a material for use as a skeletal implant. These are the mechanical properties of the structures to be replaced and the ability of the replacement materials to coexist with the native tissue. Initially, we will compare the mechanical properties of bone to the mechanical properties of replacement materials. Secondly, the biocompatibility of these materials will be explored; both in the attempts to create a better osseointegrated hip implant and reduce the negative effect of wear particles on the survival of implants.

The Mechanical Properties of Bone

The mechanical properties of bone are defined in relationship to the forces that act upon that bone. Forces in action upon any body have only 2 potential effects: a change in the velocity of the body (external effect) or the shape of the body (internal effect). Force, or load, is a measurable vector property, indicating that it has a magnitude, direction, and point of application. There are 3 basic types of forces: tension, compression, and shear. The response of any body to a force is dependent on the properties of the body itself and is referred to by the terms *stress* and *strain*. Stress is the internal resistance of a body to the forces in action upon it. In bone, stress arises from the forces or bonds between components of the tissue, primarily collagen fibers and hydroxyapatite crystals. The primary unit of stress is the Pascal (Pa), which is 1 Newton of force distributed over 1 square meter (1 N/m^2), typically a very small unit. Strain is the geometric response of a material to force application. The change in dimension of a body in response to a force is termed *deformation*. Deformation normalized to length is the definition of strain. Strains are described by the forces that produce them: normal compressive strain, normal tensile strain, and shear strain.

Parvizi J, Klatt BA.
Essentials in Total Hip Arthroplasty (pp 47-53).

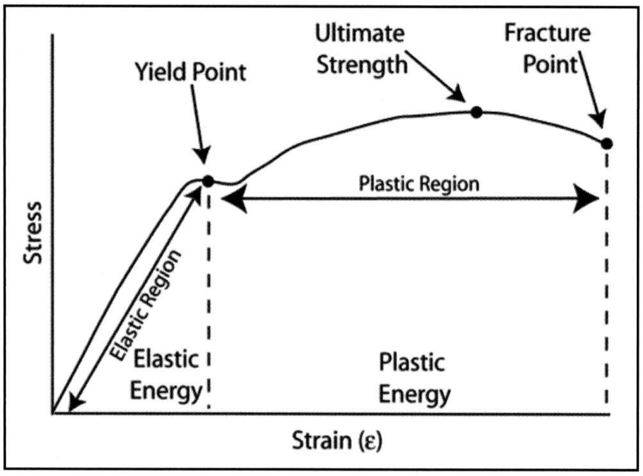

Figure 6-1. Stress-strain curve. When stress is plotted against strain, a number of parameters are calculable from the resultant curve. These include yield point, fracture point, and the ultimate strength of the material, as well as the elastic and plastic energy absorbable by the material.

Strains can be measured in several ways, including strain gauges directly bonded to materials, extensometers, brittle lacquer coatings, or birefringent coatings.[1] When mechanical properties of bone, or any material, are measured, the data generate a stress-strain curve (Figure 6-1). As can be seen from Figure 6-1, several properties of a material can be determined from this graph. The first defined point is the yield point. Up to this point, any strain on the material is recoverable. This strain is referred to as elastic deformation. Once pushed past the yield point from the elastic region into the plastic region, the deformation is permanent. The yield point is also referred to as the elastic limit, which is the limit to the amount of energy that can be adsorbed by the material without permanent deformation. The final point on the graph is the fracture point, which is the point at which there is catastrophic failure of the material. The upper stress limit is referred to as the ultimate stress, or ultimate strength. It may or may not be coincident with the failure point. The slope of the line in the elastic region is referred to as the elastic modulus of the material, while the area underneath the elastic region is the amount of energy that can be adsorbed by that material during elastic deformation, or elastic energy. Similarly, the area under the plastic region is the plastic energy of a material.

Bone is a heterogeneous composite material, made up of multiple tissues with different mechanical properties. Bone is also characterized as elastic, or capable of reversible deformations, and anisotropic, indicating greater strength in one direction. The mechanical properties of bone are determined by its density, its porosity, and its microscopic structure. Density includes the effects of both the organic and inorganic phases of bone. Porosity is determined primarily by the presence of the vascular component of bone, including the haversian canals in cortical bone and the marrow space in cancellous bone. In contrast, the microscopic structure of bone is the most variable. The orientation of haversian systems in bone play a dramatic role in the strength of cortical bone, as the systems themselves are strongest when the force applied is normal (in parallel with the haversian system). The characteristics of the trabecular bone that impact the mechanical properties of bone are orientation, bone volume, and connectivity. In addition, the orientation of collagen fibers in bone can also affect the strength of bone. Both cortical bone and cancellous bone are strongest under compression. Thus, the tensile strength of cortical bone is approximately 66% of its compressive strength and the torsional strength is approximately 35% of its compressive strength. Similarly, the tensile strength of cancellous bone is approximately 60% of its compressive strength. The ultimate strength of cortical bone is much in excess of cancellous bone; thus, human cortical bone is approximately 200 MPa,[2] while the ultimate strength of human cancellous bone ranges between 6 and 10 MPa.[3] Similarly, the elastic modulus of cortical bone ranges from 5 to 21 GPa,[4] while average values for cancellous bone elastic modulus are several hundred MPa.[5]

These, therefore, are the mechanical parameters that any prospective implant must match. It is important, however, to mention that by the vital nature of bone, it is capable of an active response to fatigue that no metal will ever be able to reproduce. Consequently, an appropriate replacing metal should exhibit a considerably greater strength than cortical bone. For this reason primarily, implant materials frequently exceed the strength and modulus of native materials by many orders of magnitude, as will be seen in the sections to follow. However, those very responsive properties of bone require that a replacing metal not too greatly exceed the modulus of the bone itself, less the bone resorb and disappear, a process referred to as stress shielding.

Mechanical Properties of Orthopedic Materials

In choosing a material for use in orthopedic applications, the first issue that must be addressed is failure. The consequences of failure in an implanted device are catastrophic. The patient is as crippled as if the native tissue had failed. However, as the implant has no capacity for self-repair, surgery is the only option and success rates for revision surgeries lag far behind those of the initial surgery. There are 4 primary causes of implant failure. These are excessive deformation, fracture, wear, and corrosion. There are several properties in materials that determine the ability of these materials to resist failure. These include ductility, toughness, hardness, and corrosion resistance.[6] These characteristics of materials are important in 2 arenas. The first, of course, is in its usage in vivo. The material must be capable of resisting the repetitive loading of the skeleton over a considerable lifespan. The other arena, however, is the process of manufacture itself. The shape of a hip implant is highly specialized and the methods by which it is formed must not negatively impact the final shape of the implant.

Ductility is a property that describes the ability of materials to undergo plastic deformation without fracturing. A high level of ductility indicates a considerable ability to deform under tensile stress. A similar term, *malleability,* refers to the similar capacity under compressive stress. Ductile and malleable metals will be much more resistant to fracture than more brittle ones. A further advantage to these materials is their manufacture. Ductile and malleable metals have more options in their manipulation, including hammering, rolling, drawing, stamping, or pressing. More brittle materials must usually be molded. However, one consequence of these methods of metal forming is the process of work hardening. Simply put, work hardening describes the process whereby subjecting a material to continued plastic deformation actually makes it more resistant to plastic deformation. This does strengthen the material while at the same time decreasing its ductility, making it more brittle. The ductility of many metals can be varied by changing the constituents in its alloys.

Toughness is the ability of a material to resist fracture when it is subjected to stress. The value for toughness is specifically calculated as the area underneath the stress-strain curve. Similarly, the term *hardness* refers to a material's ability to resist plastic deformation. As mentioned above, as a material moves into plastic deformation, the change in shape can become permanent. Hardness is known to increase with the grain size of the material, up to a point, beyond which the relationship is inverted. The strength of the intermolecular bonds of a material imparts the degree of hardness to that material.

Corrosion is a significant problem for any device asked to reside in the human body for decades. All metallic implants experience corrosion to some degree. The consequences of corrosion are 2-fold. Corrosive degradation compromises the structural integrity of the implant and the products of degradation may cause a reaction in the patient. Electrochemical corrosion can be uniform or localized. Localized corrosion can occur at locations shielded from the generalized environment as crevice corrosion, or randomly on the surface as pitting corrosion. The sensitivity of an orthopedic biomaterial to corrosion is dependent on its geometry, the composition and microstructure of its material, the stress environment, and the chemical environment. Corrosion resistance on the part of a material can be an intrinsic factor of its composition or a result of treatments applied during that product's manufacture. One such treatment is passivation, where a thin oxide layer is deposited on the surface of a metal. Titanium, for example, will actually form an effective oxide layer in air or water. However, the thickness of an oxide layer can be increased through electrolytic passivation, creating an anodized surface. A number of orthopedic devices use this to create a corrosion resistant surface.

Orthopedic Biomaterials

Titanium Alloys

Pure titanium (Ti) and titanium alloys including aluminum and vanadium (Ti-6Al-4V) were originally designed for generalized structural applications, including aircraft construction. Only later were these materials utilized for biomedical applications. As discussed above, it is advisable that the mechanical properties of a biomaterial match those of the surrounding tissue to prevent stress shielding. In this sense, titanium is the best choice for the structural components of the hip implant (stem and cup base) as its elastic modulus is lower than many other potential materials for use in implants, including stainless steel (SS) and cobalt-chrome (Co-Cr) (Table 6-1).[7] However, as the rigidity of titanium still far exceeds that of cortical bone, the search for less rigid titanium alloys continues. In addition to its advantageous moduli in comparison to other metals, Ti and Ti-6Al-4V demonstrate better biocompatibility.[8]

Cobalt-Chromium Alloys

Like titanium, chromium forms a compact oxide layer on its surface, making it remarkably resistant to corrosion. Chromium is readily soluble in cobalt, making a large number of Co-Cr alloys available. There are 3 primary forms of these alloys, also referred to as Vitallium (DENTSPLY, York, PA). The first, consisting of ~62% cobalt, ~29% chromium, with small percentages of molybdenum, nickel, and iron must be cast as it exhibits a high level of work-hardening, making it difficult to machine. The second, with ~55% cobalt, 20% chromium, 10% nickel, and 15% tungsten, is more easily machined. It has superior

Table 6-1

Mechanical Properties of Orthopedic Biomaterials

Material	Compressive Strength (MPa)	Tensile Strength (MPa)	Modulus (GPa)
Bone—cortical	0.137 [a]	0.069 [a]	13.8 [a]
Bone—cancellous	0.041 to 0.062 [a]	0.00345 [a]	-
Stainless steel	200 [b]	0.552 to 0.997 [a]	200 [b]
Cobalt chromium	700 [b]	0.669 [a]	230 [b]
Titanium	800 [b]	0.345 [a]	110 [b]
Alumina	>500 [b]	-	380 [b]
Zirconia	900 to 1200 [b]	-	210 [b]
Porous calcium phosphate	0.0069 to 0.069 [a]	0.0025 [a]	-
Dense calcium phosphate	0.21 to 0.896 [a]	0.069 to 0.193 [a]	0.345 to 0.103 [a]

[a] Jarcho M. Calcium phosphate ceramics as hard tissue prosthetics. *Clin Orthop Relat Res.* 1981;(157):259-278.
[b] Piconi C, Maccauro G. Zirconia as a ceramic biomaterial. *Biomaterials.* 1999;20(1):1-25.

mechanical properties to the first alloy but is less resistant to crevice corrosion. The final alloy, consisting of 35% cobalt, 20% chromium, 35% nickel, and 10% molybdenum, is superior to the other 2 in terms of strength and biocompatibility but also work hardens when machined, making its manufacture problematic.

Ultra-High Molecular Weight Polyethylene

UHMWPE is made up of chains of ethylene groups. As the number of ethylene groups approaches 35,000, its molecular weight exceeds 1 million, and at that point is referred to as ultra-high molecular weight polyethylene (the UHMWPE used in joint replacements generally varies between 4 and 6 molecular weight). At this molecular weight, the mechanical properties of this material exhibit considerable impact strength, exceeding that of all other plastics. In addition, it has a very low coefficient of friction, is resistant to abrasion, and is resistant to corrosion. All of these factors make UHMWPE an excellent candidate for an articulating surface. A recent improvement on the technology has been the introduction of highly cross-linked UHMWPE. Gamma or electron beam radiation is used to crosslink these materials, followed by thermal processing to improve oxidation resistance. These treatments have been predicted to reduce wear.

Alumina and Zirconia Ceramics

The most commonly used ceramics in hip implants, alumina and zirconia, unlike classic ceramics like china and porcelain, are referred to as oxide ceramics, consisting of essentially pure metal oxides. Aluminum and zirconium exhibit exceptional chemical stability and a high level of biocompatibility.[11,12] As oxide ceramics originate as fine powders, they must be initially formed by isostatic compression for medical devices. The final shape of the devices is achieved by turning and grinding, with the shaped powder agglomerate fired into a polycrystalline solid by a heating process called sintering. Alumina ceramics, for example, are entirely made up of corundum crystals. Corundum is one of the hardest materials seen in nature, exceeded only by diamond. A critical component of this sintering process is the management of grain growth. Grain growth refers to the increase in size of the crystallites within the solid as a whole. Most materials display a higher yield stress when grain size is reduced. Thus, in medical devices, where failure can be catastrophic, grain size is kept to a minimum. Alumina and zirconia ceramics share the basic difference of all ceramics as compared to metals. They are much less ductile and more brittle than metals. Both are relatively sensitive to highly localized mechanical stress application like shocks. For this reason, working on them with iron hammers is strictly avoided. However, with the increase in brittleness comes a dramatic increase in strength; for this reason, the ceramics demonstrate significant reductions in wear over traditional metal against polyethylene combinations. As a brittle material, the risk of catastrophic fracture exists; however, it has been dramatically reduced recently with the development of yttria-doped zirconia (known as tetragonal zirconia polycrystals, TZP) and magnesia doped zirconia (known a partially stabilized zirconia, PSZ). Nearly all commercially produced hip ball heads are produced from TZP, with more than 300,000 produced against 2 reported failures.[10]

Surface Modifications

While metallic hip implants have shown very good tissue interaction almost from their initiation, work has continually attempted to increase the direct attachment of bone to the implant, or osseointegration. The simplest method to promote bony ongrowth is to use an implant made of grit blasted titanium. Bone can grow onto this surface, and there are a number of implants still using this surface modification. To increase the osseointegration of implants, a number of surface coatings have been developed. The 2 most common methods for increasing osseointegration are creation of porosity and addition of a hydroxylapatite (HA) coating.

Porous metals most commonly are created in cobalt-chrome or titanium alloys. The potential for crevasse corrosion has eliminated stainless steel from possible use in these cases. As porosity is a compromise between the strength of the metal and the need to provide space for bone ingrowth, 30% porosity is rarely exceeded. Bone ingrowth can occur into pores exceeding 25 microns in diameter, with the fastest rates of ingrowth occurring into pores of 50 to 400 microns.[13,14] The thickness of a porous layer is important only in the presence of tension; shear and compression only require a thin porous layer. Porous coatings are frequently applied to the osseointegrative portion of the cup and can be applied to the entire length of the stem; however, frequently, only the most proximal portion of the stem is porous coated. There are several methods of creating porous metal. Initially, such porosity was introduced during the casting process. However, this can pose significant metallurgical problems and result in late stem failure. Microknurling is a process where a knife edge tool under high pressure makes a basket weave pattern on the surface of metal, creating up to 45% porosity, with open pores between 300 and 600 microns in diameter and depth. The advantages of this approach include minimal damage to the substrate and considerable cost savings. With plasma spraying, a coating material is heated and sprayed onto implants. This will be discussed in some detail next. Like microknurling, this process leaves the underlying substrate unchanged. However, the coating itself may be theoretically subject to potential delamination. Pure titanium wire mesh can be diffusion bonded to the surface of titanium alloy, creating changes in surface roughness. The most common method of applying a porous coating, however, is the sintering of metal beads to the surface of the implant. Metal beads are glued to the surface of an implant and allowed to dry. Successive layers of beads are glued to the initial layer. The implant with the attached beads is then heated until the metal and beads coalesce. The porosity of the coating is determined by the size of the beads themselves.

HA is exceptionally biocompatible, especially in association with bone. HA is nontoxic, nonallergenic, and elicits no inflammatory response. HA is a naturally occurring component of both bone and teeth. However, as an implant material, HA is highly unsuitable. HA is brittle, has a low impact resistance, and exhibits low tensile strength (see Table 6-1). To utilize the positive characteristics of HA while minimizing the negative, it can be applied as a surface coating to metallic substrates. This allows the composite to retain the mechanical properties of the metal, while the surface HA coating can be directly bonded to bone. This bonding to bone occurs without the characteristic fibrous coating seen at the bone-implant interface. There are a number of methods for applying bioactive coatings, including dipping, sputter-coating, electrophoresis, and plasma spraying. Plasma spraying is the most common method for the application of HA coatings. Dense, well attached coatings can rapidly be deposited onto metallic implants. One major theoretical concern with HA coatings is the possibility of delamination between the coating and the implant serving as a fracture site. Clinically, few examples of such delamination have been observed and, as their consequences are of minimal significance as the HA itself, is quite biocompatible. Despite the wide use of HA-coated implants, their ability to prevent revisions through enhanced osseointegration remains unclear. A recent study indicated that HA-coated implants imparted no significant reduction in the risk of revision.[15]

Tribology

The term *tribology* refers to the study of interacting surfaces in motion. While the material properties of bone under load are fairly simple to replace, the properties of the joint itself are much more difficult to duplicate. The 3 factors at the surface of the joint that must be taken into account are friction, wear, and lubrication. Friction is the force resisting the relative motion of surfaces in contact. Materials are characteristically described using the coefficient of friction, which is the ratio of the force of friction between 2 bodies and the force pressing them together. Wear is the consequence of friction; the erosion of material from a surface due to the action of another. Lubrication is the process employed to reduce wear by introducing a lubricant between the 2 sliding bodies. The human articular joint is well designed to minimize these factors. The coefficient of friction of human synovial joints varies from 0.025 to 0.003.[16] In addition, the living tissue has the capacity for self-repair. To create artificial bearing surfaces in replacement joints, 3 forms of articulations have been used. From Dr. Charnley's original work, metal balls have articulated against cups of UHMWPE. This combination remains the most popular to this day. As discussed before, UHMWPE has a number of properties making it a good bearing surface. However, the process of UHMWPE wear produces wear particles that have been implicated in osteolysis surrounding the implant. Efforts to increase the strength of UHMWPE, such as crosslinking have reduced wear. However, the characteristic amount of wear in a metal-on-polyethylene (PE) joint remains approximately 0.20 to 0.25 mm/year. One possible option for bearing surfaces is the ceramic-on-ceramic design. As ceramics are stronger than PE, it was expected that wear of this joint would be far reduced. In fact, the characteristic wear rate of ceramic-on-ceramic hip replacements is 0.016 mm/year, roughly 10% of the metal-on-PE numbers. However, as mentioned above, ceramics have an elevated fracture risk over both metals and PE. A second option is the metal-on-metal design. While metal-on-metal bearing surfaces were first used widely in the 1960s, poor materials and design resulted in high failure rates. A second generation of metal-on-metal hips showed good survival and an absence of PE induced osteolysis.[17] A consequence of metal-on-metal wear, however, is the systemic release of metal ions. In fact, a recent study indicated significant elevation of metal ions in blood, urine, and erythrocytes. Consequently, wear remains a significant problem in the replacement of the hip joint and further advances in the material science will be required to alleviate them.

Summary

Only a small number of materials are used in the creation of the hip implants that are used on a daily basis. This is the result of both rigorous trial and error over the past 50 years, as well as hard economic factors that make innovation expensive and rarely cost-effective. However, even at this point in the genesis of the modern hip replacement, a number of areas of innovation remain to be optimized. These include the stimulation of osseointegration with a concomitant prevention of aseptic loosening. In addition, the possibility remains open to create new generations of so-called "smart" implants that actively prevent infection. Finally, the problem of bearing surface wear is still unresolved, and, with the consequences of wear particles so well linked to implant failure, this may be the most vital innovation needed in orthopedic biomaterials.

References

1. Frankel VH, Burstein AJ. *Orthopaedic Biomechanics.* Philadelphia, PA: Lea & Febiger; 1970.
2. Burstein AH, Reilly DT, Martens M. Aging of bone tissue: mechanical properties. *J Bone Joint Surg Am.* 1976;58(1):82-86.
3. Martens M, Van Audekercke R, Delport P, De Meester P, Mulier JC. The mechanical characteristics of cancellous bone at the upper femoral region. *J Biomech.* 1983;16(12):971-983.
4. Currey JD. The effect of porosity and mineral content on the Young's modulus of elasticity of compact bone. *J Biomech.* 1988;21(2):131-139.
5. Goldstein SA. The mechanical properties of trabecular bone: dependence on anatomic location and function. *J Biomech.* 1987;20(11-12):1055-1061.
6. Mears DC, Rothwell GP. The mechanical behavior of real materials. In: *Materials and Orthopaedic Surgery.* Mears DC, ed. Baltimore, MD: Williams & Wilkins; 1979:75-106.
7. Niinomi M, Hattori T, Niwa S. Material Characteristics and biocompatibility of low rigidity titanium alloys for biomedical applications. In: *Biomaterials in Orthopaedics.* Yaszemski MJ, Trantolo DJ, Lewandrowski K-U, Hasirci V, Altobelli DE, Wise DL, eds. New York, NY: Marcel Dekker, Inc; 2004:41-62.
8. Head WC, Bauk DJ, Emerson RH Jr. Titanium as the material of choice for cementless femoral components in total hip arthroplasty. *Clin Orthop Relat Res.* 1995;(311):85-90.
9. Jarcho M. Calcium phosphate ceramics as hard tissue prosthetics. *Clin Orthop Relat Res.* 1981;(157):259-278.
10. Piconi C, Maccauro G. Zirconia as a ceramic biomaterial. *Biomaterials.* 1999;20(1):1-25.
11. Griss P, Andrian-Werburg HV. Biological activity and histocompatibility of dense Al 2 O 3 -MgO ceramic implants in rats. *J Biomed Mater Res.* 1973;7(3):453-462.
12. Mittelmeier H. Fixing endoprostheses without cement using the principle of "weightbearing ribbing." *Z Orthop Ihre Grenzgeb.* 1974;112(1):27-33.
13. Bobyn JD, Cameron HU, Abdulla D, Pilliar RM, Weatherly GC. Biologic fixation and bone modeling with an unconstrained canine total knee prosthesis. *Clin Orthop Relat Res.* 1982;(166):301-312.
14. Bobyn JD, Pilliar RM, Cameron HU, Weatherly GC. The optimum pore size for the fixation of porous-surfaced metal implants by the ingrowth of bone. *Clin Orthop Relat Res.* 1980;(150):263-270.

15. Paulsen A, Pedersen AB, Johnsen SP, Riis A, Lucht U, Overgaard S. Effect of hydroxyapatite coating on risk of revision after primary total hip arthroplasty in younger patients: findings from the Danish Hip Arthroplasty Registry. *Acta Orthop.* 2007;78(5):622-628.

16. Freeman MAR. *Adult Articular Cartilage.* London, England: Pittman Medical; 1979.

17. Brown SR, Davies WA, DeHeer DH, Swanson AB. Long-term survival of McKee-Farrar total hip prostheses. *Clin Orthop Relat Res.* 2002;(402):157-163.

7

Polyethylene

Steven Kurtz, PhD and Michael Manley, PhD

Ultra-high molecular weight polyethylene (hereafter, polyethylene) is a polymer with outstanding impact strength, wear properties, and low friction characteristics. For 5 decades, polyethylene has been a very successful bearing material for use in joint replacements, and it continues in clinical use as the dominant bearing technology for orthopedics. The durability of polyethylene is partly responsible for the rapid expansion of total hip replacement procedures in the United States.[1]

Although polyethylene is the polymeric material of choice in total joint replacements, concerns about polyethylene wear debris-induced osteolysis in the 1990s[2,3] led to the search for alternative bearing solutions.[4] Chapters 23 and 28 provide further information on osteolysis. By analyzing published studies from the literature, Dumbleton et al[5] showed that in the hip, osteolysis could be expected in patients with head penetration into the bearing of more than 0.1 mm/year, but was unlikely in patients with head penetration of less than 0.05 mm/year. As traditional polyethylene could wear at or above these rates, alternative bearings were sought to reduce wear and secondary osteolysis, thereby allowing improvement of long-term survivorship of the replacement.

To address concerns about the wear of polyethylene, highly cross-linked and thermally treated polyethylene (hereafter, cross-linked polyethylene) was clinically introduced in the United States during the late 1990s. Since that time, cross-linked polyethylene has steadily replaced conventional polyethylene for hip arthroplasty.[6] According to recent surveys, approximately 70% of hip replacements performed in the United States employ a cross-linked polyethylene acetabular liner.[7] Furthermore, based on recent projections,[8] around 315,000 primary and revision hip total procedures will be performed in the United States during 2008. Therefore, an estimated 220,000 American total hip arthroplasty patients are currently expected to benefit every year from cross-linked polyethylene technology. Considering the historical trends of increased adoption since cross-linked polyethylene was commercialized in 1998,[7] combined with the projected growth in hip arthroplasty,[8] over 1 million hip replacement patients received a cross-linked liner in the United States by 2007, less than a decade after its clinical introduction. Therefore, cross-linked polyethylene is now widely accepted by surgeons as the main alternative to hard-on-hard bearings for improving the wear resistance of hip arthroplasty.[9]

In this chapter, we focus on applications of cross-linked polyethylene in the hip. Our goal is to provide the practicing surgeon or resident with an overview of the current concepts related to cross-linked polyethylene for hip arthroplasty. Readers interested in a more detailed treatment of cross-linked polyethylene technology are referred to the *UHMWPE Biomaterials Handbook, Second Edition*[4] or a frequently updated online resource dedicated to this subject, www.uhmwpe.org. We begin with an overview of the basic science concepts and terminology surrounding cross-linked polyethylene and conclude with a critical assessment of the clinical literature on the subject of femoral head penetration and wear in commercially available cross-linked materials.

Parvizi J, Klatt BA.
Essentials in Total Hip Arthroplasty (pp 55-61).

Chemical Structure and Molecular Weight

Polyethylene is a polymer of ethylene (CH2CH2) and consists of a carbon backbone chain with pendant hydrogen atoms. Ultra-high molecular weight polyethylene (UHMWPE), used in orthopedic hip and knee applications starting in 1962, has a molecular weight ranging from 2 to 6 million Daltons. By virtue of its molecular weight, UHMWPE has the desirable attributes of wear and impact resistance, together with ductility and toughness. These attributes make UHMWPE highly suitable as a bearing material.

Crystallinity

Crystallinity is an important attribute of all polyethylene, including cross-linked polyethylene. The molecular chains in polyethylene have a natural tendency (driven by thermodynamics) to preferentially fold up against themselves, although this behavior is hindered by the considerable crowding and thermal jostling presented by adjacent molecules. Regions of the polymer with folded chains are referred to as "crystallites," and make up some 60% of the bulk material. The remainder of the bulk is known as the amorphous region with few folded chains. To the eye, crystalline regions diffract visible light, giving polyethylene its white appearance.

Crystallinity is an important structural attribute of polyethylene, as it plays a major role in the mechanical behavior of the material. Crystals are stiffer than the amorphous regions; therefore, the elastic modulus and yield stress of polyethylene will increase directly related to the amount of crystals present. The crystalline content and mechanical properties of polyethylene rods and sheets may be tailored by thermal processing. Different polyethylene manufacturers use proprietary combinations of pressure, temperature, and time to optimize the crystallinity and material properties of the stock material. Many of the processing steps for clinical polyethylene are also tailored specifically to optimize the crystalline structure, and thereby tune its material properties.

Cross-Linking

Cross-linking, the foundation of all modern polyethylene total hip bearings, is defined as the joining of 2 independent polymer molecules by a chemical covalent bond. Cross-linking of polyethylene molecular chains can be achieved by peroxide chemistry, silane chemistry, or by high energy radiation. Of these, only radiation cross-linking has been commercialized by orthopedic device manufacturers.

The extent of cross-linking in polyethylene is proportional to the absorbed dose of radiation. Historically, polyethylene bearings were gamma-treated at a dose of 25 to 40 kGy to sterilize the material. This dose resulted in the formation of some cross-links. Saturation of cross-linking is achieved at around 100 kGy of absorbed dose. Today, cross-linked polyethylene is processed with a total dose ranging from 50 to 105 kGy, depending on the manufacturer.[4] In general, increasing the dose provides a proportional improvement in wear resistance, as quantified by a hip simulator, with diminished benefits in wear resistance observed above 100 kGy.[10,11] The choice of irradiation source (gamma or e-beam) does not substantially influence wear resistance of the resulting polymer, and commercial materials are made using either methodology. Although cross-linking is highly beneficial from the perspective of wear resistance, it comes at the price of less molecular mobility, lower material ductility, and reduced fatigue and fracture resistance due to the cross-linking of the molecular chains.[12] Thus, cross-linking improves certain properties at the expense of others, so developers of orthopedic implants must balance the amount of cross-linking achieved with the maintenance of mechanical properties and/or oxidation resistance.

The final tuning step used in the production of cross-linked polyethylene is thermal processing of the irradiated material. Thermal processing below the melt transition (~137° C) is known as annealing whereas remelting refers to thermal processing above the melt transition. The choice of thermal treatment has a significant impact on the crystallinity and mechanical properties of cross-linked polyethylene.[13] It can also influence the resistance of a material to in vivo oxidation. Although the virtues of annealing and remelting have been debated in the literature,[11,14] ultimately the overall clinical performance of cross-linked polyethylene materials is the final arbiter of success.

Clinical Studies Comparing Cross-Linked and Conventional Polyethylene

Today, several formulations of cross-linked polyethylene are available clinically (eg, Crossfire [Stryker Orthopaedics, Mahwah, NJ], Longevity [Zimmer, Inc, Warsaw, IN], Marathon [DePuy Orthopaedics, Warsaw, IN], XLPE,

Table 7-1

FORMULATIONS OF CLINICALLY AVAILABLE CROSS-LINKED POLYETHYLENES FOR TOTAL HIP ARTHROPLASTY WITH PUBLISHED CLINICAL DATA

	CROSSFIRE	DURASUL	MARATHON	LONGEVITY
Manufacturer	Stryker Orthopaedics	Zimmer, Inc	DePuy Orthopaedics	Zimmer, Inc
Clinical introduction	1998	1998	1998	1999
Total dose (kGy)	105	95	50	100
Thermal treatment	Annealed	Remelted	Remelted	Remelted
Sterilization method	Gamma in nitrogen	Ethylene oxide	Gas plasma	Gas plasma
Detectable free radicals?	Yes	No	No	No
Longest average published clinical follow-up	4.9 years[16]	5 years[21]	5.7 years[26]	3.3 years[22]

Adapted from Kurtz SM. *The UHMWPE Biomaterials Handbook: Ultra-High Molecular Weight Polyethylene in Total Joint Replacement and Medical Devices.* 2nd ed. Burlington, MA: Academic Press; 2009.

Durasul [Zimmer, Inc], X3 [Stryker Orthopaedics], ArCom XL, Acumatch XL, and E-Poly [Biomet Orthopaedics, Warsaw, IN]). Of these, published clinical data are only available concerning 4 formulations and are summarized in Table 7-1. As our objective is to summarize the recent clinical evidence reported for cross-linked as compared with conventional polyethylene, we have excluded those formulations with no track record in the peer-reviewed scientific literature from our discussion. Published clinical studies are given (in alphabetic order) for Crossfire, Durasul, Marathon, and Longevity.

Crossfire

Crossfire, an annealed highly cross-linked polyethylene, was developed by Stryker Orthopaedics for use in the hip.[4] Four clinical studies of Crossfire[15-18] have been published to date, including a 2-year prospective randomized multicenter trial.[15] All of these studies employ 28-mm diameter cobalt-chromium (Co-Cr) femoral heads. These 4 studies report a reduction in head penetration for Crossfire compared to gamma-sterilized in nitrogen controls ranging between 42% and 85%.

The study with the longest follow-up, up to 5.8 years (on average, 4.9 years), is a multicenter retrospective series of 56 arthroplasties incorporating Crossfire and 53 controls (109 hips total). D'Antonio[16] reported a 72% reduction in overall 2D femoral head penetration associated with Crossfire liners as compared with control polyethylene liners. Radiolucent lines were observed around 37.7% of the acetabular components with control polyethylene and 8% of the acetabular components with Crossfire. Femoral osteolysis was noted in 14 control polyethylene hips (14 patients) and in 2 Crossfire hips (1 patient).

Durasul

Durasul was clinically introduced in 1998 and is currently produced by Zimmer, Inc.[4] Four clinical studies of Durasul[19-22] have been published, including the results of a 3-year prospective randomized trial.[19] For 3 of these studies, which compare Durasul to a gamma-sterilized control liner, the reduction in head penetration ranged between 20% and 94%. In the 3 comparative studies, the controls were either gamma-sterilized in air, in nitrogen, or in a low oxygen package. Three of these studies employ 28-mm Co-Cr femoral heads, whereas a study by Geller[22] investigated the clinical performance of 38-mm Co-Cr heads.

Dorr and colleagues[21] have reported on the 5-year follow-up for Durasul, the longest series currently available. Although the data from the 37 arthroplasties in the Durasul group were prospectively collected, the control group was retrospectively matched from a group of patients who were implanted 6 months prior to the implantation of Durasul.

The implants used in the control group were identical to those in the Durasul group, with the exception of a conventional liner (gamma-sterilized in nitrogen) being used for the controls. Dorr[21] reported a 45% reduction in overall 2D femoral head penetration associated with Durasul liners as compared with control polyethylene liners.

Marathon

Marathon was clinically introduced by DePuy Orthopaedics in 1998.[4] Four clinical studies have been published with Marathon.[23-26] The reduction in head penetration for Marathon reported in these studies ranged between 56% and 95% compared with controls that were either uncross-linked (gas plasma-sterilized) or gamma-sterilized in air. All of these studies employ 28-mm Co-Cr femoral heads. However, a study by Heisel[24] also includes the results for 7 Marathon hips with 32-mm head sizes. In addition, 3 out of 34 (9%) of the femoral heads in Heisel's study[24] were ceramic (the majority, 31 out of 34 [91%], were Co-Cr).

In a comprehensive study, Engh and coworkers[26] conducted a prospective randomized trial of Marathon with up to 7.2 years follow-up (average, 5.6 years). The control material in this series was uncross-linked, gas-plasma sterilized polyethylene. Engh[26] reported a 95% reduction in overall 2D femoral head penetration associated with Marathon liners as compared with control polyethylene liners. Although there were no revisions or cases of loosening in either the Marathon or control liners, the authors noted a significant difference in the incidence of osteolysis between the 2 groups: 57.8% of the control patients exhibited radiographic evidence of osteolysis of the pelvis or femur, as compared to an osteolysis incidence of 24.0% in the Marathon patients ($p < 0.001$). It should be noted, however, that patient satisfaction was excellent and indistinguishable between the Marathon (96.2% satisfied with results) and control (99%) groups at the longest follow-up period.

Longevity

Longevity was developed by Zimmer, Inc and clinically introduced in 1999.[4] Three clinical studies of Longevity[19,20,22] have been reported. In 2 of these studies,[19,20] a head penetration reduction of 31% and 90% was reported relative to gamma-sterilized in air or nitrogen controls. Two studies employed 28-mm Co-Cr femoral heads,[19,20] whereas the third investigated the use of 36- and 40-mm Co-Cr heads.[22]

Manning et al[20] have published the longest-term radiographic wear study comparing Longevity to conventional, gamma air-sterilized polyethylene, with up to 3.7 years follow-up (2.6 years, average). Manning[20] reported a 90% reduction in overall 2D femoral head penetration associated with Longevity liners as compared with control polyethylene liners.

"Second-Generation" Cross-Linked Polyethylene

Given the broad range of cross-linked materials currently available for hip arthroplasty, controversies remain regarding the relevance of in vivo oxidation[27] and the risk of rim impingement damage and fracture.[28] The controversies surrounding the importance of in vivo oxidation and rim fracture continue to be debated in scientific circles and have lead to the development of additional, "second-generation" cross-linked polyethylene. Examples of these materials include X3 and E-Poly. The intent of these second-generation materials is to reduce the potential for material oxidation in the long term while preserving the bulk mechanical properties necessary to use cross-linked polyethylene in higher stress applications such as thin acetabular liners and stabilized knee designs. Laboratory testing suggests that material design goals have been satisfied in these new polymer formulations. However, due to clinical introduction within the past 2 years, clinical data regarding the performance of these new formulations are not yet available.

Summary

The available literature provides sufficient information to address 4 key clinical questions regarding the suitability of first-generation cross-linked polyethylene in hip arthroplasty.

Have Mechanical Properties Proven to Be Important?

Cross-linked materials were clinically introduced at a time when 28-mm femoral heads were widely used, whereas today there is a demand for larger diameter articulations for hip arthroplasty. With the incorporation of highly cross-linked polyethylene into new large-diameter cup designs, modes of clinical failure other than wear may become new limiting factors for the long-term clinical performance of cross-linked polyethylene. These factors include component fracture associated with rim loading, thin liners, and impingement-related damage due to component malpositioning. The clinical introduction of thin acetabular liners incorporating highly cross-linked UHMWPE raises new questions regarding the mechanical properties of these thin liner designs being able to withstand structural fatigue loading.

Over the past 8 years, a few anecdotal reports of rim fracture of remelted cross-linked liners have surfaced in the literature, as well as in the United States Food and Drug Administration's Manufacturer and User Facility Device Experience reports of adverse events involving medical devices (see www.accessdata.fda.gov/scripts/cdrh/cfdocs/cfMAUDE/search.CFM). These anecdotal reports are usually associated with thin liners associated with acetabular shells implanted with a high abduction angle.

Due to the small numbers reported thus far in the literature, the incidence of rim fracture necessitating revision of cross-linked polyethylene remains poorly understood. None of the numerous clinical studies of remelted polyethylene have reported rim fracture as a clinically relevant failure mode. However, the few rare cases of rim fracture have provided motivation for improving the mechanical behavior of cross-linked polyethylene, especially for thin liners.

Does Cross-Linked Polyethylene Reduce In Vivo Head Penetration Rates?

The clinical studies published to date for 4 commercially available materials strongly support the hypothesis that cross-linked polyethylene reduces the clinical head penetration (so-called wear) rate in patients. This finding is almost entirely based on clinical studies employing 28-mm diameter Co-Cr femoral heads, but early clinical results are available with larger head sizes. We find no data in the literature to support the hypothesis that ceramic femoral heads provide any further reduction in penetration rates for cross-linked polyethylene.

The magnitude of the reduction in penetration rates, however, varies widely even among studies employing the same material. Some of the variability in wear rates displayed by studies of same material may be due to differences in radiographic wear measurement techniques, as well as differences in the way penetration rates are reported, which change from study to study.

Another difficulty is that the magnitude of the head penetration, especially at short-term follow-up periods and with cross-linked polyethylene, is extremely small, and borders on the detection limit of digitized radiographs. Hence, it is not uncommon for short-term wear studies with cross-linked polyethylene to sometimes observe a "negative wear rate," corresponding to a shift of the femoral head out of rather than into the polyethylene socket. These artifacts further complicate measurement of the low wear rates encountered with cross-linked polyethylene.

Standardized methods for measuring and reporting radiographic head penetration would be helpful for performing future comparison of cross-linked polyethylenes. Efforts are underway to standardize radiographic wear measurement protocols at the American Society of Testing and Materials, and a working group was formed by the F04.22 Committee on Arthroplasty in 2003 for this purpose. However, to date, no standards on this subject have been published.

Do Certain Cross-Linked Polyethylene Formulations Reduce In Vivo Head Penetration Rates More Than Others?

The ability to compare the reported reduction in penetration rate among different cross-linked polyethylene remains extremely limited. In addition to the reasons outlined above, the initial penetration rate of liners is design-dependent, with certain shells accommodating greater "settling in" of the polyethylene component than others. In addition, different cross-linked polyethylene formulations have varying time-dependent mechanical properties. These properties influence the early creep performance of the liner in the shell. It becomes almost impossible to compare head penetration across studies when different "control" polyethylene materials are employed by different groups of investigators. For example, studies that employ uncross-linked, gas sterilized control liners, which have approximately 2 times the wear rate of gamma-sterilized control liners,[29] will tend to overemphasize the difference between the cross-linked and control situation when compared to studies that employ a gamma-sterilized liner control.

Thus, we are unable, with the data published thus far, to find evidence to support the hypothesis that one manufacturer's formulation of cross-linked polyethylene has a significantly lower radiographic femoral head penetration rate as compared with another manufacturer's formulation. At best, we can reasonably assert that published data strongly support the hypothesis that cross-linked polyethylene exhibits lower radiographic head penetration than conventional control materials, whether the controls are gamma-sterilized in an inert environment or simply gas sterilized (eg, gas plasma or ethylene oxide). The precise magnitude of the reduction in head penetration associated with a particular material remains the subject of scientific debate.

Does Cross-Linked Polyethylene Reduce In Vivo Wear Rates?

It would be difficult, based on short-term radiographic penetration studies alone, to conclude that simply because cross-linked polyethylene exhibits reduced head penetration, it also exhibits reduced wear in vivo. However, support for this latter "wear reduction" hypothesis is reflected in the penetration histories for cross-linked polyethylene over time. Cross-linked polyethylene generally shows a decelerating head penetration rate over time. This is consistent with lower in vivo wear rate as compared with conventional polyethylene. Further support comes from published retrieval studies of annealed[27,30] and remelted[31] cross-linked polyethylene. These short-term retrieval studies confirm a similar adhesive/abrasive wear mechanism, but a lower magnitude of wear than would be expected from conventional materials.

Stronger support for the "wear reduction" hypothesis comes from recent intermediate-term clinical studies,[16,26] showing a lower incidence of osteolysis with both annealed and remelted cross-linked polyethylene. Only one of the studies[26] published thus far, which is a prospective randomized trial in which only the liner material was exchanged, provides Level I scientific evidence of reduced osteolysis associated with the use of a cross-linked polyethylene liner after up to 7.2 years of implantation. This finding is particularly encouraging because the experimental Marathon liners involved in the study are cross-linked with the lowest radiation dose among commercial products. Hence, other cross-linked materials treated with a higher radiation dose are expected to be even more wear resistant.

In summary, the available body of intermediate term clinical literature currently provides some encouraging support for the hypothesis that cross-linked polyethylene, when coupled with a 28-mm Co-Cr femoral head, reduces in vivo wear, as well as femoral head penetration. As wear reduction can be expected to reduce revisions due to osteolysis, a more definitive conclusion awaits the longer-term clinical follow-up data.

References

1. Kurtz S, Ong K, Lau E, Mowat F, Halpern M. Projections of primary and revision hip and knee arthroplasty in the United States from 2005 to 2030. *J Bone Joint Surg Am.* 2007;89(4):780-785, 2007.
2. Harris WH. The problem is osteolysis. *Clin Orthop.* 1995;311:46-53.
3. Willert HG, Bertram H, Buchhorn GH. Osteolysis in alloarthroplasty of the hip. The role of bone cement fragmentation. *Clin Orthop Relat Res.* 1990;(258):108-121.
4. Kurtz SM. The UHMWPE *Biomaterials Handbook: Ultra-High Molecular Weight Polyethylene in Total Joint Replacement and Medical Devices.* 2nd ed. Burlington, MA: Academic Press; 2009.
5. Dumbleton JH, Manley MT, Edidin AA. A literature review of the association between wear rate and osteolysis in total hip arthroplasty. *J Arthroplasty.* 2002;17(5):649-661.
6. Kurtz SM, Muratoglu OK, Evans M, Edidin AA. Advances in the processing, sterilization, and crosslinking of ultra-high molecular weight polyethylene for total joint arthroplasty. *Biomaterials.* 1999;20(18):1659-1688.
7. Mendenhall S. Hospital resources and implant cost management–a 2006 update. *Orthopaedic Network News.* 2007;18(3):13-19.
8. Kurtz S, Lau E, Ong K, Zhao K, Kelly M, Bozic K. Future young patient demand for primary and revision joint replacement: national projections from 2010 to 2030. *Clin Orthop Relat Res.* 2008;33:1784.
9. Jasty M, Rubash HE, Muratoglu O. Highly cross-linked polyethylene: the debate is over--in the affirmative. *J Arthroplasty.* 2005;20(4 suppl 2):55-58.
10. Wang A, Essner A, Polineni VK, Stark C, Dumbleton JH. Lubrication and wear of ultra-high molecular weight polyethylene in total joint replacements. *Tribology International.* 1998;31(1-3):17-33.
11. Muratoglu OK, Kurtz SM. Alternative bearing surfaces in hip replacement. In: Sinha R, ed. *Hip Replacement: Current Trends and Controversies.* New York, NY: Marcel Dekker; 2002:1-46.
12. Gencur SJ, Rimnac CM, Kurtz SM. Fatigue crack propagation resistance of virgin and highly cross-linked, thermally treated ultra-high molecular weight polyethylene. *Biomaterials.* 2006;27(8):1550-1557.
13. Kurtz SM, Villarraga ML, Herr MP, Bergstrom JS, Rimnac CM, Edidin AA. Thermomechanical behavior of virgin and highly cross-linked ultra-high molecular weight polyethylene used in total joint replacements. *Biomaterials.* 2002;23(17):3681-3697.
14. Kurtz SM, Manley M, Wang A, Taylor S, Dumbleton J. Comparison of the properties of annealed cross-linked (Crossfire) and conventional polyethylene as hip bearing materials. *Bull Hosp Jt Dis.* 2002-2003;61(1-2):17-26.
15. Martell JM, Verner JJ, Incavo SJ. Clinical performance of a highly cross-linked polyethylene at two years in total hip arthroplasty: a randomized prospective trial. *J Arthroplasty.* 2003;18(7 suppl 1):55-59.
16. D'Antonio JA, Manley MT, Capello WN, Bierbaum BE, Ramakrishnan R, Naughton M, Sutton K. Five-year experience with Crossfire highly cross-linked polyethylene. *Clin Orthop Relat Res.* 2005;441:143-150.
17. Krushell RJ, Fingeroth RH, Cushing MC. Early femoral head penetration of a highly cross-linked polyethylene liner vs a conventional polyethylene liner. *J Arthroplasty.* 2005;20(7 suppl):73-76.

18. Rohrl S, Nivbrant B, Mingguo L, Hewitt B. In vivo wear and migration of highly cross-linked polyethylene cups a radiostereometry analysis study. *J Arthroplasty.* 2005;20(4):409-413.
19. Digas G, Karrholm J, Thanner J, Malchau H, Herberts P. Highly cross-linked polyethylene in total hip arthroplasty: randomized evaluation of penetration rate in cemented and uncemented sockets using radiostereometric analysis. *Clin Orthop.* 2004;429(429):6-16.
20. Manning DW, Chiang PP, Martell JM, Galante JO, Harris WH. In vivo comparative wear study of traditional and highly cross-linked polyethylene in total hip arthroplasty. *J Arthroplasty.* 2005;20(7):880-886.
21. Dorr LD, Wan Z, Shahrdar C, Sirianni L, Boutary M, Yun A. Clinical performance of a Durasul highly cross-linked polyethylene acetabular liner for total hip arthroplasty at five years. *J Bone Joint Surg Am.* 2005;87(8):1816-1821.
22. Geller JA, Malchau H, Bragdon C, Greene M, Harris WH, Freiberg AA. Large diameter femoral heads on highly cross-linked polyethylene: minimum 3-year results. *Clin Orthop Relat Res.* 2006;447:53-59.
23. Hopper RH Jr, Young AM, Orishimo KF, McAuley JP. Correlation between early and late wear rates in total hip arthroplasty with application to the performance of marathon cross-linked polyethylene liners. *J Arthroplasty.* 2003;18(7 suppl 1):60-67.
24. Heisel C, Silva M, dela Rosa MA, Schmalzried TP. Short-term in vivo wear of cross-linked polyethylene. *J Bone Joint Surg Am.* 2004;86-A(4):748-751.
25. Heisel C, Silva M, Schmalzried TP. In vivo wear of bilateral total hip replacements: conventional versus cross-linked polyethylene. *Arch Orthop Trauma Surg.* 2005;125:555-557.
26. Engh CA Jr, Stepniewski AS, Ginn SD, et al. A randomized prospective evaluation of outcomes after total hip arthroplasty using cross-linked marathon and non-cross-linked Enduron polyethylene liners. *J Arthroplasty.* 2006;21(6 suppl 2):17-25.
27. Kurtz SM, Hozack WJ, Purtill JJ, et al. Significance of in vivo degradation for polyethylene in total hip arthroplasty. *Clin Orthop Relat Res.* 2006;453:47-57.
28. Halley D, Glassman A, Crowninshield RD. Recurrent dislocation after revision total hip replacement with a large prosthetic femoral head. A case report. *J Bone Joint Surg Am.* 2004;86-A(4):827-830.
29. Hopper RH Jr, Young AM, Orishimo KF, Engh CA Jr. Effect of terminal sterilization with gas plasma or gamma radiation on wear of polyethylene liners. *J Bone Joint Surg Am.* 2003;85-A(3):464-468.
30. Kurtz SM, Hozack W, Turner J, et al. Mechanical properties of retrieved highly cross-linked Crossfire liners after short-term implantation. *J Arthroplasty.* 2005;20(7):840-849.
31. Muratoglu OK, Greenbaum ES, Bragdon CR, Jasty M, Freiberg AA, Harris WH. Surface analysis of early retrieved acetabular polyethylene liners: a comparison of conventional and highly cross-linked polyethylenes. *J Arthroplasty.* 2004;19(1):68-77.

8

Polymethylmethacrylate Bone Cement

Manny Porat, MD and Javad Parvizi, MD, FRCS

While the origins of polymethylmethacrylate (PMMA) bone cement can be traced as far back as the 19th century, the earliest applications in medicine were in the 1930s in the field of dentistry. In orthopedics, Herschell and Judet are credited with some of the early documented applications of PMMA in 1945 and 1950. Early forms of acrylic bone cement were used as femoral head prostheses.[1] In 1953, Haboush used PMMA, in a similar fashion as seen today, as a grout to enhance fixation of implants. However, it is Charnley, in the early 1970s, who is often credited with pioneering the current usages of PMMA during cemented total hip arthroplasty. Bone cement, also known as acrylic acid for its very recognizable smell, is used not as an adhesive or glue but rather as a grout relying on fixation by interlocking fit between surfaces, bone-to-cement and cement-to-metal prosthesis.

The PMMA used in modern orthopedic surgery is a polymer that is often stored in 2 separate states, as both a liquid and powder form. The liquid typically contains a methylmethacrylate (MMA) monomer, hydroquinone, and dimethyl para-toluidine. The hydroquinone is a stabilizer that inhibits premature polymerization of the MMA from heat or light prior to mixing with the powder. The dimethyl para-toluidine is used to accelerate the polymerization process once the powder is added. The powder portion of PMMA, usually doubling the amount of the liquid, contains polymerized PMMA mixed with comonomers of styrene, methyl acrylate, or butyl methacrylate, which adds to the strength of the final product. To visualize the final product on radiographs, a radiopaque material such as barium sulfate or zirconia is added to the powder solution. Finally, a dye like chlorophyll is added to distinguish its color from that of bone. The powder and liquid solutions are mixed to form the final PMMA product ready for use during an operation.

Polymerization Process

Bone cement is packaged in its powder and liquid forms intended to be mixed during the operation. Mixing the separated components initiates the polymerization process. This process would normally take hours and would be unreasonably long during a surgical procedure. However, the process is accelerated by the activators added to the solution. Pure MMA has a very low viscosity and if introduced prior to polymerization, could seep into the blood system and possibly cause cardiorespiratory distress.[2] Mixing the liquid MMA and powder PMMA increases the viscosity during polymerization and allows the final product to remain where it is placed. The polymerization process begins by creating benzoyl free radicals, which break the original carbon-to-carbon double bonds of the MMA. That initiates a free radical chain propagation that results in new carbon-to-carbon single-bond long-chain polymers.

The polymerization process can be observed by the members of the operative team in 4 stages: the mixing period, waiting period, working period, and hardening period. The mixing period is characterized by combining the liquid and powder substrates. Even at this early stage, the polymerization process has initiated as the room temperature and ambient air are catalysts for the free radical chain reaction.

Parvizi J, Klatt BA.
Essentials in Total Hip Arthroplasty (pp 63-68).

An obvious change in the viscosity of the material can be visualized as the prepolymerized beads swell during the mixing of the solutions. This process can be performed in a vacuum or in the open air. An air-free environment can potentially decrease bubbles associated with mixing the cement in open air adding to the overall volumetric shrinkage.[3] The formation of a homogenous mass in the mixing bowl heralds the waiting period. The polymerization process continues during the waiting period as the increasing viscosity changes the once liquid PMMA to that of a doughy texture. The PMMA is subsequently transferred to a cement gun. The timing of this process is quite variable and depends upon the concentration of the accelerator, molecular weight of the MMA, presence of stabilizers, and temperature of the room.

At the beginning of the working period, the consistency of PMMA is like sticky dough, allowing the cement to be easily applied to the femur or desired location. When ready, the PMMA will not stick to the surgical gloves. PMMA that is applied too early lacks the recommended viscosity, allowing for previously mentioned large leakage into the blood stream. Anesthesia needs to maintain normovolemia and avoid hypotension for the introduction of the PMMA, as the monomer can cause a transient hypotension. There can also be a fat embolism from the introduction and pressurization of the cement.

Perfusion pressures in the body will allow blood to intermix with the solution if it is delivered prematurely, weakening the final product.

The final stage is the hardening period during which the PMMA will take its final shape and solidify in approximately 10 to 20 minutes. The polymerization process is an exothermic reaction that releases considerable heat. In vitro studies have recorded temperature ranges from 70°C to 120°C. However, most in vivo studies have not found temperature elevations that extreme. Prolonged exposures to temperature above 56°C cause collagen to denature while bone thermal necrosis is seen at temperatures above 47°C. This was initially a concern with the use of PMMA. However, decreasing the amount of monomer as well as prepolymerized PMMA beads in the powder decrease the amount of heat released. No thermal injury from PMMA has been demonstrated in the literature and is currently not considered a major complication. As the viscosity increases during this period, there is a compensatory volumetric shrinkage of about 2% to 7%.[4]

Each step in the polymerization process of PMMA is critical for the porosity and final strength of the product. The literature demonstrates that fracture strength is directly related to the porosity of the bone cement and thus an increase in macropores can make it susceptible to fracture and propagation of a crack. Air can be a source of macropore formation in the bone cement, so modern techniques actively try to eliminate its presence in the final product. It can be dissolved within the powder or trapped in the liquid during the mixing process. Air can also be entrapped during transfer to the delivery gun or even during the filling of the medullary canal. In addition to air molecules affecting porosity, evaporation of volatile monomers from the heat can create larger pores. Unfused beads of PMMA during the polymerization process can also increase porosity of the final product. In order to combat these potential complications, several techniques have been shown to reduce overall pore size in bone cement. Centrifugation of the hand-mixed liquid and powder PMMA was found to be effective in reducing the pore size as the air-filled pores have a lower density and rise to the surface. One potential side effect of this process is that the denser radiopaque particles in the bone cement may lead to an inhomogenous mixture. Vacuum mixing methods have been found to decrease the pore size and improve ultimate fatigue strength of the bone cement. In addition to mixing techniques, prechilling the monomer can reduce boiling at low vapor pressures, which helps to reduce porosity of the final product. The location of the micropores can also adversely affect the cemented component as large pores at the cement metal interface can be a site for stress and potentially propagate a fracture of the cement mantle.[5]

Mechanical Properties

Cemented implants can transmit loads over a larger area than uncemented prostheses. PMMA is a brittle material and the modulus of elasticity is approximately 10 times lower than that of the surrounding cortical bone and 100 times lower than that of the metal implant, which allows it to act as an elastic layer between the stiffer layers around it. PMMA is 50% weaker in compression and shear than cortical bone and, when used in load bearing, must be supported by bone to avoid fracture of the cement. Bone cement is a viscoelastic material that demonstrates the properties of creep and stress relaxation. These characteristics have been important in stem design and in the ability to protect the overall interface and longevity of the prosthesis.

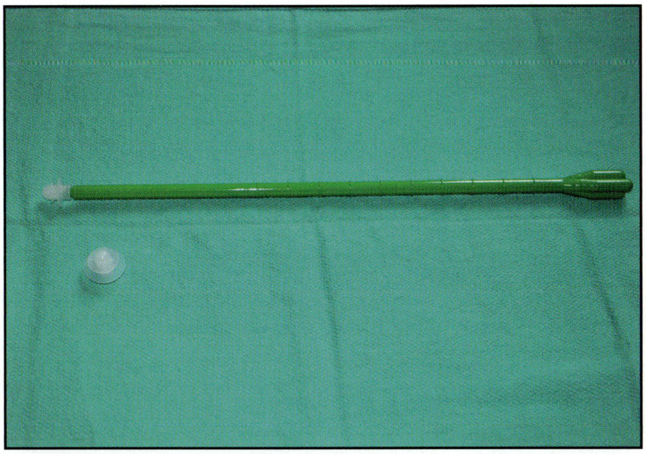

Figure 8-1. Canal plug and inserter.

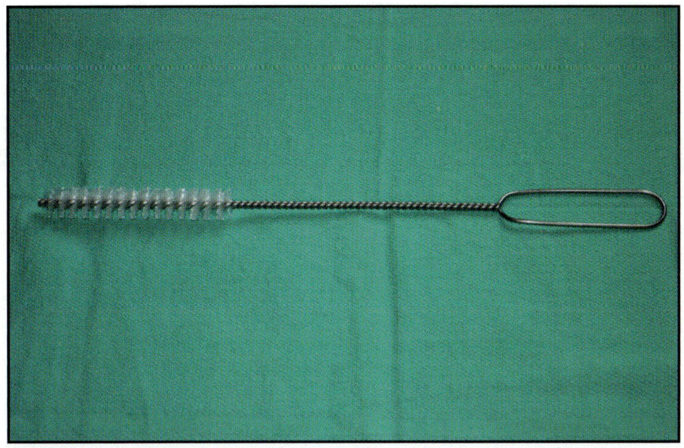

Figure 8-2. Femoral canal brush.

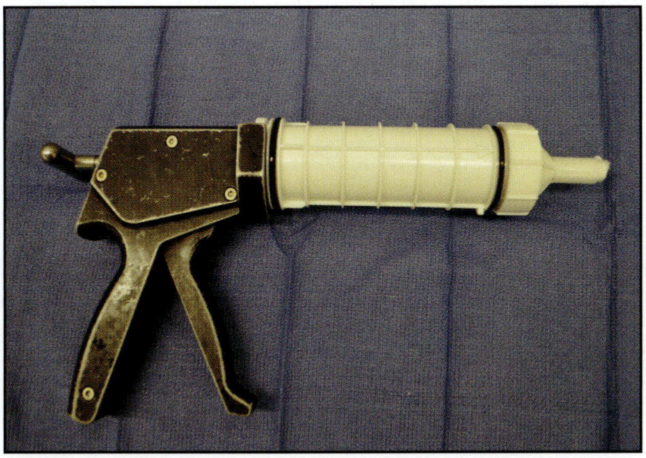

Figure 8-3. Cement gun.

Cement Techniques

Cemented fixation in joint arthroplasty has undergone several major developments in technique to improve the cement mantle and failure rate.

The first generation of modern day cement techniques was originated by Charnley in the 1970s. During the early phases, acrylic bone cement was mixed in the open air with a spatula or blade to a doughy consistency and subsequently packed into the native femoral canal. Implants were made of stainless steel with sharp unpolished edges and a narrow border. Large variances in surgeon techniques and inferior prosthesis led to higher failure rates in the cement mantle. Reported radiographic loosening of the prosthesis using first-generation techniques were 20% to 24% at 5-year follow-up and increased to 30% to 40% at 10 years.[6] High early failure rates led to a demand for improvements in cement methodology.

In the mid 1970s, advancements in arthroplasty brought a second generation of cement techniques. The following improvements led to dramatic reduction in failures of early arthroplasty implants. To increase pressure within the femoral canal during cementing, a bone block or plastic plug (Figure 8-1) was introduced 2 to 3 cm distal to the femoral component. This advancement increased the cement intrusion into the surrounding cancellous bone. Prior to placing the femoral plug, a canal brush (Figure 8-2) and pulsatile lavage of the femoral canal aided in removing any marrow, fat, blood, or loose bodies from the broaching of the canal. Irrigation of the canal dramatically increased cement intrusion and ultimately improved the shear strength of the hardening cement mantle around the prosthesis. The use of a cement gun (Figure 8-3) during delivery of PMMA allowed surgeons to apply the cement to the broached canal in a retrograde fashion instead of finger packing the cement. This allowed a more standard delivery of the cement, permitting a more complete filling of the canal and avoiding gaps and laminations in the cement mantle. In addition to improvements in implants such as super alloys with broad medial borders and rounded edges, there were reductions in failure rates reported 3% to 10%.[6]

Third-generation techniques, beginning in the early 1980s, included improved mixing techniques for the PMMA. Mixing of the cement in open air bowels by hand was supplemented by vacuum mixing and centrifugation, which helped reduce the porosity of the PMMA prior to loading the cement gun. Cement pressurization (Figure 8-4) was also found to be helpful in improving the interface between the PMMA and bone. After pressurization, the cement mantle was found to have a greater interdigitation with the surrounding bone, thus improving the shear strength. Optimal depth of cement penetration was found to be 4 mm.[7] In 2002, the Swedish National

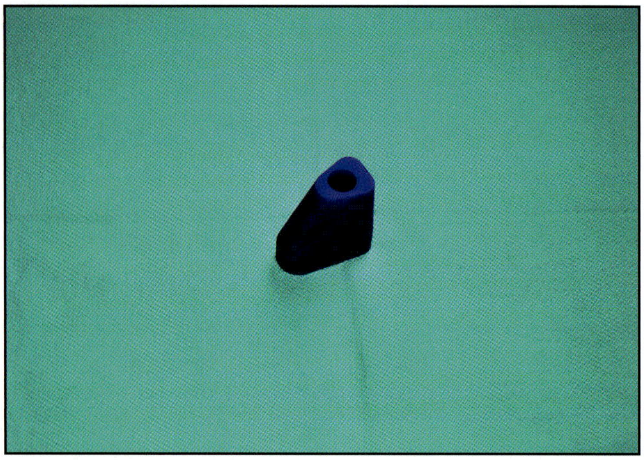

Figure 8-4. Femoral canal pressurizer.

Hip Arthroplasty Register noted that pressurization of the femoral canal resulted in a reduction in revision rates from aseptic loosening.[8]

The currently used fourth-generation techniques incorporate the improvements of earlier generations and stem centralization. Increased rates of cemented femoral prosthesis failures due to deficient cement mantle thickness is supported by the literature.[9] Optimal thickness of the cement mantle is 2.5 to 5 mm around the prosthesis. Excessive varus or valgus positioning of the femoral component has also been associated with higher failure rates.[10] In order to combat these potential mishaps, the addition of a stem centralizer, either prefabricated on the stem or placed on the stem during surgery, in theory aids in a more universal cement mantle around the prosthesis and helps with prosthesis alignment. Possible complications of the centralizers have been reported and include fracture with some designs. Early follow-up studies are promising but additional long-term studies are needed to determine how effective stem centralizers are.

Radiographic Analysis of Cement Mantle

To effectively evaluate the cement mantle by radiographic means after arthroplasty, Barrack et al proposed a grading system from A to D.[6] Grade "A" is defined by complete filling of the medullary cavity with what was described initially as "white-out" of the cement bone interface. Grade "B" involves slight radiolucency of the cement-bone interface and has near complete filling of the medullary canal. Grade "C" mantles have radiolucencies greater than 50% of the bone cement interface or have incomplete cement mantles with implant opposition against the cortex. A grade "D" mantle has gross radiolucencies and/or failure to surround the tip of the stem. Chambers et al in 2001 demonstrated that grade C or D cement mantles have a 9-fold increased failure risk.[11]

At long-term follow-up, radiographic analysis of the cement mantle is usually described by Gruen zone analysis. He defined 7 zones around the stem. According to Harris, if there is a continuous lucency around the stem, it is considered "probably" loose. If there is lucency around 50% to 99%, it is considered "possibly" loose. A cemented femoral stem is definitely loose if it subsides, debonds (has new lucency at implant/cement mantle that was not present on initial postoperation x-rays), has a cement mantle fracture, or has an implant breakage.

Antibiotics in Cement

Infection after total joint arthroplasty is a devastating complication that occurs in 1% to 2% of primary surgeries. Infection rates are higher after revision surgery and is often a challenging problem requiring a multidisciplinary approach. Antibiotics are the mainstay of treatment. Buchholz and Engelbrecht, in 1970, first introduced the notion of loading acrylic bone cement with antibiotics for primary arthroplasty patients.[12] Antibiotics are released from the surface of the cement and from voids within. Only 10% of the antibiotics impregnated in the cement effectively reach the tissue due to the hydrophobicity of the bone cement.

For an antibiotic to be effective in PMMA, it must meet several criteria. It must be water soluble and heat stable. The exothermic reaction during the hardening of PMMA is destructive to many antibiotics. The antibiotic must have bactericidal effect at the tissue levels attained and must be able to escape the bone cement and elute to the surrounding tissue. It must evoke minimal local inflammatory or allergic reactions and cannot compromise the mechanical integrity of the cement around it. Many antibiotics meet these requirements for addition into bone cement. The most commonly used antibiotic added to bone cement in the United States is tobramycin (Figure 8-5). It is heat stable, efficiently eluted to surrounding tissue, and has an effective track record against common offending organisms such as *Staphylococcus aureus* and *Staphylococcus epidermidis.* Tobramycin levels peak around 48 hours and are detectable at 9 weeks after implantation. Other antibiotics commonly impregnated into bone cement include gentamicin, vancomycin, and, less frequently, cephalosporins.[12]

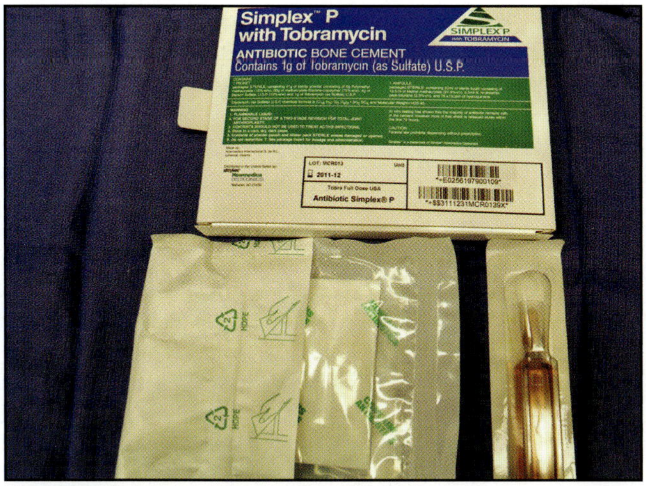

Figure 8-5. Antibiotic cement powder and liquid.

The cement concentration of the antibiotic is critical during the mixing process as doses that are too low will not be effective and higher doses can potentially weaken the cement, making it susceptible to fatigue or cracking. Prophylaxis dosing requires smaller doses of antibiotics, around 1 g or less of powdered antibiotic per 40 g of bone cement. Treatment doses are needed at larger amounts for effective therapeutic levels. At least 3.6 g of antibiotic per 40 g of cement is needed and can range as high as 6 to 8 g per 40 g.[13]

The current literature supports the use of antibiotics in bone cement as a means of prophylaxis. Results from the Norwegian Arthroplasty Register reveal that patients treated with only systemic antibiotic prophylaxis had a 1.8 times higher rate of infection than patients who received combined systemic and antibiotic-impregnated cement. While these results have been confirmed in additional studies, opponents have cited that there is an overall decrease in infection rates, a result of multifactorial improvements in arthroplasty practices. The use of antibiotic-loaded cement has also been advocated in revision hip surgery based on data from the Swedish Joint Registry. Currently, the literature does not have studies demonstrating the superiority of one antibiotic over another for prophylaxis.[13]

There are several potential disadvantages to the addition of antibiotics to acrylic bone cement. The overaddition of certain antibiotics can decrease the compressive strength. The most widely studied antibiotic is gentamicin. Caution should be used when adding large amounts of gentamicin; however, studies have shown no large change in compressive or tensile strength of the cement.[14] There are reports of decreases in strength when antibiotics are hand mixed into acrylic cement as compared to using commercially prepared solutions.[15] Several studies have looked into the possible toxicity to osteoblasts when using large quantities of antibiotics. In some studies, large doses decreased replication rates of these cells and caused cell death in in vitro studies.[13] The clinical literature does not contain cases of systemic toxicity or adverse events caused by antibiotics. Another concern of the continued use of antibiotic-loaded acrylic cement is the potential for antimicrobial resistance as it is already an ongoing dilemma. Some studies have looked into the concern of reimplantation of new prosthesis in a previously infected arthroplasty patient. The results demonstrated a higher reinfection rate with resistant microorganisms in patients originally treated with antibiotic-loaded cement.

Osteolysis

Osteolysis of bone after arthroplasty, once termed *cement disease,* has been shown to be a cause of prosthetic aseptic loosening. Histologic examination of the lytic lesions demonstrates inflammatory cells among the macrophages and giant cells. Macrophages have been shown to be activated by debris from polymethylmethacrylate, polyethylene, and various metals after placement of prosthesis. PMMA particles 1 to 300 μm have been shown to stimulate macrophages in vitro.[16] Particle debris from PMMA activates an inflammatory cascade with elevated levels of interleukin-1, tumor necrosis factor, and prostaglandins. These elevated markers have been associated with local bone resorption and may play a role in osteolysis. Other studies have examined the effects of hydrostatic pressure from particle debris on bone and the increased rates of osteolysis. These studies speculate that PMMA particles caused local osteolysis and loosening of implants from elevated hydrostatic pressures in bone.[17]

Summary

The use of PMMA in modern hip arthroplasty began with Sir Charnley in the 1970s. His initial success paved the way for further improvements in both prosthesis development and the acrylic cement process. Advances in acrylic bone cement mixing techniques and application have improved outcomes of cemented total hip prosthesis. The use of PMMA in total hip arthroplasty has become more limited since the introduction and widespread use of ingrowth stems, but PMMA is still widely used. It is important that the surgeon has a good understanding of PMMA and its proper use.

References

1. Webb JC, Spencer RF. The role of polymethylmethacrylate bone cement in modern orthopaedic surgery. *J Bone Joint Surg Br.* 2007;89(7):851-857.
2. Orsini EC, Byrick RJ, Mullen JB, Kay JC, Waddell JP. Cardiopulmonary function and pulmonary microemboli during arthroplasty using cemented or non-cemented components. The role of intramedullary pressure. *J Bone Joint Surg.* 1987;69:822-832.
3. Schreurs BW, Spierings PTJ, Huiskes R, Siooff TJ. Effects of preparation techniques on the porosity of acrylic cements. *Acta Orthop Scand.* 1988;54(4):403-409.
4. Callaghan JJ, Rosenberg AG, Rubash HE. *The Adult Hip.* Volumes I and II. Philadelphia, PA: Lippincott Williams & Wilkins; 2007.
5. Jafri AA, Green SM, Partington PF, McCaskie AW, Muller SD. Pre-heating of components in cemented total hip arthroplasty. *J Bone Joint Surg Br.* 2004;86(8):1214-1219.
6. Barrack R, Mulroy R, Harris W. Improved cementing techniques and femoral componenet loosening in young patients with hip arthroplasty. A 12-year radiographic review. *J Bone Joint Surg Br.* 1992;74(3):385-389.
7. Askew MJ, Steege JW, Lewis JL, Ranieri JR, Wixson RL. Effect of cement pressure and bone strength on polymethylmethacrylate fixation. *J Orthop Res.* 1984;1(4):412-420.
8. Swedish Arthroplasty Register. 2002 Annual Report. Goteborg, Sweden: Swedish Arthroplasty Register; 2002.
9. Ahmed AM, Raab S, Miller JE. Metal/cement interface strength in cemented stem fixation. *J Orthop Res.* 1984;2(2):105-118.
10. Berger RA, Seel MJ, Wood K, Evans R, D'Antonio J, Rubash HE. Effect of a centralizing device on cement mantle deficiencies and initial prosthetic alignment in total hip arthroplasty. *J Arthroplasty.* 1997;12(4):434-443.
11. Chambers IR, Fender D, McCaskie AW, et al. Radiological features predictive of aseptic loosening in cemented Charnley femoral stems. *J Bone Joint Surg.* 2001;83(6):838-842.
12. Joseph T, Chen A, Di Cesare P. Use of antibiotic-impregnated cement in total joint arthroplasty. *J Am Acad Orthop Surg.* 2003;11(1):38-47.
13. Jiranek WA, Hanssen AD, Greenwald AS. Antibiotic-loaded bone cement for infection prophylaxis in total joint replacement. *J Bone Joint Surg.* 2006;88(11):2487-2500.
14. Marks KE, Nelson CL, Lautenschlager EP. Antibiotic impregan-ted acrylic bone cement. *J Bone Joint Surg.* 1976;(3)58(3):358-364.
15. Deluise M, Scott CP. Addition of hand-blended generic tobramycin in bone cement: effect on mechanical strength. *Orthopedics.* 2004;27:1289-1291.
16. Holt G, Murnaghan C, Reilly J, Meek RM. The biology of aseptic osteolysis. *Clin Orthop Relat Res.* 2007;460:240-252.
17. Skogland B, Aspenberg P. PMMA particles and pressure: a study of the osteolytic properties of two agents proposed to cause prosthetic loosening. *J Orthop Res.* 2001;21:196-201

9

Nonsurgical Management of Hip Osteoarthritis

Eric L. Grossman, MD, FAAOS; S.M. Javad Mortazavi, MD; and Peter F. Sharkey, MD

Currently there are 208,600 total hip arthroplasties (THAs) performed for a variety of indications in the United States yearly. These numbers are projected to increase approximately 174% by 2030 with a total of 572,000 THAs performed annually. Despite these projections, only a small fraction of patients with osteoarthritis (OA) will require operative intervention. Before a patient is considered for a surgical procedure, all nonoperative measures of management should be exhausted; this process can often continue over several years. Therefore, orthopedic surgeons must be skilled in the early diagnosis of OA and well versed in the use of established and current nonoperative treatments.

The goal of nonoperative management of OA is limited to symptomatic relief for the patient. Nonoperative management allows for continued function, while making living with the disease tolerable. Ultimately, the major goals in the treatment of OA include pain relief, maintenance of mobility through preservation of muscle strength and range of motion, minimization of disability, and reducing the risk of disease progression.

A diagnosis of hip OA can be associated with anxiety and depression due to the patient's concerns about the disease progression and the impact this will have on his or her ability to perform activities of daily living and the eventual need for a wheelchair or major surgery. The severity of symptoms in OA is influenced greatly by the patient's attitude, anxiety, depression, and daily activity level. Symptom relief, particularly in the early stages, may need to consider these factors in addition to pain, stiffness, and muscle weakness.

Considering the wide age range of patients with OA and the above mentioned variables suggests that the needs of affected patients are heterogeneous and for this reason treatment of patients with OA of the hip should be individualized and tailored to the severity of the disease. Both nonpharmacologic and pharmacologic measures should be used in the treatment of hip OA, keeping in mind that nonpharmacologic measures are the keystone. For mildly symptomatic patients, treatment may be limited to reassurance, patient education, instruction about joint protection, physical and occupational therapy, and other nonpharmacologic modalities. For this group, occasionally analgesics may be required. In patients with more severe OA that is unresponsive to nonpharmacological modalities, treatment requires a comprehensive program using a spectrum of nonpharmacologic measures in addition to appropriate pharmacologic agents for a given patient. Patients with severe symptomatic OA of the hip require an aggressive approach to decreasing pain, increasing mobility, and improving function. However, before narcotic addiction occurs or stiffness and weakness become irreversible, patients benefit from surgical consultation and evaluation for joint reconstruction.[1] Skill and extensive understanding of the patients and their needs is required to select the most appropriate interventions at the correct time.

Parvizi J, Klatt BA.
Essentials in Total Hip Arthroplasty (pp 69-77).

Nonpharmacological Management of Osteoarthritis

International guidelines advocate nonpharmacological treatments as the first-line of management for patients with OA.[1-10] Nonpharmacological treatments currently considered to have a sufficient level of scientific evidence are education, exercise, assist devices (canes, insoles), weight reduction, and nutritional counseling and supplements.[2,9,10] It is critically important that patients understand that nonoperative care may not appear miraculously effective to them and that it will likely only insidiously improve OA symptoms. Conversely, it must be emphasized that if nonoperative interventions are consistently used by the patient, they are effective.

Patient Education

In view of the chronic nature of OA, effective management of the disease requires that the patient understand the condition. A patient needs to understand the natural history of the disease and modalities that will alter the progression of OA. Therefore, the patient is responsible for the majority of disease care and management under the supervision of the physician working closely with him or her. Patient education programs aim to impart a thorough understanding of the disease process and provide knowledge and skills to individuals so that they may better manage their arthritis. The patient should understand the progressive nature of OA. Education should emphasize that the patients have got a central role in managing their disease. Furthermore, patients should learn both nonpharmacological and pharmacological methods for the management of OA. Education should highlight that abuse and overuse of the joint will aggravate symptoms and accelerate disease progression. It is very important to prevent overuse and to use the joints in the most adequate way. A variety of self-management programs have been developed for patients with OA,[11-18] such as the Arthritis Self-Management Program that is sponsored in the United States by the Arthritis Foundation.[1,8,19,20] Participation in a structured, community-based education intervention led by trained lay leaders, can result in significant improvement in the psychological well-being of participants.[12] Patients who participate in such programs report enhanced performance of self-management behaviors (eg, taking their medication properly and communicating with their health care providers). Furthermore, the benefits may endure for years, even with no reinforcement of the intervention. Regular patient-physician contact has also been shown to be valuable in the management of OA. Periodic telephone-support interventions by lay personnel may also promote self-care in patients with OA.[21,22]

Exercise

Exercise is a commonly prescribed and effective treatment for patients with hip OA. Therapeutic exercise has been recommended in several treatment guidelines for patients with OA of the hip. Exercise therapy involves the prescription of muscular contraction and bodily movement ultimately to improve the overall function, strength, and flexibility of the individual and to help meet the demands of daily living.[23,24]

Disuse of the OA joint secondary to pain will lead to muscle atrophy, which in turn causes altered biomechanics, resulting in increased joint loading and localized stress. Strengthening exercises of the periarticular muscles are very important as they play a major role in protecting the articular cartilage from stress and progression of OA of the hip or knee.[25]

However, the benefits of therapeutic exercise extend beyond slowing joint deterioration. Improved muscle strength in OA patients is correlated to the patient's functional level. In addition, muscle rehabilitation is associated with improved psychological status. Improvement in lower extremity strength, endurance, proprioception, and functional status has been shown to be associated with decreased anxiety and depression.[26]

Participation in conditioning exercises can safely improve the fitness and health of patients with hip OA without increasing their pain. Arthritis is a major reason that elderly individuals have a limited activity level and often restricts activity more than heart disease, hypertension, blindness, or diabetes. OA of the hip limits physical activity and the amount of exercise that an individual can perform. Patients are at an increased risk for diseases related to their inactivity (ie, hypertension, obesity, diabetes, cardiovascular disease). Therefore, it is of paramount importance that OA sufferers remain vibrant and active so as to limit the development or progression of medical comorbidities. This is possible by choosing appropriate exercises for the patient. The amount of aerobic conditioning (eg, walking, cycling, aquatic exercise) necessary for cardiovascular fitness is not so great that it cannot be achieved by those with OA. Patients with OA of lower extremity joints who perform low-impact moderate to vigorous exercise at least 3 days per week (ie, 70% to 85% of maximal heart rate) at an intensity that permits an individual to talk while exercising continuously for 20 to 60 min improve their fitness and health without exacerbating their joint pain or increasing their need for analgesia. It has been

Table 9-1

EXERCISE PRESCRIPTION FOR LOWER-LIMB OSTEOARTHRITIS

The program should be individualized after considering the following:

- Severity of pain
- Joint stability
- Patient's resources (time, money, facilities, equipment)
- Patient's interests

The program should include the following:

- Warm up 5 minutes
- Range-of-movement exercises
- Flexibility exercises
- Daily stretching and range-of-movement exercises
- Strengthening exercises
- Isometric exercises (static muscle contraction that does not move a joint or alter muscle length) up to twice daily during acute inflammatory periods
- Isotonic exercises (resistance training exercises, often with weights) maximum 2 days per week
- Endurance/fitness exercises
- Walking, swimming, dancing, aquarobics, or cycling 3 to 4 times per week

The intensity, duration, and frequency of exercise should be specified and graded to allow for progression. Tactics to improve compliance:

- Set specific, realistic, positive goals which should be written down
- Start slowly and build up gradually
- Keep a diary
- Plan to exercise at a time when least tired and sore
- Exercise with a friend

reported that those who exercise consistently experience a decrease in their joint pain and disability while improving their cardiovascular muscular fitness (strength and endurance).[27,28] Exercise therapy can incorporate physiotherapists that can customize the exercise program by altering the content (eg, muscle strengthening exercises, functional task-oriented exercises), dosage (eg, frequency, intensity, duration), and delivery mode (eg, individualized, group-based, home-based). While physiotherapists choose the delivery mode, content, and dosage of exercise therapy, many questions remain regarding the type and format of exercise that should be prescribed.[29] OA has the unique ability to effect single or multiple joints within an individual, and those joints affected may be in varying stages of progression. For this reason, it is essential that each patient be treated in an individualized manner regarding his or her exercise therapy regimen[30] (Table 9-1).

The positive post-treatment effects of exercise therapy on pain and function in patients with OA of the hip and/or knee are not sustained long-term unless exercise becomes routine. Therefore, additional booster sessions after therapy are needed to maintain the beneficial effects of exercise therapy. This illustrates the importance of exercise therapy in OA and the fact that patients with OA should perform exercises routinely.[31]

Weight Reduction and Diet

Obesity is an important risk factor for lower extremity joint deterioration and disability caused by knee and hip OA.[32,33] Fortunately for the patient, being overweight or obese is for the most part a modifiable risk factor for OA. The biological mechanisms for the role of obesity in the development of OA are not entirely clear, although there are those who believe it results from changes in joint forces. In addition, there is also evidence that obesity is associated with systemic changes that cause OA. It was shown that obese patients were at risk of both weight and non-weight-bearing joints.[32] Therefore, obesity should be treated aggressively to limit its role in OA disease progression, as well as to provide better overall health. Weight loss may prevent arthritic disease, especially in the knees, and those who are overweight are at high risk of disease progression and are likely to have a course that leads to disability and knee replacement.[34]

There is evidence to support the benefits of weight reduction for hip OA. Nevertheless, despite the absence of trial data, interventions that reduce adverse mechanical forces across a compromised hip joint have obvious intuitive validity.

There is no evidence for the involvement of any specific dietary factor in the etiology-pathogenesis of hip OA.[35] However, analysis of data derived from the Framingham study points to the value of an overall well-balanced diet.[36] Fruits and vegetables are an excellent source of antioxidants. Oxidative agents play a role in inflammation and data have demonstrated that patients who consume high amounts of fruits and vegetables are much less likely to develop OA. Additionally, loss of cartilage increases localized stress transmitted to the exposed bone and this can lead to a clinical situation analogous to a stress fracture. These lesions can be seen with magnetic resonance imaging (MRI) and have been referred to as bone marrow lesions (BMLs). Information from Framingham suggests that while patients who consume large quantities of vitamin D and calcium are no less likely to develop OA, they have a substantially reduced risk of having symptoms associated with OA.[37]

Assistive Devices and Mechanical Aids

Despite the absence of trial data, interventions that reduce mechanical forces across a compromised hip joint have obvious validity.[9] Assistive devices and shoe modification seem to be helpful in decreasing symptoms in patients with OA and improving their function.[38] Many individuals with OA of the spine or lower limb are more comfortable wearing cushioned shoes with good shock-absorbing properties versus more traditional footwear.[39] Cushioned shoes may help through a variety of mechanisms based on their type of modifications including reduction of vertical impact, increased shock absorption, and improvements in balance. Additionally, they may reduce the vertical impact of the feet, which is increased in older individuals,[40] and help them improve the balance, which is reduced due to knee or hip pain.[41]

Assistive devices such as canes can make a dramatic difference for an osteoarthritic patient. When used appropriately, it has the ability to reduce loading on the hip joint by 20% to 30%. However, careful attention must be given to the cane's length, characteristics, and use.[42] The top of the cane's handle should reach the patient's proximal wrist crease when the patient is standing with arms at the side.[39,43] In patients with unilateral OA of the hip, the cane should be held on the unaffected side. In patients with bilateral hip involvement, canes may be less effective and the patient may opt for the use of crutches, a walker, or even a wheelchair.[1]

Pharmacologic Therapy

As mentioned earlier, the cornerstone of nonoperative OA management should be nonpharmacologic therapy and all pharmacologic interventions should be considered as an adjunct that may be intermittently used or maintained throughout treatment. Pharmacologic and nonpharmacologic therapies are most effective when used in combination.[5]

Acetaminophen

Acetaminophen is considered a front-line pharmacologic treatment for most patients with OA.[4,9,10,44,45] This is mainly due to its favorable side effect profile as well as to the perception that it is equally as effective as nonsteroidal anti-inflammatory drugs (NSAIDs).[46,47] In patients with mild or moderate pain, acetaminophen has been shown to be as effective as NSAIDs. However, in more severely symptomatic patients with significant inflammation, NSAIDs are believed to be more efficacious than acetaminophen. In addition, the results of recent epidemiological studies raised some concerns that high-dose administration of acetaminophen may have a similar risk profile to NSAIDs regarding upper gastrointestinal (GI) complications.[48,49] Nevertheless, a recent meta-analysis did not demonstrate an increased risk of GI bleeding with acetaminophen with a dose of 2 to 4 g daily.[45] Currently, there is not enough evidence to demonstrate that long-term use of acetaminophen causes renal toxicity.[50] However, acetaminophen should be avoided in patients with excessive alcohol consumption and active liver disease. Acetaminophen has been shown to compromise existing liver function in these patients.[4]

Nonsteroidal Anti-Inflammatory Drugs

For decades, NSAIDs have been widely used for the management of pain associated with OA.[51] Nonselective NSAIDs usually provide analgesia at lower doses but have both increased analgesic and anti-inflammatory effects at higher recommended doses. Their mechanism of action is via the inhibition of cyclooxygenase isoforms 1 and 2 (COX-1 and COX-2). Patients with OA who have failed to respond to full doses of acetaminophen should be considered as candidates for NSAID therapy.[2,4,9,52] Currently there is no evidence to suggest that one NSAID is superior to another in relieving pain in patients with OA.[53] The GI toxicity and side effect profile of all NSAIDs remains a major concern particularly for patients of advanced age.[54] Patients over 65 years with a history of a peptic ulcer or a GI bleed, concomitant use of tobacco or alcohol, the presence of comorbid conditions such as heart disease, coadministration of glucocorticoids, or anticoagulation therapy are at an increased risk of significant adverse GI events.[4,7,53] GI side effects are dose dependent; therefore, NSAIDs should be prescribed in the smallest possible dose that provides acceptable symptomatic relief.[55] To diminish potential GI adverse effect, misoprostol (a PGE2 analogue) or a proton pump inhibitor can be added to the therapeutic regimen.[56,57] Over-the-counter doses of histamine receptor 2 (H-2) blockers and antacids have not been shown to reduce serious clinical GI events.[58,59]

Highly Selective Nonsteroidal Anti-Inflammatory Drugs

The use of COX-2-specific inhibitors has been proposed as a method for reducing the GI adverse event profile of

NSAID therapy.[60] The COX-2 inhibitors have been found to be more effective than placebo and comparable in efficacy to nonselective NSAIDs in patients with hip or knee OA.[61-64] Endoscope studies have demonstrated that COX-2 inhibitors are associated with a lower incidence of gastroduodenal ulcer disease than comparable NSAID and similar to that of placebo interventions. This improvement in GI profile makes the COX-2 inhibitor better suited for the patient that is at increased risk for serious GI complications.[64] In addition, they have no clinically significant effect on platelet aggregation or bleeding time when used in the pharmacologic doses in patients with OA.[4] The COX-2 inhibitors are not completely without risk and have been shown to cause renal toxicity comparable to nonselective NSAIDs. They must be administered with caution in patients with mild to moderate renal insufficiency.[53] There continues to be serious concerns regarding the COX-2 inhibitors' cardiovascular effects, particularly in the light that several of these agents were removed from the marketplace. Investigations are ongoing and currently there is no consensus on this matter, but the major area of concern is the cardiovascular safety profile, which is still under investigation.[60,65] Nonetheless, it has been demonstrated that there is some increased risk of adverse cardiovascular events in patients using these agents.[66]

Narcotic Agents

Narcotic agents are only rarely used to treat pain associated with OA.[4] A narcotic analgesic should be considered only if the patient has failed to tolerate or respond to nonselective or highly selective NSAIDs and is not a surgical candidate. The efficacy of tramadol, an atypical opiod that activates opiod receptors and inhibitory pain systems, has been shown to be comparable to NSAIDs in treatment of hip OA.[67] Tramadol is currently recommended for the treatment of moderate to severe pain in patients who are intolerant of or unresponsive to nonselective NSAIDs or COX-2 inhibitors.[68] Tramadol is thought not to have the potential for significant addictive tendencies. Possible adverse effects are nausea, constipation, lightheadedness, dizziness, seizure, and sedation.[4] Patients who do not respond to or cannot tolerate tramadol and who continue to have severe pain may be considered for more potent opiod therapy.[5] Analgesics, such as codeine and propoxyphene, have been effectively used in treating patients with OA,[69] especially in combination with non-narcotic analgesics like acetaminophen. The combination of codeine and acetaminophen has been shown to achieve significantly improved pain relief in hip OA than acetaminophen alone, but was poorly tolerated. The most frequent side effects of this combination are nausea, constipation, and somnolence.[70] Narcotics should only be used if the patient is unlikely to have surgical intervention. Their long-term use makes pain management after arthroplasty much more difficult.

Topical Agents

Topical agents can be used in the management of OA and include capsaicin-based and NSAID-based agents. The first group is preparations containing capsaicin and act through a reversible depletion of substance P stores, a neurotransmitter of peripheral pain sensations. The second types of topical preparations are those containing NSAIDs. Although there is little evidence to support the use of topical agents in the treatment of OA of deep joints, they have been shown to be effective in superficial joints like hand and knee.[71-74] There is no evidence to recommend their administration for hip OA.

Intra-Articular Agents

Injection procedures of the hip joint are technically difficult to perform and ultrasonographic or fluoroscopic guidance is needed. The efficacy of injection in the hip joint using hyaluronic acid or corticosteroids is questionable. Although some studies that were uncontrolled with short-term follow-up have suggested efficacy,[75] there is evidence that injections of hyaluronic acid did not significantly reduce pain on walking (assessed by means of visual-analogue scale) as compared with placebo injection.[76] In addition, this preparation is not approved for treatment of OA of the hip in the United States.[20] Intra-articular corticosteroid injection has shown only a small short-term benefit in pain reduction in patients with OA of the knee in a randomized trial.[52] However, there is not enough evidence to support the efficacy of steroid injection for hip OA, irrespective of its increased technical difficulty.[74] Therefore, these approaches are not routinely used in clinical practice for the treatment of hip OA.

Nutraceutical

Glucosamine and Chondroitin Sulfate

A number of systematic reviews have been undertaken to support the use of these agents in OA, but none of them are specific for the hip.[77-81] Controlled trials have shown that these agents are efficacious for pain relief in patients with

OA of the hip or knee. However, in a recent large trial sponsored by the National Institutes of Health involving patients with OA of the knee, the use of glucosamine hydrochloride and chondroitin sulfate, either alone or in combination, was not superior to that of placebo in an intention-to-treat analysis[82]; this trial did not assess OA of the hip. Evidence of a structure-modifying effect of these oral supplements is lacking, and the mechanism by which they might work is unclear.[20] Further studies, particularly addressing efficacy at higher pain levels, will help in additionally defining their utility in the OA treatment paradigm.[83]

Fish Oils and Omega-3 Polyunsaturated Fatty Acids

There is extensive documentation on the beneficial anti-inflammatory affects of high-dose fish oil in the reduction of joint pain from rheumatoid and OA. However, there is no clinical trial that specifically investigated their effects in patients with hip OA.

Several mechanisms have been proposed to explain the beneficial effects of these compounds in the symptomatic relief of pain in patients with arthritis. They may affect the lipid composition of bone marrow. An excess of marrow fat can cause weakening or necrosis of medullary bone, resulting in collapse and joint destruction.[84] Studies showed that lipid-lowering medications like statins and fibrates as well as fish oils and omega-3 polyunsaturated fatty acids may protect bone marrow from the effect of excess marrow fat.[84,85] They are also shown to change the composition of joint lipids from more to less saturated.[86] Unsaturated phospholipids have a greater surface area and better lubricant characteristics. They also affect inflammation at the cellular level. Incorporation of omega-3 fatty acids into articular cartilage chondrocyte membranes results in a dose-dependent reduction in the expression and activity of proteoglycan degrading enzymes (aggrecanases), inflammatory cytokines (IL-1b), tumor necrosis factor, and COX-2.[87-89]

References

1. Hochberg MC, Altman RD, Brandt KD, et al. Guidelines for the medical management of osteoarthritis. Part I. Osteoarthritis of the hip. American College of Rheumatology. *Arthritis Rheum.* 1995;38(11):1535-1540.
2. Pendleton A, Arden N, Dougados M, et al. EULAR recommendations for the management of knee osteoarthritis: report of a task force of the Standing Committee for International Clinical Studies Including Therapeutic Trials (ESCISIT). *Ann Rheum Dis.* 2000;59(12):936-944.
3. Guidelines for the diagnosis, investigation and management of osteoarthritis of the hip and knee. Report of a Joint Working Group of the British Society for Rheumatology and the Research Unit of the Royal College of Physicians. *J R Coll Physicians Lond.* 1993;27(4):391-396.
4. Recommendations for the medical management of osteoarthritis of the hip and knee: 2000 update. American College of Rheumatology Subcommittee on Osteoarthritis Guidelines. *Arthritis Rheum.* 2000;43(9):1905-1915.
5. Panel on Chronic Pain in Older Persons. The management of chronic pain in older persons. *J Am Geriatr Soc.* 1998;46:635-651.
6. Altman RD, Lozada CJ. Practice guidelines in the management of osteoarthritis. *Osteoarthritis Cartilage.* 1998;(6 suppl A):22-24.
7. Hochberg MC. What a difference a year makes: reflections on the ACR recommendations for the medical management of osteoarthritis. *Curr Rheumatol Rep.* 2001;3(6):473-478.
8. Lane NE, Thompson JM. Management of osteoarthritis in the primary-care setting: an evidence-based approach to treatment. *Am J Med.* 1997;103(6A):25S-30S.
9. Zhang W, Doherty M, Arden N, et al. EULAR evidence based recommendations for the management of hip osteoarthritis: report of a task force of the EULAR Standing Committee for International Clinical Studies Including Therapeutics (ESCISIT). *Ann Rheum Dis.* 2005;64(5):669-681.
10. Zhang W, Moskowitz RW, Nuki G, et al. OARSI recommendations for the management of hip and knee osteoarthritis, part I: critical appraisal of existing treatment guidelines and systematic review of current research evidence. *Osteoarthritis Cartilage.* 2007;15(9):981-1000.
11. Barlow JH, Turner AP, Wright CC. Long-term outcomes of an arthritis self-management programme. *Br J Rheumatol.* 1998;37(12):1315-1319.
12. Goeppinger J, Armstrong B, Schwartz T, Ensley D, Brady TJ. Self-management education for persons with arthritis: managing comorbidity and eliminating health disparities. *Arthritis Rheum.* 2007;57(6):1081-1088.
13. Lorig K, González VM, Laurent DD, Morgan L, Laris BA. Arthritis self-management program variations: three studies. *Arthritis Care Res.* 1998;11(6):448-454.
14. Lorig K, Ritter PL, and Plant K. A disease-specific self-help program compared with a generalized chronic disease self-help program for arthritis patients. *Arthritis Rheum.* 2005;53(6):950-957.
15. Lorig KR, Sobel DS, Stewart AL, et al. Evidence suggesting that a chronic disease self-management program can improve health status while reducing hospitalization: a randomized trial. *Med Care.* 1999;37(1):5-14.
16. Osborne RH, Spinks JM, Wicks LP. Patient education and self-management programs in arthritis. *Med J Aust.* 2004;180(5 suppl):S23-6.
17. Osborne RH, Wilson T, Lorig KR, McColl GJ. Does self-management lead to sustainable health benefits in people with arthritis? A 2-year transition study of 452 Australians. *J Rheumatol.* 2007;34(5):1112-1117.

18. Warsi A, LaValley MP, Wang PS, Avorn J, Solomon DH. Arthritis self-management education programs: a meta-analysis of the effect on pain and disability. *Arthritis Rheum.* 2003;48(8):2207-2213.
19. Hochberg MC, Perlmutter DL, Hudson JI, Altman RD. Preferences in the management of osteoarthritis of the hip and knee: results of a survey of community-based rheumatologists in the United States. *Arthritis Care Res.* 1996;9(3):170-176.
20. Lane NE. Clinical practice. Osteoarthritis of the hip. *N Engl J Med.* 2007;357(14):1413-1421.
21. Rene J, Weinberger M, Mazzuca SA, Brandt KD, Katz BP. Reduction of joint pain in patients with knee osteoarthritis who have received monthly telephone calls from lay personnel and whose medical treatment regimens have remained stable. *Arthritis Rheum.* 1992;35(5):511-515.
22. Thomas KS, Muir KR, Doherty M, Jones AC, O'Reilly SC, Bassey EJ. Home based exercise programme for knee pain and knee osteoarthritis: randomised controlled trial. *BMJ.* 2002;325(7367):752.
23. Bartels EM, Lund H, Hagen KB, Dagfinrud H, Christensen R, Danneskiold-Samsøe B. Aquatic exercise for the treatment of knee and hip osteoarthritis. *Cochrane Database Syst Rev.* 2007;(4):CD005523.
24. Fransen M, McConnell S, Bell M. Exercise for osteoarthritis of the hip or knee. *Cochrane Database Syst Rev.* 2003;(3):CD004286.
25. Roddy E, Zhang W, Doherty M, et al. Evidence-based recommendations for the role of exercise in the management of osteoarthritis of the hip or knee--the MOVE consensus. *Rheumatology (Oxford).* 2005;44(1):67-73.
26. van Baar ME, Dekker J, Oostendorp RA, et al. The effectiveness of exercise therapy in patients with osteoarthritis of the hip or knee: a randomized clinical trial. *J Rheumatol.* 1998;25(12):2432-2439.
27. Philbin EF, Groff GD, Ries MD, Miller TE. Cardiovascular fitness and health in patients with end-stage osteoarthritis. *Arthritis Rheum.* 1995;38(6):799-805.
28. Ries MD, Philbin EF, Groff GD. Relationship between severity of gonarthrosis and cardiovascular fitness. *Clin Orthop Relat Res.* 1995;(313):169-176.
29. Grainger R, Cicuttini FM. Medical management of osteoarthritis of the knee and hip joints. *Med J Aust.* 2004;180(5):232-236.
30. Exercise prescription for older adults with osteoarthritis pain: consensus practice recommendations. A supplement to the AGS Clinical Practice Guidelines on the management of chronic pain in older adults. *J Am Geriatr Soc.* 2001;49(6):808-823.
31. Pisters MF, Veenhof C, van Meeteren NL, et al. Long-term effectiveness of exercise therapy in patients with osteoarthritis of the hip or knee: a systematic review. *Arthritis Rheum.* 2007;57(7):1245-1253.
32. Nevitt MC. Obesity outcomes in disease management: clinical outcomes for osteoarthritis. *Obes Res.* 2002;10(suppl 1):33S-37S.
33. Felson DT, Zhang Y, Anthony JM, Naimark A, Anderson JJ. Weight loss reduces the risk for symptomatic knee osteoarthritis in women. The Framingham Study. *Ann Intern Med.* 1992;116(7):535-539.
34. Felson DT. Does excess weight cause osteoarthritis and, if so, why? *Ann Rheum Dis.* 1996;55(9):668-670.
35. Segal L, Day SE, Chapman AB, Osborne RH. Can we reduce disease burden from osteoarthritis? *Med J Aust.* 2004;180(5 suppl):S11-7.
36. McAlindon TE, Jacques P, Zhang Y, et al. Do antioxidant micronutrients protect against the development and progression of knee osteoarthritis? *Arthritis Rheum.* 1996;39(4):648-656.
37. McAlindon TE, Felson DT, Zhang Y, et al. Relation of dietary intake and serum levels of vitamin D to progression of osteoarthritis of the knee among participants in the Framingham Study. *Ann Intern Med.* 1996;125(5):353-359.
38. Buckwalter JA, Stanish WD, Rosier RN, Schenck RC Jr, Dennis DA, Coutts RD. The increasing need for nonoperative treatment of patients with osteoarthritis. *Clin Orthop Relat Res.* 2001;(385):36-45.
39. Dieppe P. Management of hip osteoarthritis. *BMJ.* 1995;311(7009):853-857.
40. Robbins S, Waked E, Krouglicof N. Vertical impact increase in middle age may explain idiopathic weight-bearing joint osteoarthritis. *Arch Phys Med Rehabil.* 2001;82(12):1673-1677.
41. Messier SP, Glasser JL, Ettinger WH Jr, Craven TE, Miller ME. Declines in strength and balance in older adults with chronic knee pain: a 30-month longitudinal, observational study. *Arthritis Rheum.* 2002;47(2):141-148.
42. Blount WP. Don't throw away the cane. *J Bone Joint Surg Am.* 1956;38-A(3):695-708.
43. Manek NJ, Lane NE. Osteoarthritis: current concepts in diagnosis and management. *Am Fam Physician.* 2000;61(6):1795-1804.
44. Neame R, Zhang W, Doherty M. A historic issue of the annals: three papers examine paracetamol in osteoarthritis. *Ann Rheum Dis.* 2004;63(8):897-900.
45. Zhang W, Jones A, Doherty M. Does paracetamol (acetaminophen) reduce the pain of osteoarthritis? A meta-analysis of randomised controlled trials. *Ann Rheum Dis.* 2004;63(8):901-907.
46. Altman RD, Zinsenheim JR, Temple AR, Schweinle JE. Three-month efficacy and safety of acetaminophen extended-release for osteoarthritis pain of the hip or knee: a randomized, double-blind, placebo-controlled study. *Osteoarthritis Cartilage.* 2007;15(4):454-461.
47. Towheed TE, Maxwell L, Judd MG, Catton M, Hochberg MC, Wells G. Acetaminophen for osteoarthritis. *Cochrane Database Syst Rev.* 2006(1):CD004257.
48. Garcia Rodriguez LA, Hernandez-Diaz S. Relative risk of upper gastrointestinal complications among users of acetaminophen and nonsteroidal anti-inflammatory drugs. *Epidemiology.* 2001;12(5):570-576.
49. Garcia Rodriguez LA, Hernandez-Diaz S. The risk of upper gastrointestinal complications associated with nonsteroidal anti-inflammatory drugs, glucocorticoids, acetaminophen, and combinations of these agents. *Arthritis Res.* 2001;3(2):98-101.
50. Fored CM, Ejerblad E, Lindblad P, et al. Acetaminophen, aspirin, and chronic renal failure. *N Engl J Med.* 2001;345(25):1801-1808.

51. Towheed T, Shea B, Wells G, Hochberg M. Analgesia and non-aspirin, non-steroidal anti-inflammatory drugs for osteoarthritis of the hip. *Cochrane Database Syst Rev.* 2000;(2):CD000517.

52. Dieppe P, Brandt KD. What is important in treating osteoarthritis? Whom should we treat and how should we treat them? *Rheum Dis Clin North Am.* 2003;29(4):687-716.

53. Hochberg MC, Dougados M. Pharmacological therapy of osteoarthritis. *Best Pract Res Clin Rheumatol.* 2001;15(4):583-593.

54. Hernandez-Diaz S, Rodriguez LA. Association between nonsteroidal anti-inflammatory drugs and upper gastrointestinal tract bleeding/perforation: an overview of epidemiologic studies published in the 1990s. *Arch Intern Med.* 2000;160(14):2093-2099.

55. Lewis SC, Langman MJ, Laporte JR, Matthews JN, Rawlins MD, Wiholm BE. Dose-response relationships between individual nonaspirin nonsteroidal anti-inflammatory drugs (NANSAIDs) and serious upper gastrointestinal bleeding: a meta-analysis based on individual patient data. *Br J Clin Pharmacol.* 2002;54(3):320-326.

56. Leandro G, Pilotto A, Franceschi M, Bertin T, Lichino E, Di Mario F. Prevention of acute NSAID-related gastroduodenal damage: a meta-analysis of controlled clinical trials. *Dig Dis Sci.* 2001;46(9):1924-1936.

57. Lanas A, García-Rodríguez LA, Arroyo MT, et al. Effect of antisecretory drugs and nitrates on the risk of ulcer bleeding associated with nonsteroidal anti-inflammatory drugs, antiplatelet agents, and anticoagulants. *Am J Gastroenterol.* 2007;102(3):507-515.

58. Rostom A, Wells G, Tugwell P, Welch V, Dubé C, McGowan J. The prevention of chronic NSAID induced upper gastrointestinal toxicity: a Cochrane collaboration metaanalysis of randomized controlled trials. *J Rheumatol.* 2000;27(9):2203-2214.

59. Rostom A, Wells G, Tugwell P, Welch V, Dube C, McGowan J. Prevention of chronic NSAID induced upper gastrointestinal toxicity. *Cochrane Database Syst Rev.* 2000;(3):CD002296.

60. Deeks JJ, Smith LA, Bradley MD. Efficacy, tolerability, and upper gastrointestinal safety of celecoxib for treatment of osteoarthritis and rheumatoid arthritis: systematic review of randomised controlled trials. *BMJ.* 2002;325(7365):619.

61. Bensen WG, Fiechtner JJ, McMillen JI, et al. Treatment of osteoarthritis with celecoxib, a cyclooxygenase-2 inhibitor: a randomized controlled trial. *Mayo Clin Proc.* 1999;74(11):1095-1105.

62. Clemett D, Goa KL. Celecoxib: a review of its use in osteoarthritis, rheumatoid arthritis and acute pain. *Drugs.* 2000;59(4):957-980.

63. Cannon GW, Caldwell JR, Holt P, et al. Rofecoxib, a specific inhibitor of cyclooxygenase 2, with clinical efficacy comparable with that of diclofenac sodium: results of a one-year, randomized, clinical trial in patients with osteoarthritis of the knee and hip. Rofecoxib Phase III Protocol 035 Study Group. *Arthritis Rheum.* 2000;43(5):978-987.

64. Bombardier C, Laine L, Reicin A, et al. Comparison of upper gastrointestinal toxicity of rofecoxib and naproxen in patients with rheumatoid arthritis. VIGOR Study Group. *N Engl J Med.* 2000;343(21):1520-1528, 2 p following 1528.

65. Bresalier RS, Sandler RS, Quan H, et al. Cardiovascular events associated with rofecoxib in a colorectal adenoma chemoprevention trial. *N Engl J Med.* 2005;352(11):1092-1102.

66. Solomon DH, Avorn J, Stürmer T, Glynn RJ, Mogun H, Schneeweiss S. Cardiovascular outcomes in new users of coxibs and nonsteroidal antiinflammatory drugs: high-risk subgroups and time course of risk. *Arthritis Rheum.* 2006;54(5):1378-1389.

67. Roth SH. Efficacy and safety of tramadol HCl in breakthrough musculoskeletal pain attributed to osteoarthritis. *J Rheumatol.* 1998;25(7):1358-1363.

68. Cepeda MS, Camargo F, Zea C, Valencia L. Tramadol for osteoarthritis: a systematic review and metaanalysis. *J Rheumatol.* 2007;34(3):543-555.

69. Peloso PM, Bellamy N, Bensen W, et al. Double blind randomized placebo control trial of controlled release codeine in the treatment of osteoarthritis of the hip or knee. *J Rheumatol.* 2000;27(3):764-771.

70. Kjaersgaard-Andersen P, Nafei A, Skov O, et al. Codeine plus paracetamol versus paracetamol in longer-term treatment of chronic pain due to osteoarthritis of the hip. A randomised, double-blind, multi-centre study. *Pain.* 1990;43(3):309-318.

71. Banning M. The use of topical diclofenac for pain in osteoarthritis of the knee: a review. *Br J Community Nurs.* 2006;11(11):487-492.

72. Ergun H, Külcü D, Kutlay S, Bodur H, Tulunay FC. Efficacy and safety of topical nimesulide in the treatment of knee osteoarthritis. *J Clin Rheumatol.* 2007;13(5):251-255.

73. Widrig R, Suter A, Saller R, Melzer J. Choosing between NSAID and arnica for topical treatment of hand osteoarthritis in a randomised, double-blind study. *Rheumatol Int.* 2007;27(6):585-591.

74. Zhang W, Doherty M, Leeb BF, et al. EULAR evidence based recommendations for the management of hand osteoarthritis: report of a Task Force of the EULAR Standing Committee for International Clinical Studies Including Therapeutics (ESCISIT). *Ann Rheum Dis.* 2007;66(3):377-388.

75. Fernandez Lopez JC, Ruano-Ravina A. Efficacy and safety of intraarticular hyaluronic acid in the treatment of hip osteoarthritis: a systematic review. *Osteoarthritis Cartilage.* 2006;14(12):1306-1311.

76. Qvistgaard E, Christensen R, Torp-Pedersen S, Bliddal H. Intra-articular treatment of hip osteoarthritis: a randomized trial of hyaluronic acid, corticosteroid, and isotonic saline. *Osteoarthritis Cartilage.* 2006;14(2):163-170.

77. Felson DT, McAlindon TE. Glucosamine and chondroitin for osteoarthritis: to recommend or not to recommend? *Arthritis Care Res.* 2000;13(4):179-182.

78. McAlindon, TE, LaValley MP, Felson DT. Efficacy of glucosamine and chondroitin for treatment of osteoarthritis. *JAMA.* 2000;284(10):1241.

79. McAlindon TE, LaValley MP, Gulin JP, Felson DT. Glucosamine and chondroitin for treatment of osteoarthritis: a systematic quality assessment and meta-analysis. *JAMA.* 2000;283(11):1469-1475.

80. Towheed TE, Anastassiades TP, Shea B, Houpt J, Welch V, Hochberg MC. Glucosamine therapy for treating osteoarthritis. *Cochrane Database Syst Rev.* 2001;(1):CD002946.
81. Leeb BF, Schweitzer H, Montag K, Smolen JS. A metaanalysis of chondroitin sulfate in the treatment of osteoarthritis. *J Rheumatol.* 2000;27(1):205-211.
82. Clegg DO, et al. Glucosamine, chondroitin sulfate, and the two in combination for painful knee osteoarthritis. *N Engl J Med.* 2006;354(8):795-808.
83. Altman RD, Reda DJ, Harris CL, et al. Commentary: osteoarthritis of the knee and glucosamine. *Osteoarthritis Cartilage.* 2006;14(10):963-966.
84. Pritchett JW. Statins and dietary fish oils improve lipid composition in bone marrow and joints. *Clin Orthop Relat Res.* 2007;456:233-237.
85. Hills BA. Synovial surfactant and the hydrophobic articular surface. *J Rheumatol.* 1996;23(8):1323-1325.
86. Pritchett, JW. Statin therapy decreases the risk of osteonecrosis in patients receiving steroids. *Clin Orthop Relat Res.* 2001;(386):173-178.
87. Curtis CL, Hughes CE, Flannery CR, Little CB, Harwood JL, Caterson B. N-3 fatty acids specifically modulate catabolic factors involved in articular cartilage degradation. *J Biol Chem.* 2000;275(2):721-724.
88. Cleland L, James M, Proudman S. Fish oil: what the prescriber needs to know. *Arthritis Res Ther.* 2005;8(1):202.
89. Kremer JM, Lawrence DA, Petrillo GF, et al. Effects of high-dose fish oil on rheumatoid arthritis after stopping nonsteroidal antiinflammatory drugs. *Arthritis Rheum.* 1995;38(8):1107-1114.

10

Hip Arthroscopy

Junaid Makda, MD; Eric B. Smith, MD; Khalid M. Yousuf, MD, MS; and Javad Parvizi, MD, FRCS

As the understanding of the etiology of hip disease has progressed, improvements in both nonsurgical and surgical treatments have been made. The choice of appropriate treatment depends on patient age, the cause and extent of the disease, the anticipated rate of progression, and the expected durability of the procedure.

Hip arthroscopy was first proposed and described in the 1930s. However, it was not until the 1980s that it became a standard procedure to treat hip pathology. Hip arthroscopy allows for a minimally invasive visualization and treatment of intra-articular pathology. It is an alternative to arthrotomy to treat conditions such as labral tears, femoroacetabular impingement (FAI), cartilage lesions, and loose bodies. As the etiology of hip pain is better understood, the indications for hip arthroscopy will continue to expand.

Over the last few decades, the number of hip arthroscopy procedures has been increasing annually.[1] It is important to recognize that hip arthroscopy is a technically demanding procedure with a steep learning curve. The osseous anatomy, large soft tissue envelope, and proximity of neurovascular structures make access to the joint difficult. Additional training should be sought by the surgeon prior to performing this procedure. Furthermore, special distraction tools, proper arthroscopic instrumentation, and education of the support staff are needed for the success of the procedure.

This chapter will discuss the indications, general setup, complications, and outcomes of hip arthroscopy.

Clinical Evaluation

A complete history and physical examination are necessary in determining the source and cause of hip pain. The hip is intimately associated with the pelvis, and pain may arise from intra-articular and extra-articular abnormalities as well as from lower back and intra-abdominal pathologies. The differential diagnosis of hip pain is quite broad (Table 10-1) and a thorough evaluation can avoid unnecessary interventions.

History

A general history should include the age of the patient, overall health and associated comorbidities, birth history, medications, previous treatment and surgeries, history of trauma, and relevant family history. The physician should clarify the location of the pain, timing and onset of symptoms, alleviating and exacerbating factors, and specific pattern of symptoms. Position and activity-related symptoms can be highly suggestive of the source.

Patients with a labral injury generally have a history of a twisting injury or describe a degenerative process. Symptoms often include a sharp stabbing pain or catching and locking of the involved hip. Arthritic pain will, in general, worsen with activity and will lead to decreased and painful range of motion. Pain after prolonged sitting is associated with FAI. Patients complaining of groin discomfort with a gradual

Parvizi J, Klatt BA.
Essentials in Total Hip Arthroplasty (pp 79-84).

Table 10-1

DIFFERENTIAL DIAGNOSIS OF HIP PAIN

Traumatic causes • Subluxation or dislocation • Fracture or stress fracture • Hematoma • Contusion Labral pathology • Femoroacetabular impingement • Hypermobility • Trauma • Dysplasia Infectious/tumorous/metabolic conditions • Septic arthritis • Osteomyelitis • Benign neoplasms of bone or soft tissue • Malignant neoplasms of bone or soft tissue • Metastatic disease of bone • Inflammatory conditions • Rheumatoid arthritis • Reiter syndrome • Psoriatic arthritis Chondral pathology • Lateral impaction • Osteonecrosis • Loose bodies • Chondral shear injury • Osteoarthritis	Capsule pathology • Laxity • Adhesive capsulitis • Synovitis or inflammation Synovial proliferative disorders • Pigmented villonodular synovitis • Synovial chondromatosis • Chondrocalcinosis Extra-articular pathology • Coxa saltans (internal or external) • Psoas impingement • Abductor tears (rotator cuff tears of the hip) • Athletic pubalgia • Trochanteric bursitis • Ischial bursitis • Osteitis pubis • Piriformis syndrome • Sacroiliac pathology • Tendonitis (hip flexors, abductors, adductors)

Adapted from Shindle MK, Voos JE, Heyworth BE, et al. Hip arthroscopy in the athletic patient: current techniques and spectrum of disease. *J Bone Joint Surg Am.* 2007;89(suppl 3):29-43.

onset that is worse with vigorous activities may be associated with a synovial pathology. Catching, locking, giving-way, or other mechanical symptoms following a traumatic event should raise suspicion of loose or foreign bodies.

Physical Examination

Basic principles of a physical examination, inspection, and palpation are essential to narrow down the differential diagnosis. Observation of gait and posture as the patient enters the room can provide information on abductor strength and leg length discrepancy. Physical exam and hip range of motion, both active and passive, should be tested while the patient is standing and lying supine. A thorough evaluation of neurovascular status, palpation of areas of gross atrophy and tenderness, and provocative testing are useful in delineating the etiology of pain.

Logrolling of the leg isolates the hip joint and is a specific test for intra-articular pathology.[2] Patients with a labral tear often demonstrate normal motion and strength, but have pain with flexion/internal rotation or abduction/external rotation. Patients with FAI usually have limited internal rotation and adduction while the hip is flexed. A sensitive tool in screening for FAI is the anterior impingement test, which is performed while the patient is supine; the hip is internally rotated as it is passively flexed to 90 degrees and

Table 10-2

PATHOLOGY THAT MAY BENEFIT FROM HIP ARTHROSCOPY

Foreign body/loose bodies	Avascular necrosis
Labral tears	Impinging osteophytes
Joint sepsis	Post-traumatic conditions
Chondral injuries	Ruptured ligamentum teres
Synovial chondromatosis	Status post total hip arthroplasty

adducted.[3] A positive test reproduces pain secondary to the abnormal contact of the femoral neck and the acetabular rim. Individuals with symptomatic loose bodies will have pain and catching with rotation.

INDICATIONS

The indications of hip arthroscopy continue to evolve. With better instrumentation and a thorough understanding of hip pathology, a variety of hip conditions can be treated with hip arthroscopy (Table 10-2). Careful patient selection and reasonable patient expectations are essential for a successful outcome.

CONTRAINDICATIONS

Since hip arthroscopy requires access to the intra-articular space, any condition precluding distraction of the joint is a contraindication to the procedure. Absolute contraindications include ankylosis and relative contraindications are comorbidities, poor bone quality, open wounds or wound infections around the site of surgery, and obesity.

SETUP/PREOPERATIVE PLANNING

Performing the Procedure

General anesthesia is commonly used for hip arthroscopy. Muscle relaxant helps to allow distraction of the joint during the procedure. Some authors recommend additional anesthesia with femoral nerve block, spinal, or epidural. Though infection is rare (<1%), an appropriate antibiotic with broad spectrum coverage should be administered within 1 hr of the start of the procedure.

Operating Room Setup

Special equipment is necessary to smoothly perform the procedure. Both fluoroscopic and arthroscopic equipment are needed, so a relatively large operating room is necessary for the procedure. Though the procedure can be performed with a standard fracture table, this often does not allow for visualization while actively moving the joint and evaluating for impingement. A special hip arthroscopy operating room table allows for the appropriate exposure of the joint during both static and dynamic portions of the case. During the procedure, the hip must initially be distracted and locked into position to allow for safe, easy access to the central compartment. Then, distraction will be released and access to the peripheral compartment is necessary to visualize the joint during range of motion to evaluate for impingement and the presence of cam and/or pincer impingement lesions.

Equipment

Since there are numerous pieces of equipment, designing a detailed diagram for the operating room personnel can be very beneficial. Considering the surgeon is positioned at the operative side of the hip, the order of equipment from head to toe on the contralateral side is as follows:

- Arthroscopic monitor
- Arthroscopic unit
- Fluid management system/suction
- Fluoroscopic C-arm
- Fluoroscopic monitor

Obviously, the setup can and should be adjusted by the surgeon; however, this positioning allows for easier access by the circulating nurse and unobstructed sight lines during the case whether the C-arm is in position or pulled back away from the patient (Figure 10-1).

In addition to the room equipment, the following special arthroscopic equipment is also necessary:

- 70- and 30-degree arthroscopes
- Extra-length, rigid, flexible, and slotted canulas
- Scope bridge to allow moving camera between portals without removing portal
- Extra-length straight and/or curved arthroscopic shavers
- Flexible electrothermal probes

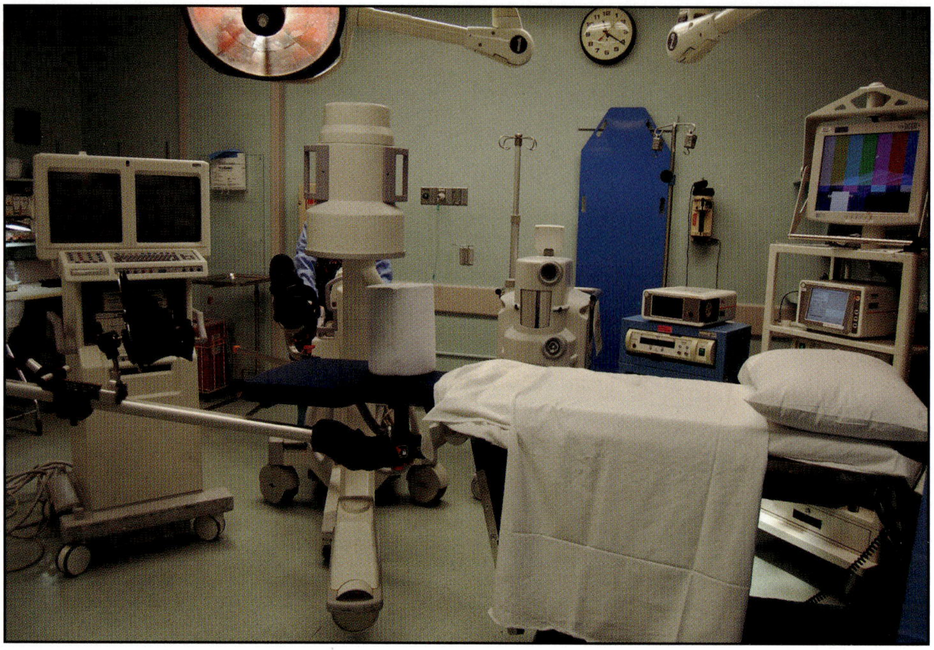

Figure 10-1. Operating room setup.

- Extra-length arthroscopic instruments (ie, biters, graspers)

Patient Positioning

Depending on surgeon preference and comfort, the procedure can be performed with the patient in the supine or lateral positions. Supine positioning is reliable and reproducible—the orientation is familiar to orthopedic surgeons and the anesthesiologists have more comfort with airway control. Prepping the surgical site in this position is easy and once the scope is inserted into the joint, it is often so stable that you can let go of it with your hand, if necessary.[4] Some surgeons, especially those who perform hip replacements via a posterior approach, prefer the lateral decubitus position. Though the fluoroscopic image intensifier may interfere with the surgeon, this position may allow easier access in obese patients and may also allow improved access to the posterior portion of the joint.[5,6] Regardless of the positioning technique, special leg holders that allow for distraction are attached to the end of the bed.

Once anesthesia is induced, the patient is slid distally on the bed such that his or her groin rests on a well-padded peroneal post. The post can be slightly off center, directed into the proximal medial thigh of the operative hip. Ensure the genitalia are not being compressed or pinched. The legs can temporarily be placed in the leg holders or held by an assistant while the arms are secured. Place a pillow on the patient's chest and wrap his or her arms around the front of it. Secure a draw sheet around the arms with towel clips. Then secure the well-padded feet into the leg holders. Since it is imperative to have continuous distraction of the operative hip, ensure the foot is placed tightly into the holder and reinforce with Coban (3M, St. Paul, MN). Thick cushioning of the peroneal post and the operative foot are imperative to prevent skin breakdown, pressure sores, and neuropraxias of the pudendal and peroneal nerves. Ensure the contralateral leg is securely placed in the leg holder. Keep the attachment for the contralateral leg unlocked to allow for distal and proximal motion (when traction is applied to the operative side, dangerous compressive or distractive forces can unknowingly be transferred to the nonoperative limb and lead to injury). Tilting the nonoperative side of the table down approximately 10 to 20 degrees will actually result in level positioning of the patient once traction is applied to the leg.

Once the patient is in position, perform a preliminary "time out" prior to distracting the hip. Bring the fluoroscopic C-arm into position. Smooth yet forceful traction is then applied. With general anesthesia and appropriate muscle relaxation, the majority of hip arthroscopies can be done with distraction forces between 25 and 100 pounds. Higher forces can result in direct groin injury and/or neuropraxia.[7-9] The hip position angles should be abduction approximately 20 to 25 degrees, neutral rotation (it may be necessary to slightly internally rotate the foot), and neutral flexion. Utilizing general anesthesia with appropriate muscle relaxation, apply ion and lock the limb into place. Confirm with fluoroscopy that the femoral head is distracted approximately 1 cm. If the joint is tight, allow a few minutes for the capsule to relax and try again. Once the vacuum seal of the joint is released, distraction should be easily achieved. Note the time. To avoid neuropraxia and/or peroneal skin damage, traction longer than 2 hours should be avoided.[8-10] Please note that some surgeons like an unscrubbed assistant to distract the hip after sterile draping.

Draping and Equipment Setup

Draping is relatively straightforward. After prepping the area, apply a down sheet over the contralateral limb. Then place towels or sticky drapes surrounding the operative site and draw out your landmarks: greater trochanter and the anterior-superior iliac spine (ASIS). Apply the sticky portion of a shower curtain-type drape directly to the hip. Simply open the drape and lay over the patient's body. To shield the anesthesiologist, attach a vertical drape to 2 IV poles on the operative side of the patient at the head of the bed. Then place a mayo stand between this drape and the surgeon. Place the scopes, shavers, and cautery on the mayo stand and hand off all cords across the abdomen of the patient to the circulating nurse. Due to the placement of the patient's arms and the peroneal post, it is not necessary to secure the cords to the drapes. While the surgeon is handing off the cords, the scrub nurse can drape the fluoroscopic C-arm.

Establishing the Portals

Two or 3 portals are used routinely for hip arthroscopy: anterior, anterolateral, and posterolateral. Poor portal placement can drastically increase the complexity and difficulty of the case. Portal placement requires a thorough understanding of the anatomy, particularly the neurovascular bundle and the lateral femoral cutaneous nerve. After inspection and palpation, the bony landmarks of the greater trochanter and ASIS should be identified and marked. A line should be drawn distally from the ASIS and a second line medially from the anterior proximal edge of the greater trochanter until the 2 lines intersect.

The first portal typically established is the anterolateral. A spinal needle is placed 1 cm medial to the anterior proximal edge of the greater trochanter and directed horizontally. Using fluoroscopy, the tip of the needle can be visualized entering the superolateral hip joint. Be certain not to scrape the femoral head with the needle and avoid placing it through the labrum. Remove the inner needle trocar and inject 20 to 30 cc of saline. Remove the syringe and the saline should stream out of the needle canula, confirming it is intra-articular. Insert a Nitinol wire and remove the needle canula. Make a small oblique incision of the skin only and insert the scope trocar and canula. Use fluoroscopy to confirm that the wire is not bending or getting caught in the joint. Once the canula is in place, remove the wire and trocar and insert the 70-degree scope. Turn on the fluid and irrigate the joint.

Establish the anterior portal next. Following the line medially from the first portal, insert the spinal needle just lateral to the line drawn distally from the ASIS. Placing the portal medial to this line endangers the femoral nerve. Direct the needle approximately 45 degrees cephalad and 30 degrees medially to enter the anterior medial aspect of the joint.[4] Fluoroscopy can assist in establishing this portal, but use the arthroscope to visualize the needle penetrating the capsule. Remove the needle trocar and insert a Nitinol wire through and then remove the needle canula. To avoid injuring the lateral femoral circumflex nerve, make a very superficial (skin only) incision obliquely in line with the path of the nerve (ie, from proximal medial to distal lateral). Insert the scope canula and trocar. Keep the tip of the wire in view with the arthroscope until the canula is safely placed intra-articularly. Remove the Nitinol wire and trocar. At this point it is beneficial to insert an arthroscopic scalpel carefully through the anterior portal and make a capsulotomy. This significantly increases the mobility of instruments passed through the anterior portal. Then insert a probe and perform the diagnostic arthroscopy.

Most, if not all, of the arthroscopy can be performed using the anterior and anterolateral portals alone. If it is necessary (ie, posterior labral tear, posterior loose body), the posterolateral portal can be utilized. This portal is in line laterally with the other 2 portals. The entry point is 1 cm posterior to the posterolateral edge of the proximal greater trochanter. Aim the spinal needle slightly cephalad and anteriorly. Aiming posteriorly can cause injury to the sciatic nerve. Additionally, care must be taken when initially positioning the patient as hip flexion or external hip rotation can place the sciatic nerve at higher risk of injury.[4,8,9] Once the needle is visualized in the posterior aspect of the joint, use the Nitinol wire technique for inserting the canula.

Complications

The reported complication rate of hip arthroscopy is between 1.3% and 6.4%.[11] Most complications are minor and transient; however, major complications have been reported (Table 10-3). Traction neurapraxia of the pudendal and sciatic nerves is associated with prolonged transaction and improper positioning. A well-padded perineum post

Table 10-3

COMPLICATIONS OF HIP ARTHROSCOPY

Neurovascular traction injury
Perineum injuries
Fluid extravasation
Heterotopic ossification
Infection
Avascular necrosis
Instrument breakage

placed laterally into the medial thigh can reduce the risk of neurapraxia. Damage to the terminal branches of the lateral femoral cutaneous nerve can occur when placing the anterior portal.[12] The surgeon should explain this risk to the patient and that damage to the nerve will cause loss of sensation in the lateral thigh. A case of death has been reported attributed to fluid extravasation in a patient with an acetabular fracture.[13] The most common complications are iatrogenic. Damage to the labrum and scuffing of the articular cartilage are commonly caused by portal placement. Proper technique and careful attention by the surgeon can drastically reduce these complications.

SUMMARY

Hip arthroscopy can be a successful procedure with proper patient selection, realistic patient expectations, and correct indications for surgery. Meticulous attention to patient positioning and portal placement by the surgeon can reduce iatrogenic complications. Hip arthroscopy is a technically demanding procedure with a steep learning curve. In the proper hands, it is an excellent minimally invasive technique to visualize and treat diseases of the hip.

With continued research and a better understanding of hip pathology, alternative treatments to total hip arthroplasty are at the forefront of care for young adults. Appropriate physical examination and diagnostic imaging are crucial to obtain the right diagnosis and thereby the appropriate treatment options. Nonoperative management is appropriate in patients with mild to moderate symptoms or those who are reluctant for operative intervention. Surgical management, which has been shown to be successful in the literature, is practical only when operated on patients with proper indications. Many of the procedures have a steep learning curve and should only be utilized after appropriate training. These treatment options can delay or eliminate the need for a hip replacement in young patients.

REFERENCES

1. Shindle MK, Voos JE, Heyworth BE, et al. Hip arthroscopy in the athletic patient: current techniques and spectrum of disease. *J Bone Joint Surg Am.* 2007;89(suppl 3):29-43.
2. Byrd JW. Hip arthroscopy. *J Am Acad Orthop Surg.* 2006;14(7):433-44.
3. Sierra RJ, Trousdale RT, Ganz R, Leunig M. Hip disease in the young, active patient: evaluation and nonarthroplasty surgical options. *J Am Acad Orthop Surg.* 2008;16(12):689-703.
4. Byrd JW. Hip arthroscopy by the supine approach. *Instr Course Lect.* 2006;55:325-336.
5. Edwards D, Villar R. Arthroscopy of the hip joint. *Practitioner.* 1992;236:924, 926, 929.
6. Glick JM, Sampson TG, Gordon RB, Behr JT, Schmidt E. Hip arthroscopy by the lateral approach. *Arthroscopy.* 1987;3:4-12.
7. Arthroscopy of the Hip. In: Callaghan J, Rubash H, Rorabeck C, editors. *The Adult Hip.* Vol 1. Philadelphia, PA: Lippincott Williams & Wilkins; 1998:721-736.
8. Ilizaliturri VM Jr. Complications of arthroscopic femoroacetabular impingement treatment: a review. *Clin Orthop Relat Res.* 2009;467(3):760-768.
9. Griffin DR, Villar RN. Complications of arthroscopy of the hip. *J Bone Joint Surg Br.* 1999;81(4):604-606.
10. Mason JB, McCarthy JC, O'Donnell J, et al. Hip arthroscopy: surgical approach, positioning, and distraction. *Clin Orthop Relat Res.* 2003;(406):29-37.
11. Sampson TG. Complications of hip arthroscopy. *Clin Sports Med.* 2001;20(4):831-835.
12. Byrd JW, Pappas JN, Pedley MJ. Hip arthroscopy: an anatomic study of portal placement and relationship to the extra-articular structures. *Arthroscopy.* 1995;11(4):418-423.
13. Bartlett CS, DiFelice GS, Buly RL, Quinn TJ, Green DS, Helfet DL. Cardiac arrest as a result of intraabdominal extravasation of fluid during arthroscopic removal of a loose body from the hip joint of a patient with an acetabular fracture. *J Orthop Trauma.* 1998;12(4):294-299.

11

Femoroacetabular Impingement

Benjamin Bender, MD; Ashok Gowda, MD; and Javad Parvizi, MD, FRCS

Femoroacetabular impingement (FAI) is a condition in which structural abnormalities of the femoral head-neck junction and/or the acetabulum result in early degenerative changes in the nondysplastic hip. FAI has been recognized as a source of hip discomfort in many patients with no other known cause and with only subtle abnormalities on plain radiographs.[1-6] The presence of abnormal morphology involving the proximal femur and/or the acetabulum resulting in repetitive microtrauma from the neck abutting against the acetabular rim can lead to labral lesions and acetabular cartilage delamination. The early chondral and labral lesions continue to progress and result in osteoarthritis.[2,3]

Typical conditions seen to cause FAI include post-traumatic deformities, coxa profunda, acetabular protrusion, acetabular retroversion, developmental causes such as Legg-Calvé-Perthes disease and slipped capital femoral epiphysis, and extra-articular impingement.

The majority of patients who present with FAI are young, active, and complain of activity-related groin pain. Hips that have structural abnormalities have decreased range of motion (ROM) secondary to FAI; however, some patients who perform extreme range of hip motion (ballet dancers, yoga practitioners, mountain climbers, martial artists) may have completely normal or increased ROM.

Degeneration and tearing of the labrum has been detected on magnetic resonance imaging (MRI) and is associated with progressive damage to the adjacent cartilage. This may be the result of impingement of the anterior and anterosuperior femoral head-neck junction against that portion of the acetabular labrum adjacent to it. This type of impingement is thought to be one of the precursors of osteoarthritis.[7] The causative link between FAI and degenerative joint disease remains unknown, though several studies have shown an association between labral tears and osteoarthritis in the setting of impingement.[3,4,8]

The diagnosis of FAI is based on the patient's clinical history and physical examination and is further supported by findings on radiography, computed tomography (CT), and MRI. Differential diagnosis may include hip dysplasia with joint instability, intra-articular hip diseases without impingement, and referred pain originating outside the hip joint.

Various Impingements

The pattern and stages of chondral and labral hip injuries and the findings at the time of surgery define the 2 types of FAI: cam and pincer. In an epidemiological study of 149 hips with impingement, 26 (17.4%) had isolated cam impingement, 16 (10.7%) had isolated pincer impingement, and 107 (71.8%) had combined cam-pincer impingement.[9]

Cam Impingement

Cam impingement is more common in young athletic men and is caused by an abnormal femoral head-neck

Parvizi J, Klatt BA.
Essentials in Total Hip Arthroplasty (pp 85-93).

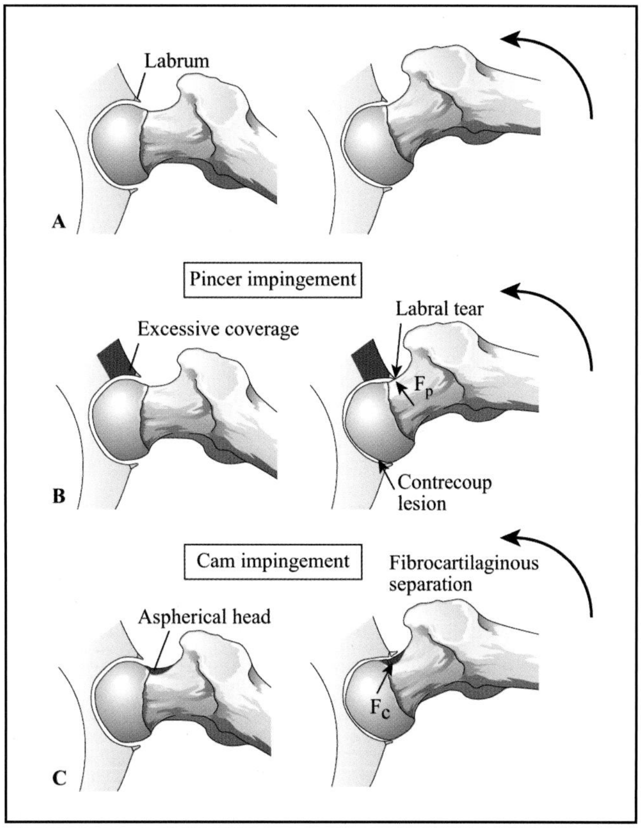

Figure 11-1. A normal hip (A) has an impingement-free range of motion within the physiologic amplitudes of joint motion. In pincer impingement (B), the main impact force (Fp) is directed tangential to the joint surface, leading to a full tear of the labrum (mainly resulting from the acetabular overcoverage). In cam impingement (C), the aspherical portion of the femoral head–neck junction is jammed into the acetabulum. The main impact force (Fc) is perpendicular to the joint surface, leading to a fibrocartilaginous separation (undersurface tear of the labrum). (Adapted from Tannast M, Siebenrock KA. Conventional radiographs to assess femoroacetabular impingement. *Instr Course Lect.* 2009;58:203-212.)

junction. The aspherical head-neck junction is jammed into the acetabulum, leading to a labro-cartilaginous separation and shearing off of the cartilage from the subchondral bone (Figure 11-1). In pure cam impingement of the hip, the predominant abnormality is in the contour of the anterosuperior femoral head-neck junction with normal acetabular morphology.

Traditionally, the anterosuperior femoral head–neck junction has a concave configuration. In cam impingement, this junction is either flattened or convex. This morphologic abnormality can cause the femoral head to become somewhat aspherical and during forceful motion, particularly flexion, the nonspherical portion of the femoral head can be squeezed under the acetabular rim. This abnormal contact results in damage primarily to the acetabular cartilage at the anterosuperior acetabular rim.[3-5,8] This chondral abrasion or avulsion subsequently leads to a tear or detachment of the acetabular labrum. Repetitive impingement can result in osteophyte formation on the anterior femoral neck, further exacerbating the problem and limiting the ROM of the hip.

Evidence suggests a developmental abnormality due to aberrant separation of the common physis of the femoral head and the greater trochanter may result in the decreased femoral head-neck offset and a nonspherical appearance of the femoral head.[10] Patients with cam FAI often have an abnormally shaped proximal femur with insufficient head-neck offset, such as those seen in abnormalities leading to head tilt or pistol grip deformities, slipped capital femoral epiphysis (SCFE), post-traumatic deformities, malunited femoral neck fractures, femoral retroversion, coxa vara, or femoral head necrosis with flattening. Cam impingement is characterized by deeper cartilage lesions and more extensive labral tears due to the greater degree of articular compression from nonspherical femoral head rotation.[5,10]

Pincer Impingement

Pincer impingement is most common in middle-aged athletic women as a result of linear contact between a prominent anterior aspect of the acetabular rim and the femoral head or femoral head-neck junction. In a normal hip, the acetabulum is anteverted; that is, the anterior wall is medial to the posterior wall. Pincer impingement results from abnormal contact between the acetabular rim and the femoral neck as seen in abnormalities of acetabular morphology, such as acetabular retroversion and abnormalities of anterior and/or lateral overcoverage such as coxa profunda and acetabular protrusion. These conditions increase either the relative depth of the acetabulum or the circumferential overcoverage of the femoral head (see Figure 11-1). In pure pincer impingement, the predominant abnormality is the morphology of the acetabulum.

Contre-coup lesions of the posteroinferior acetabulum[3] are seen with repetitive abutments but are limited to a small region on the acetabular rim and are typically more benign than the lesions seen in cam impingement.

Clinical Presentation

History

Classically, impingement presents in a young or middle-aged patient who at the time of presentation describes the gradual onset of unilateral hip pain predominantly in the groin. Patients with anterior FAI commonly present with activity-related anterior inguinal groin pain, pain overlying

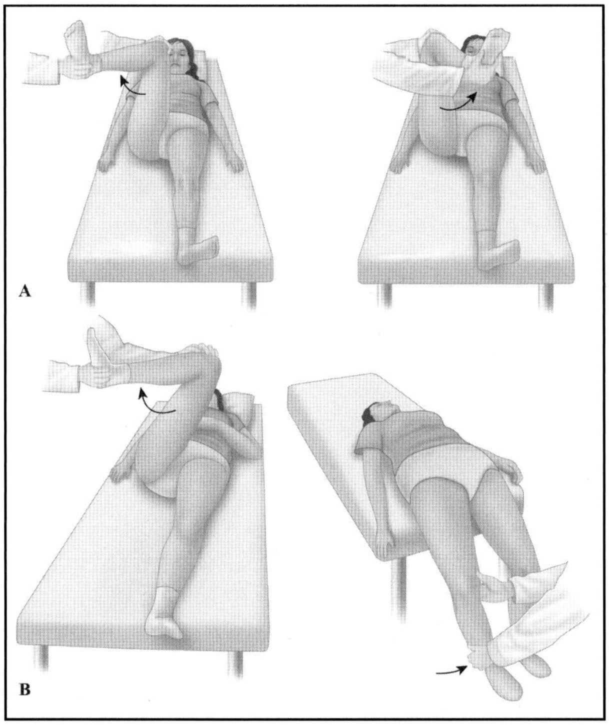

Figure 11-2. (A) Impingement test. Forced flexion, internal rotation, and adduction of the involved extremity reproduces symptoms related to femoroacetabular impingement. (B) Posterior impingement test. Pain is reproduced posteriorly in patients with involvement of the posterior acetabulum as the extremity is forcefully externally rotated. (Adapted from Hozak WJ, Parvizi J, Bender B. *Surgical Treatment of Hip Arthritis: Reconstruction, Replacement, and Revision.* Philadelphia, PA: Elsevier, Inc; 2009.)

the trochanters, and pain with flexion and internal rotation. Associated lateral and posterior hip pain is also common. The patient may report mechanical symptoms (locking, catching, giving-way) indicative of a labral tear or a delamination injury of the articular cartilage. Prior to presentation to an orthopedist, patients often have been seen by multiple physicians and have been given a wide range of diagnoses, including sports hernia, tendonitis, and synovitis. Most patients have failed conservative treatment including nonsteroidal anti-inflammatory drugs (NSAIDs) and physical therapy due to the structural nature of the pain.

Prior radiographs have often been read as negative as deformities are often subtle and patients can present with a history of extensive diagnostic work-up testing and potentially inappropriate surgical therapeutic modalities, including laparoscopy, laparotomy, knee arthroscopy, lumbar spine decompression, and inguinal hernia repair.

The acetabular labrum, similar to the meniscus of the knee, is known to carry proprioceptive and nociceptive nerve fibers, and compression or disruption of the labrum is a well-documented source of pain.[11] Typical patients present approximately 30 years earlier than the typical osteoarthritis patient (ie, third, fourth, and fifth decades rather than the sixth to ninth decades of life). Symptoms of impingement are most frequently unilateral, though bilateral FAI can occur in individuals who have connective tissue or other disorders resulting in hip joint laxity.

Initially, hip pain is intermittent and may be exacerbated by athletic activities, prolonged walking, prolonged sitting, or driving. Mechanical symptoms such as locking, catching, or clicking are common with labral tears, but these are nonspecific for the disorder. Of note, pain is typically worse when the hip is in internal rotation or at least 70 degrees of flexion.[12]

Clinical Evaluation

A detailed patient evaluation is focused on identifying the specific etiology of the patient's symptoms, carefully defining the structural anatomy of the hip joint, and assessing the extent of joint degeneration. Patient-specific factors such as age, activity level, comorbidities, and physical condition are also important determinants in the final treatment plan. Examination of the hip often reveals limitation of motion, particularly in internal rotation and adduction in flexion. The impingement test is almost always positive (Figure 11-2). This test is done with the patient supine. The hip is internally rotated as it is passively flexed to approximately 90 degrees and adducted. Flexion and adduction leads to the approximation of the abnormal contact of the femoral neck and the acetabular rim with recreation of the pain most reliably when there is a chondral lesion. Posteroinferior impingement also may exist.

The posterior impingement test is a provocative test to elicit posteroinferior impingement. It is performed by having the patient lie supine on the edge of the bed and having the legs hang free from the end of the bed in order to produce maximum hip extension. External rotation with the hip in extension that gives rise to severe, deep-seated groin pain by shear or compression of the acetabular labrum is indicative of posteroinferior impingement. A positive impingement test has been correlated with acetabular rim lesions as visualized on magnetic resonance (MR) arthrogram of the hip.[13] If buttock pain is reproduced with this test, then posterior cartilage degeneration has occurred.[2,3,6]

A complete examination of the limb and lumbar spine is also prudent in order to rule out other common sources of hip pain, including bursitis, nerve entrapments, and referred pain. Additionally, great overlap exists in the presentation of hernias. A thorough examination of the lower abdominal musculature should be undertaken or a referral to a general

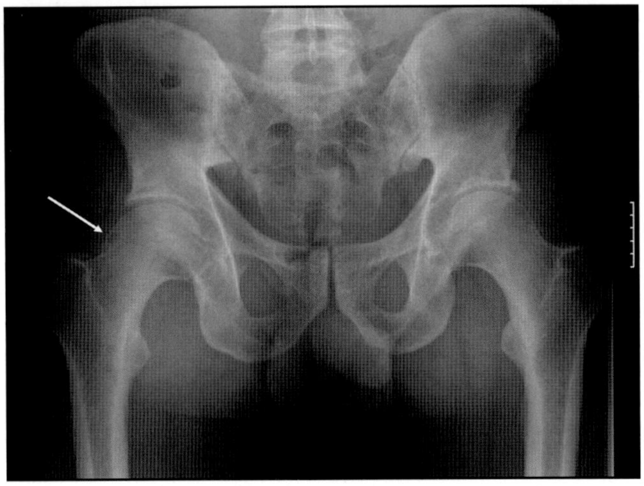

Figure 11-3. Prominence of the femoral head-neck junction in the anterosuperior portion of the proximal femur (right hip) is known as the "pistol grip deformity" due to its similarities with the smooth hand grip of many pistols.

surgeon should be considered for further work-up in cases where the diagnosis is questionable.

Imaging Studies

Plain radiographs including anteroposterior (AP) pelvis and lateral cross table view should be obtained. Acetabular orientation (anteversion, retroversion) and the depth of the acetabulum (coxa profunda, protrusion) are assessed on the AP pelvic view. Proper assessment of the acetabular shape and version is carried out when the central x-ray beam has to be centered approximately 2 cm above the symphysis pubis. Standing true AP radiograph and a lateral radiograph of the hip should be ordered for any patient with suspected FAI as this radiographic view is critical to assess version of the acetabulum. A true AP pelvic radiograph is obtained when there is symmetry of the iliac wings and of the obturator foramina and the coccyx is at a point in the midline within a distance of 0 to 2 cm above the symphysis pubis. Conventional radiography is also helpful for evaluating patients who have had prior trauma and fractures of the acetabulum or proximal femur. Residual bony deformities contributing to FAI can be adequately surveyed using conventional radiographs.

The abnormal anatomy of the proximal femur can be seen on the AP pelvic radiograph. The shape of the femoral head is classified as a pistol grip deformity (Figure 11-3) if the lateral contour of the femoral head extends in a convex shape to the base of the neck (flattening of the femoral head-neck junction) and is classified as aspheric if the epiphysis of the head protrudes laterally out of a circle around the head. The cross table lateral view may also be helpful to show the decreased femoral head-neck offset (Figure 11-4) and to detect the presence of a bony prominence or "bump" on the anterior femoral head-neck junction. The crossover sign of acetabular retroversion on the AP pelvic radiograph and rim ossification often suggests FAI.[14,15]

Coxa profunda is present when the floor of the acetabular fossa touches the ilioischial line (Kohler line) and acetabular protrusion is present when the femoral head lies medially to this line (Figure 11-5). In some patients with coxa profunda and posterior FAI, a double contour sign of the rim is present on standard radiographs. MRI images show that this results from bone apposition rather than ossification of the labrum. Fibrocystic changes (herniation pits) in the anterosuperior femoral neck junction have been reported in approximately 33% of hips with anterior FAI.[16]

Most patients with impingement require cross-sectional studies such as MRI. The use of a high-field scanner (1.5 and, recently, 3.0 Tesla) and a surface coil to improve resolution can reduce possible misses. For axial and coronal oblique images, T1-weighted spin-echo sequences and fast low-angle shot (FLASH) 2D sequence images can be used. For sagittal oblique images, T1-weighted spin-echo images and T2-weighted turbo spin-echo sequences can be used.[6,8,13]

MR arthrogram may be performed if no pathology is seen on MRI or if an articular defect is suspected. Labral separations from the anterior articular rim or labral tears can be identified. The acetabular labrum, when damaged, shows increased signal on T2-weighted images extending to the articular surface. MR arthrogram is 63% sensitive and 71% specific for diagnosing labral tears. Sensitivity increases to 92% with a small field view.[17,18] Double densities, where dye is seen between the articular cartilage and bone on magnetic resonance arteriogram, may indicate degenerative defects of the articular cartilage or delamination defects. Currently, 5 and 20 mL of gadolinium-diethylenetriaminepenta-acetate (DTPA) is injected under fluoroscopy for hip MR arthrogram.[6,8,13]

Cross-sectional evaluation based on MRI of the hip affected by FAI may show an increased alpha angle on the oblique axial images (Figure 11-6). Alpha angle detects the abnormal femoral morphology associated with cam FAI. Alpha angle represents the angle formed by a line between the center of the femoral head and the center of the femoral neck, and a line between the center of the femoral head and the point at which the femoral head-neck contour diverges from a circle drawn around the femoral head. The alpha angle is used as an objective representation of the prominence of the anterior femoral head-neck junction. The more prominent the alpha angle, the more the predilection for impingement of the anterosuperior femoral head-neck

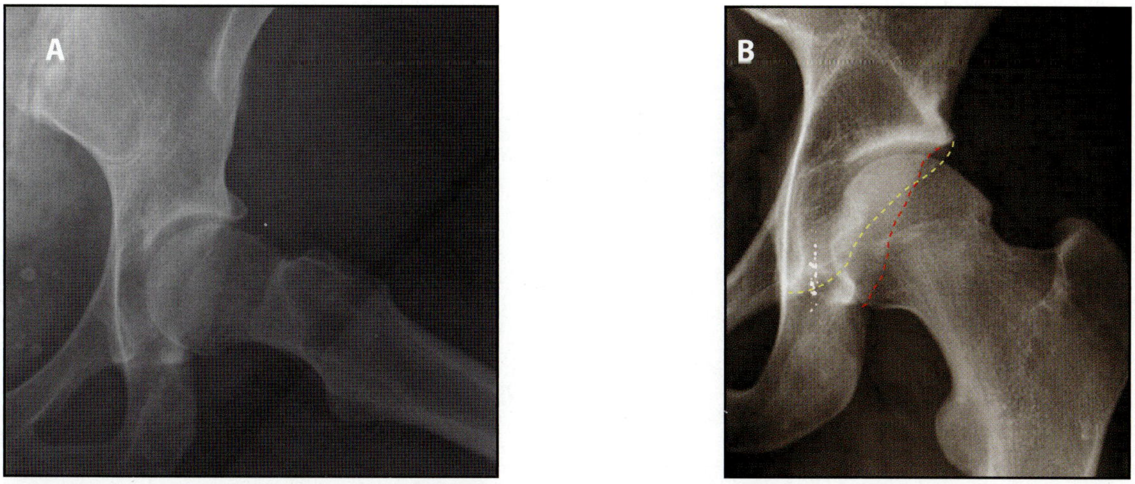

Figure 11-4. (A) Frog leg lateral view. (B) Altered offset at the femoral head-neck junction and evident acetabular retroversion, including the crossover sign between the anterior and posterior wall of the acetabulum and the ischial spine sign.

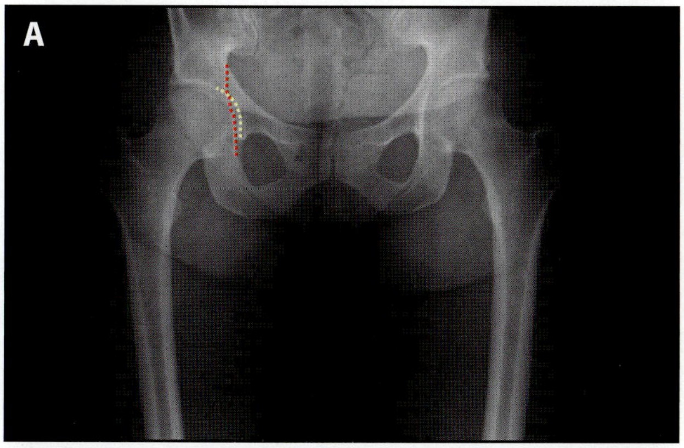

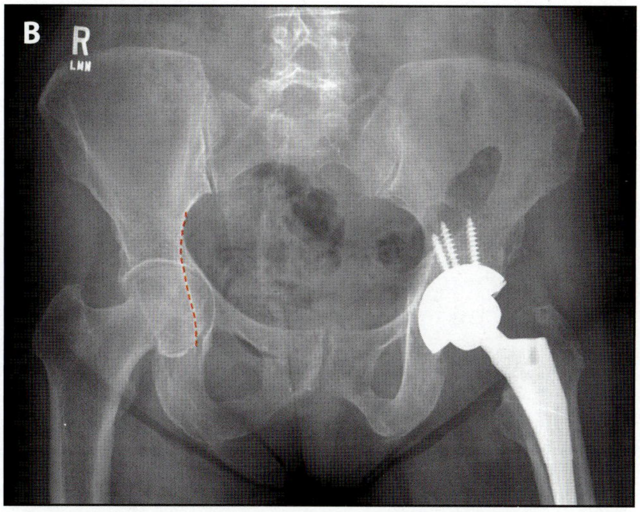

Figure 11-5. Coxa profunda/acetabular protrusion. Typically, the acetabular fossa lies lateral to the ilioischial line. The lateral center edge angle is between 25 and 39 degrees. The extrusion index is approximately 25%. The epiphyseal scar lies within the femoral head circle. The acetabular index is slightly positive. The posterior wall goes through the femoral center. (A) Coxa profunda is defined by an overcrossing of the acetabular fossa with the IL. (B) In protrusion even the femoral head line is crossing the IL.

junction against the adjacent acetabulum. Notzli et al[5] found a mean angle of 74 degrees in patients with clinical symptoms of FAI compared to 42 degrees in control groups and proposed that an alpha angle of >50 degrees may be an appropriate cross-sectional criterion in assessing for FAI. Additionally, they concluded that patients with clinical symptoms of FAI had hips with significantly less concavity at the femoral head-neck junction than did patients in the control group.

CT has less commonly been used when compared with plain radiographs and MRI for diagnosis of FAI. Conventional 2-dimensional CT imaging is deficient in displaying subtle contour deformities on the periphery of the femoral head-neck junction and has limitations in establishing the femoral head-neck axis. Additionally, confirmation of the presence of specifically oriented pathoanatomy predisposing to the dynamic states of FAI is very difficult to achieve with 2-dimensional reconstructions. Recently, however, 3-dimensional CT has been proven to represent an accurate tool to assess abnormalities of the hip in FAI.[13]

In certain circumstances, the actual process of impingement can be demonstrated with cross-sectional imaging. In open MRI units or in MRI or CT units with a large bore, the patient may flex and internally rotate his or her hip thereby producing a physiologic demonstration of FAI. Patients can subsequently be imaged with their hip in maximum flexion and internal rotation. The resulting impingement of the femoral head-neck junction on the

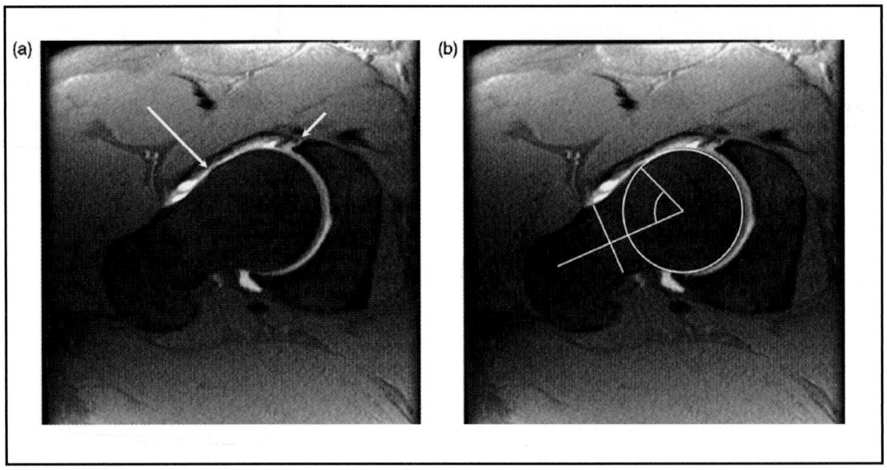

Figure 11-6. Oblique T1-weighted fat suppressed image shows abnormal anterior superior femoral head–neck offset and anterior superior labral tear and the lines used for measuring alpha angle. An angle greater than 55 degrees is considered abnormal.

acetabular labrum and acetabulum may thus be directly visualized. Although this type of view may give a representative view of what is happening biomechanically, the direct apposition of the impinged elements may create difficulty when attempting to analyze the anatomy in the region.[6,13]

Nonsurgical Treatment

Management of patients with FAI initially begins with a trial of conservative treatment ranging from anti-inflammatory medications to activity modification, restriction of athletic activities, and intra-articular cortisone injections.

A trial of nonsteroidal anti-inflammatory medications may be appropriate to relieve pain of acute onset; however, chronic use may mask symptoms of an underlying destructive process.

Physical therapy with emphasis on improving ROM or stretching is usually not productive. Aggressive maneuvers to gain hip flexion and internal rotation motion may irritate the hip and should be avoided.

For patients with moderate to advanced degenerative disease, nonoperative modalities can be considered as temporizing therapies prior to joint arthroplasty.[6,13] Conservative management is likely only to be temporarily successful as the young age of these patients and their high activity levels and/or athletic ambitions may jeopardize compliance. Conservative nonsurgical therapy should be exhausted before any decision is made for surgical intervention. The finding of a labral tear in these patients should not be a direct indication for surgical intervention.

Surgical Treatment

The primary objective of surgery, independent of the technique selected, is to address the structural impingement lesions and the associated intra-articular disease elements (labrum, articular cartilage).

Surgical management involves dislocation of the hip with preservation of the blood supply to the femoral head and femoroacetabular osteoplasty initially described by Ganz et al.[2] This technique is indicated specifically in patients with pincer impingement secondary to the retroverted acetabulum, coxa profunda, or protrusion. Dislocation allows for the potential to address the acetabular side with a resection osteoplasty, if necessary, of the entire rim. Additionally, labral repair, resection, or fixation can be performed. Surgical dislocation provides complete access to the femoral head-neck junction for resection of the prominent anterior neck or nonspherical femoral head. This approach allows excision of aspherical portions of the superior femoral head-neck junction in the area over the retinacular vessels that would otherwise be difficult to access arthroscopically. Reorientation of the proximal femur with a flexion-valgus intertrochanteric osteotomy can be performed in patients with femoral retroversion or coxa vara. Treatment of proximal femoral deformities with reorientation osteotomies of the femoral neck and relative neck lengthening with advancement of the trochanter for patients with impingement secondary to high riding trochanters and short necks can also be performed.

A lateral surgical incision and linear division of the fascia lata to approach the greater trochanter is utilized. A trochanteric flip osteotomy is then performed at the lateral border of the piriformis fossa proximally and at the vastus ridge distally. When properly performed, the trochanter segment will have a small attachment of the abductor muscles. The external rotator muscles are preserved during this approach and the medial femoral circumflex artery is protected by the intact obturator externus muscle. The osteotomized trochanter is gently retracted anteriorly and the anterior capsule is dissected free of any muscular attachment. A lazy S–shaped capsulotomy is then performed to expose the hip joint. After division of the ligamentum teres, the hip is dislocated. Prior to the formal dislocation, the FAI is confirmed and the site of impingement is identified. Femoral osteoplasty is then performed to remove the prominent area of the femoral neck. Restoration of the femoral neck clearance allows an impingement-free physiologic range of motion for the affected hip. The goal is to remove as much of the prominent area as is needed to allow flexion of 120 degrees and internal rotation of 40 degrees.

Relative femoral neck lengthening with trochanteric advancement is another possibility of increasing clearance. In this procedure, the acetabulum is inspected and the site and extent of labral and/or chondral injury is identified. If necessary, the labrum in the anterosuperior region of the rim is then dissected free of the rim and the normal portion of the labrum preserved. The torn labrum is then débrided and an osteotomy of the acetabular rim is performed. Once a stable intact chondral region is identified the remaining labrum is reattached using nonabsorbable anchor sutures. The hip is subsequently reduced and impingement-free physiologic range of motion is confirmed. The capsule is loosely closed and the soft tissues are apposed with interrupted sutures. The trochanteric osteotomy is then fixed using 2 4.5-mm cortical screws. The screws are placed in the center of the osteotomy and are aimed toward the lesser trochanter. No surgical drain is used. Of note, up to 1 cm of acetabular rim may be removed without causing instability of the hip as the chondral lesion usually extends 0.5 to 1 cm into the acetabulum.

Contraindications to open surgical management are advanced degenerative changes, patients in the fifth decade of life, and those with retroversion or poor lateral coverage (resection of the anterior overcoverage could risk turning the lateral dysplasia into a global dysplasia and risk anterior instability).[19]

Espinosa et al[20] retrospectively reviewed the clinical and radiographic results of 52 patients (60 hips) who underwent open treatment. In the first 25 hips, the torn labrum was resected (group 1); in the next 35 hips the intact portion of the labrum was reattached to the acetabular rim (group 2). At 1 and 2 years postoperatively, the Merle d'Aubigné clinical score and the Tönnis arthrosis classification system were used to compare the 2 groups. At 1 year postoperatively, both groups showed a significant improvement in their clinical scores (mainly pain reduction) compared with their preoperative values ($p = 0.0003$ for group 1 and $p < 0.0001$ for group 2). At 2 years postoperatively, 28% of the hips in group 1 had an excellent result, 48% had a good result, 20% had a moderate result, and 4% had a poor result. At 2 years postoperatively, 80% of the hips in group 2 had an excellent result, 14% had a good result, and 6% had a moderate result. Comparison of the clinical scores between the 2 groups revealed significantly better outcomes for group 2 at 1 year ($p = 0.0001$) and at 2 years ($p = 0.01$). Radiographic signs of osteoarthritis were significantly more prevalent in group 1 than in group 2 at 1 year ($p = 0.02$) and at 2 years ($p = 0.009$). They concluded that patients treated with labral reattachment recovered earlier and had superior clinical and radiographic results compared with patients who had undergone resection of a torn labrum.[20,21]

Hip Arthroscopy

Hip arthroscopy, a potentially attractive alternative, offers a minimally invasive technique for diagnostic and therapeutic management of FAI.[22-24] Arthroscopy may be useful in the treatment of labral tears generated by FAI, particularly when minimal morphologic abnormality exists. Arthroscopy also may be combined with other surgical techniques without the need for trochanteric osteotomy or intraoperative hip dislocation.[25] Combined arthroscopy with limited open femoral head-neck osteoplasty has been shown to adequately manage abnormal anatomy and pathophysiology in a manner that is less invasive than other surgical alternatives.[25]

The patient is supine or in a lateral decubitus position in hip arthroscopy. Under fluoroscopic guidance, a spinal needle is inserted into the hip joint. The joint is inflated with arthroscopic fluid. A guide wire is inserted through the spinal needle and cannulated trochars are inserted into the hip joint. Of note, care must be taken to avoid scuffing the femoral and acetabular articular cartilage. Typically, 2 or 3 portals are used: anterior, anterolateral, and posterolateral. To reduce risk to the peroneal structures, especially the pudendal nerve, and to avoid traction neurapraxia to the femoral and sciatic nerves, the duration of traction should be minimized.[26]

Despite offering a minimally invasive approach, hip arthroscopy has limitations due to maneuverability in a confined space. Removal of the bony prominence on the femoral neck, especially when it extends to the posterior neck region, may be difficult and either overresection or underresection may occur due to difficulty in assessing the depth of resection. In addition, arthroscopic resection of the impinging acetabular rim in both retroversion and pincer impingement cases cannot be performed because current arthroscopic tools do not allow access to the posterior wall for resection. Stable reattachment of the labrum is also difficult because one cannot reflect the labrum and débride the underlying surface to provide a proper bed for reattachment. Patients with coxa profunda or protrusion, severe acetabular retroversion, and the obese may prove difficult to treat arthroscopically. Finally, little can be done in arthroscopy to adequately treat the chondral lesion that may be associated with the labral tear. At this time, due to these limitations, hip arthroscopy should be reserved for simple cam impingement, though wider application of arthroscopic treatment of FAI may be possible with further improvements in the surgical technique and in instrument design.[22-24,26,27]

Surgical Treatment Without Dislocation

Alternative approaches for the treatment of FAI are being explored because of the morbidity associated with surgical hip dislocation, namely, the need for non-weight-bearing for an extended period and the potential for trochanteric osteotomy nonunion. A modified Smith-Petersen anterior approach may be used to perform an arthrotomy of the hip. Under direct visualization the prominence on the femoral neck region can be resected easily and effectively. A detached labrum also can be addressed using this approach. Reattachment of the labrum using anchor sutures is possible. Traction systems attached to the operating table can be used to subluxate the hip and examine the chondral lesion and resect the lesion when necessary.[6,20,28]

Total hip arthroplasty and total hip resurfacing in young patients are viable alternative options for unreconstructable hips with advanced or progressive degenerative disease. Successful outcomes with modern bearings of alumina-on-alumina and metal-on-metal and a new generation of highly durable cross-linked polyethylene or gamma-irradiated polyethylene may address the disabling end-stage arthritis in this younger group of patients.[27,29,30]

Although good short-term results have been reported for the surgical treatment of FAI, no long-term results are available to date.[29,31]

Periacetabular Osteotomy

Periacetabular osteotomy (PAO) is performed for correction of retroversion. It is indicated in patients with a positive anterior impingement test and findings of acetabular rim lesions on MR arthrogram. The crossover and posterior wall signs suggestive of posterolateral dysplasia are present on a pelvic radiograph.[19] Contraindication for PAO is excessive posterior wall coverage. Correction in this setting may lead to impingement in extension. Significant combined pincer and cam impingement requires surgical dislocation to address the femoral side adequately. Advanced anterior cartilage degeneration would place a degenerative segment in the weight-bearing zone after correction.

Summary

FAI is characterized by decreased clearance and abnormal contact between the femoral head-neck junction and the acetabular rim. This disorder is due to proximal femoral and/or acetabular rim deformities and is now recognized as a common cause of prearthritic hip pain and secondary osteoarthritis. Abnormal femoroacetabular abutment, particularly in positions of hip flexion and internal rotation, predispose affected patients to labral tears, articular cartilage damage, and premature osteoarthritis. Impingement abnormalities can be divided into 2 major categories: cam and pincer.

The presence of a consistent history and physical findings such as a positive impingement test should alert the physician to the possibility of hip impingement syndrome. Radiographic studies might be reported as normal unless critically reviewed by specialists familiar with the subtleties of impingement syndrome. Treatment of FAI focuses on improving hip motion and alleviating femoral abutment against the acetabular rim. Early surgical intervention provides relief of symptoms and may decelerate the progression of the degenerative process for this group of young patients.

References

1. Eijer H, Myers SR, Ganz R. Anterior femoroacetabular impingement after femoral neck fractures. *J Orthop Trauma.* 2001;15(7):475-481.
2. Ganz R, Gill TJ, Gautier E, Ganz K, Krügel N, Berlemann U. Surgical dislocation of the adult hip. *J Bone Joint Surg Br.* 2001;83(8):1119-1124.
3. Ganz R, Parvizi J, Beck M, Leunig M, Nötzli H, Siebenrock KA. Femoroacetabular impingement: a cause for osteoarthritis of the hip. *Clin Orthop Relat Res.* 2003(417):112-120.
4. McCarthy JC, Noble PC, Schuck MR, Wright J, Lee J. The role of labral lesions to development of early degenerative hip disease. *Clin Orthop Relat Res.* 2001(393):25-37.
5. Nötzli HP, Wyss TF, Stoecklin CH, Schmid MR, Treiber K, Hodler J. The contour of the femoral head-neck junction as a predictor for the risk of anterior impingement. *J Bone Joint Surg Br.* 2002;84(4):556-560.

6. Parvizi J, Leunig M, Ganz R. Femoroacetabular impingement. *J Am Acad Orthop Surg.* 2007;15(9):561-570.
7. Leunig M, Beck M, Woo A, Dora C, Kerboull M, Ganz R. Acetabular Rim degeneration: a constant finding in the aged hip. *Clin Orthop Relat Res.* 2003(413):201-207.
8. Ito K, Minka II M, Leunig M, Werlen S, Ganz R. Femoroacetabular impingement and the cam-effect. A MRI-based quantitative anatomical study of the femoral head-neck offset. *J Bone Joint Surg.* 2001;83(2):171-176.
9. Beck M, Kalhor M, Leunig M, Ganz R. Hip morphology influences the pattern of damage to the acetabular cartilage. Femoroacetabular impingement as a cause of early osteoarthritis of the hip. *J Bone Joint Surg.* 2005;87(7):1012-1018.
10. Siebenrock KA, Wahab KHA, Werlen S, Kalhor M, Leunig M, Ganz R. Abnormal extension of the femoral head epiphysis as a cause of cam impingement. *Clin Orthop Relat Res.* 2004;(418):54-60.
11. Kim YT, Azuma H. The nerve endings of the acetabular labrum. *Clin Orthop Relat Res.* 1995;(320):176-181.
12. Klaue K, Durnin CW, Ganz R. The acetabular rim syndrome. A clinical presentation of dysplasia of the hip. *J Bone Joint Surg.* 1991;73(3):423-429.
13. Tannast M, Kubiak-Langer M, Langlotz F, Puls M, Murphy SB, Siebenrock KA. Noninvasive three-dimensional assessment of femoroacetabular impingement. *J Orthop Res.* 2007;25(1):122-131.
14. Reynolds D, Lucas J, Klaue K. Retroversion of the acetabulum. *J Bone Joint Surg.* 1999;81(2):281-288.
15. Clohisy JC, Carlisle JC, Beaulé PE, et al. A systematic approach to the plain radiographic evaluation of the young adult hip. *J Bone Joint Surg.* 2008;90(suppl 4):47-66.
16. Leunig M, Beck M, Kalhor M, Kim Y, Werlen S, Ganz R. Fibrocystic changes at anterosuperior femoral neck: prevalence in hips with femoroacetabular impingement. *Radiology.* 2005;236(1):237-246.
17. Toomayan GA, Holman WR, Major NM, Kozlowicz SM, Vail TP. Sensitivity of MR arthrography in the evaluation of acetabular labral tears. *Am J Roentgenol.* 2006;186(2):449-453.
18. Leunig M, Werlen S, Ungersböck A, Ito K, Ganz R. Evaluation of the acetabular labrum by MR arthrography. *J Bone Joint Surg.* 1997;79(2):230-234.
19. Siebenrock KA, Schoeniger R, Ganz R. Anterior femoro-acetabular impingement due to acetabular retroversion. Treatment with periacetabular osteotomy. *J Bone Joint Surg.* 2003;85(2):278-286.
20. Espinosa N, Rothenfluh DA, Beck M, Ganz R, Leunig M. Treatment of femoro-acetabular impingement: preliminary results of labral refixation. *J Bone Joint Surg.* 2006;88(5):925-935.
21. Espinosa N, Beck M, Rothenfluh DA, Ganz R, Leunig M. Treatment of femoro-acetabular impingement: preliminary results of labral refixation. Surgical technique. *J Bone Joint Surg.* 2007;89(1 suppl 2):36-53.
22. Guanche CA, Bare AA. Arthroscopic treatment of femoroacetabular impingement. *Arthroscopy.* 2006;22(1):95-106.
23. Philippon MJ, Stubbs AJ, Schenker ML, Maxwell RB, Ganz R, Leunig M. Arthroscopic management of femoroacetabular impingement: osteoplasty technique and literature review. *Am J Sports Med.* 2007;35(9):1571-1580.
24. Sampson TG. Arthroscopic treatment of femoroacetabular impingement: a proposed technique with clinical experience. *Instr Course Lect.* 2006;55:337-346.
25. Clohisy JC, McClure JT. Treatment of anterior femoroacetabular impingement with combined hip arthroscopy and limited anterior decompression. *Iowa Orthop J.* 2005;25:164-171.
26. Byrd JWT. The role of hip arthroscopy in the athletic hip. *Clin Sports Med.* 2006;25(2):255-278.
27. Bare AA, Guanche CA. Hip impingement: the role of arthroscopy. *Orthopedics.* 2005;28(3):266-273.
28. Beck M, Leunig M, Parvizi J, Boutier V, Wyss D, Ganz R. Anterior femoroacetabular impingement: part II. Midterm results of surgical treatment. *Clin Orthop Relat Res.* 2004;(418):67-73.
29. Lavigne M, Parvizi J, Beck M, Siebenrock KA, Ganz R, Leunig M. Anterior femoroacetabular impingement: part I. Techniques of joint preserving surgery. *Clin Orthop Relat Res.* 2004;(418):61-66.
30. Millis MB, Kim Y. Rationale of osteotomy and related procedures for hip preservation: a review. *Clin Orthop Relat Res.* 2002;(405):108-121.
31. Zebala LP, Schoenecker PL, Clohisy JC. Anterior femoroacetabular impingement: a diverse disease with evolving treatment options. *Iowa Orthop J.* 2007;27:71-81.

12

History of Hip Surgery

Orhan Bican, MD and Lauren K. Kahl, MD

Osteoarthritis has been a problem since the beginning of time. Palaeopathologists have detected osteoarthritis of the hip with the same distributions and prevalence today as they did in the earliest human skeletons.[1] Nevertheless, the first surgical attempts to treat osteoarthritis of the hip did not occur until 200 years ago. Until the introduction of ether as an anesthetic agent in 1847, hip surgery had repelled even the most ambitious orthopedic surgeons. The first attempts began in the 18th century with amputation and joint resection, but due to lack of aseptic precautions, the success rate was very low. Most applications were limited to severe open trauma cases and tuberculous arthritis. French scientist Louis Pasteur, the first to prove germ theory, inspired Joseph Lister to introduce antisepsis during surgery to the medical community via a publication in 1867. Advances such as the introduction of rubber gloves by William Halstead in 1890 and the development of the no-touch technique by W. Arbuthnot Lane in 1902 were key steps in developing aseptic surgery. Sir John Charnley developed remarkable techniques in the control of air contamination and subsequent bacterial infection, which continues to be the most devastating complication after total hip arthroplasty (THA).[2]

The first hip resection was performed in London by Anthony White in 1822 in a patient with chronic joint abscess and dislocation of the femoral head. The patient was treated for open fracture using a long splint and regained a remarkable level of function 12 months later.[3] John Rhea Barton of Philadelphia is credited with performing the first arthroplasty in the United States in 1887. He described an osteotomy between greater and lesser trochanters of a young sailor to secure motion of an ankylosed hip secondary to trauma. His goal was to enable mobility as well as correct the deformity. He achieved this with the help of postoperative range of motion exercises.[4] Lewis Sayre of New York reportedly performed 70 hip resections by 1875 and was one of the pioneers of the procedure.[5] In a case series of 59 patients, Sayre reported a 66% survival rate and a 13% immediate postoperative mortality rate. Due to these alarming results, indications were limited to septic arthritis. Still results were poor due to the systemic burden of infection. Therefore, the optimism in undertaking a resection was debatable, and many surgeons believed it to be a poor operation. In 1940, Gathorne Girdlestone of Oxford revised the indications and techniques of joint resection in his text on bone and joint tuberculosis. He outlined the essential steps of the operation as follows:

- Complete exposure of the anterior and upper aspects of the joint
- Excision of the capsule and synovia
- Division of all structures inserted into the greater trochanter
- Dislocation of the remains of the femoral head and cleaning out of the acetabulum
- A transverse osteotomy, usually just above the lesser trochanter depending on the site of the disease

Introduction of medications to fight tuberculosis after World War II left salvage management of infected prostheses as the only indication for this technique known as the Girdlestone resection.

Parvizi J, Klatt BA.
Essentials in Total Hip Arthroplasty (pp 95-101).

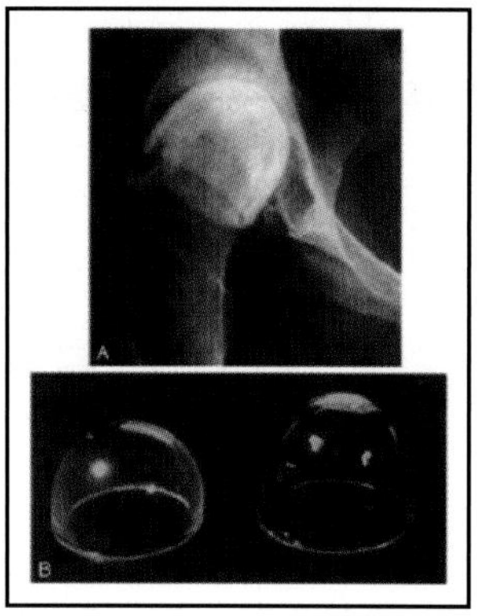

Figure 12-1. The original glass mold of Smith-Petersen is shown. (A) Radiograph of a hip obtained 2 years after arthroplasty. (B) Photographs of glass moulds. (Reprinted with permission from Calandruccio RA. Arthroplasty. In: Edmonson AS, Crenshaw AH, eds. *Campbell's Operative Orthopaedics.* 6th ed. New York, NY: Springer-Verlag; 1980:2156-2433.)

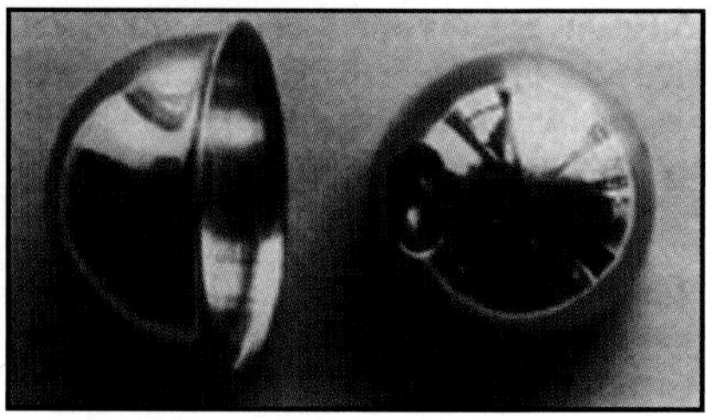

Figure 12-2. The Smith-Petersen Vitallium cup is shown. (Reprinted with permission from Shands AR. Fundamentals in hip surgery. In: Tronzo RG, ed. *Surgery of the Hip.* 2nd ed. New York, NY: Springer-Verlag; 1984:1-26.)

Resection arthroplasty removed the cause of pain, but did so at the price of stability. Attempts to provide lasting mobility at a functional level gave rise to interpositional arthroplasty. This technique is characterized by the insertion of various substances between resected joint surfaces in an attempt to prevent ankylosis. In 1840, wooden blocks were interposed in temporomandibular joints but this ultimately failed due to ankylosis.[6] Since then, muscle, fascia, and pig bladder (Baer's membrane) have all been used as interpositional material. However, nothing produced long-lasting results until Marius Smith-Petersen introduced cup arthroplasty. While still a resident in 1917, he introduced the anterior approach to the hip joint, which still to this day bears his name. Subsequently, his first arthroplasty was performed in 1923.[7] Initially, he used a cup made of glass but it was too brittle to withstand the compressive forces encountered during ambulation and eventually collapsed (Figure 12-1). The introduction of Vitallium (cast cobalt-chrome-molybdenum alloy) as a biologically inert substance in 1940 produced favorable results (Figure 12-2). Otto Aufranc continued this work and of the 1000 cup arthroplasties performed at Massachusetts General Hospital, he reported satisfactory results in 85% of patients.[8] Later attempts to improve results with the use of metallic interpositional arthroplasty were unsuccessful, and further studies concentrated on joint replacement.

Fractures of the Hip

Hip fractures were first classified in 1822 by Astley Cooper on the basis of intracapsular and extracapsular blood supply. He stated that he never treated an intracapsular fracture with conservative methods.[9] This inspired surgeons to develop open reduction internal fixation techniques with materials made of ivory and silver. Serious debates arose regarding this procedure largely due to its abandonment by prominent surgeons such as Nicholas Senn. Smith-Petersen's contributions to the procedure in 1917 resulted in great advancements. He combined the anterior and lateral incisions into one large incision, enabling exposure to the joint capsule. Through direct visualization he was able to reduce the fracture and insert a nail through the lateral cortex of the trochanter. Smith-Petersen initially designed a triflanged nail to fix these fractures. Later, this design was modified by various individuals.[10] Sven Johansson added a central hole to the nail, enabling surgeons to insert it though a small lateral incision. This later was developed into closed reduction as the standard treatment of femoral fractures.

Joint Replacement

Initially, the purpose of all hip surgeries was to alleviate pain and restore motion in ankylosed or infected joints. Joint excision and osteotomies were helpful with regards to pain but sacrificed stability. Joint replacement as a treatment method first appeared in 1891 in Berlin, Germany with Themistocles Gluck. Gluck produced an ivory ball and socket joint that he fixed to bone with nickel-plated screws and cement consisting of resin and plaster of Paris.[11] Later modifications to this procedure improved on hemiarthroplasty as treatment of intracapsular hip fractures by the introduction of an acetabular component. The second remarkable attempt at joint replacement was made 37 years later in 1938 by Philip Wiles of London. Simultaneously, Smith-Petersen was developing the cup arthroplasty in Boston, Massachusetts. Wiles implanted matched acetabular and femoral components made of stainless steel in 6 patients with Still's disease. Screw fixation prevented rotation of the acetabular while the femoral head was secured with a bolt lodged through the neck of the femur.[3] This procedure allowed previously bedridden patients to ambulate. In 1940, Hohlman introduced a short-stem Vitallium (DENTSPLY, York, PA) prosthesis, and in 1946, Drs. Jean and Robert Judet reproduced the same design using acrylic-polymethylmethacrylate. These early prostheses were unreliable as they experienced significant head erosion from stress as early as after the first 2 postoperative years. As Charnley recognized, they were designed with a defective load-bearing capacity.

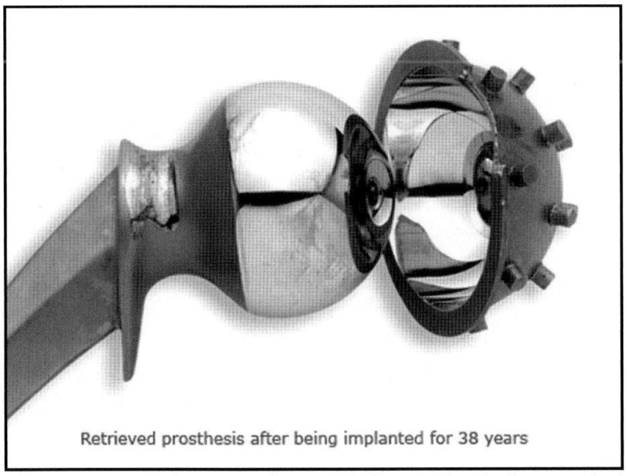

Figure 12-3. McKee-Farrar total hip replacement. The Vitallium cup had studs for fixation to the cement. The femoral vitalium component had a collar and a curved stem. (Reprinted with permission from Smith and Nephew.)

In the 1950s, long-stem femoral prostheses became popular. Various models were introduced by Dr. Austin T. Moore, Dr. Charles O. Townley, and Dr. Frederick Röeck Thompson. Moore added fenestrations to the prosthesis in order to reduce its weight. In 1961, this design was further modified to produce a self-locking stem in which bone chips were placed in the fenestrations to stimulate bone growth across them. Bipolar cups lined with Teflon (DuPont, Parkersburg, WV) were introduced in the 1950s. However, the severe biological reaction that occurred triggered a search for higher-quality material. High molecular weight polyethylene (HMWPE) was chosen by Charnley in the 1960s for its inert properties and was consequently used in many articular designs.

Two surgeons in Norvich, England, Kenneth McKee and John Watson Farrar, developed a THA using a modified Thompson's hemiarthroplasty with a metal cup that screwed into the acetabulum[2,12] (Figure 12-3). This metal-on-metal technique had mixed results, but it was the basis for Charnley's later method.

Sir John Charnley

Most of the orthopedic community agrees that Sir John Charnley is the father of modern hip arthroplasty. In James Le Fanu's book *The Rise and Fall of Modern Medicine,* Charnley's contributions are counted among the 12 definitive moments in medicine, including the discovery of penicillin.[13] Charnley's method of THA was the culmination of many years of hard work in both the laboratory and clinic. Observing patients with Judet's prosthesis convinced Charnley that a successful replacement arthroplasty would require prosthesis with low-friction bearings. During the late 1950s, he studied the friction between various materials in order to prove this theory. He had modified the McKee-Farrar prostheses by replacing the acetabular cup with the low-friction substance, Teflon. Also, by halving the diameter of the femoral head from 42 to 22.25 mm, he reduced the contact area significantly. Initially successful, the results were considered a breakthrough. Unfortunately, Teflon's high wear rate led to a severe inflammatory response from the eroded particles. Complications noted after 200 operations included prosthetic loosening, renewed hip pain, and eventually avascular necrosis and femoral head resorbtion. In 1962, a German manufacturer introduced HMWPE to Charnley. In order to prevent a recurrence of the Teflon disaster, he implanted samples of Teflon and HMWPE under his own skin. Teflon produced an initial systemic reaction, and Charnley later developed a firm tender nodule at the implantation site. HMWPE, however, was not painful and did not produce a local reaction.[14]

Between 1962 and 1965, Charnley conducted 773 total hip arthroplasties using HMWPE both in his new and old patients. He fixed both the acetabular and femoral components with self-curing acrylic cement. He published the long-term result of his low-friction arthroplasty in 1972, reporting a 90% rate of complete pain resolution (Figure 12-4). The outcome was outstanding even in very difficult revision cases.[15] At 20 years follow-up, 85% of these patients were pain-free and 80% had a near-normal range of motion. The Charnley arthroplasty spread quickly but adoption in the United States was delayed. Here, the use of acrylic cement needed to be approved by the Food and Drug Administration for use in humans.

The outcome of cemented THA is highly technique dependent. Errors in bone resection and reaming can be compensated for by the addition of more cement. This, however, can lead to component loosening. Cementation technique has improved significantly while the chemical composition has remained constant. Early techniques involved limited preparation of the bone bed. Cement was introduced anterograde, and little attempt was made at pressurization. This resulted in poor penetration into cancellous bone, inadequate cement mantles, and lamination of cement. Robin Ling, Jo Miller, and William Harris contributed to the improvement of cementation techniques and introduced low viscosity cement.[2] Present-day cementation techniques include cleaning of the endosteal bone with pulsed lavage, retrograde insertion, and sustained pressurization to optimize micro-interlock.[16] The design of the polyethylene cup

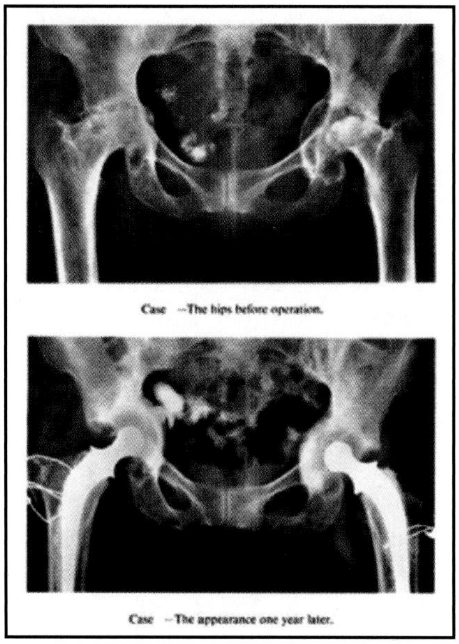

Figure 12-4. Charnley total hip replacement system. A 57-year-old female underwent bilateral total hip replacement in 1963 with an interval of 3 months. The patient underwent revision surgery on the right side due to late mechanical failure. (Reproduced with permission and copyright © of the British Editorial Society of Bone and Joint Surgery [Charnley J. The long-term results of low-friction arthroplasty of the hip performed as a primary intervention. *J Bone Joint Surg Br.* 1972;54(1):61-76].)

has changed little over the decades, although addition of a flange has enhanced pressurization. With the advancements of this technique, cementless fixation dependent on circumferential bony ingrowth into the prosthesis was becoming more feasible. This technique was appealing because it avoided failures associated with cement, decreased operation time, and improved long-term survival.

Cementless Fixation

Although providing great fixation in the short run, first-generation cementation techniques were associated with high long-term failure rates. At the time the cementation technique was improving, efforts were made to develop biological fixation. Using components with a porous interface allowed bone ingrowth and osseointegration, eliminating the need for cement. Early implant designs were cylindrical with an extensive porous coating along the length of the implant that provided good diaphyseal bone ingrowth. Superior results have been experienced with wedge-shaped femoral components with circumferential proximal porous coating. This pattern decreases the potential for femoral osteolysis by eliminating access channels for particle debris. Furthermore, it provides better bone-to-prosthesis contact. Similarly, the acetabular component in a cementless THA has a large, porous contact area. Depending on the design, spikes or screws that bite into pelvic bone keep the prosthesis in position while the reamed surface osseointegrates. Although long-term failure due to cement dysfunction is avoided with cementless arthroplasty, outcomes are dependent on the amount and the strength of bone ingrowth achieved. Many studies have shown cemented arthroplasty to be adequate in the short run but also improve over time.[16] However, larger components and longer recovery times are required for proper fixation with this technique.

The AML Total Hip Replacement (DePuy/Johnson & Johnson, Raynham, MA) was one of the early cementless designs that achieved great success. Since its introduction in 1978, this prosthesis has achieved excellent results with regards to longevity and stability. The AML was a cobalt-chrome stem with long porous coating. While the ingrowth was reliable and survival rates were good, there were concerns with thigh pain from the stiffness of the implant, proximal stress shielding, and the difficulty of removal in the revision setting. Later hips were designed to overcome some of these issues and most ingrowth hips today reflect these modifications. Current primary hip replacement stems rely on ingrowth mostly within the metaphyseal region. This decreases stress shielding of the proximal bone and reduces the thigh pain concerns. The removal of these implants is far less challenging at revision and is not as damaging to the remaining bone. Furthermore, the stems are mostly made of titanium alloys today. The modulus of titanium is closer to that of bone, and this enhances the compatibility of the implant. While THA has met the needs of many patients, there have been demands for more durability and longevity, especially in the younger generation.

Current Advancements

Since the development of successful fixation of cemented and cementless hip prosthesis, progress in THA has turned to improving bearing surfaces. Metal-on-polyethylene bearings have been one of the mainstays of THA. However, several studies have reported aseptic loosening and osteolysis secondary to wear and particulate polyethylene debris. This is especially prevalent in younger, more active patients in which more debris is generated.[17,18] For this reason, surgeons turned to hard-on-hard bearings that could avoid excessive wear and last the life of the prosthesis.

Metal-on-metal bearings solved the issue of premature wear but introduced other problems. The production of

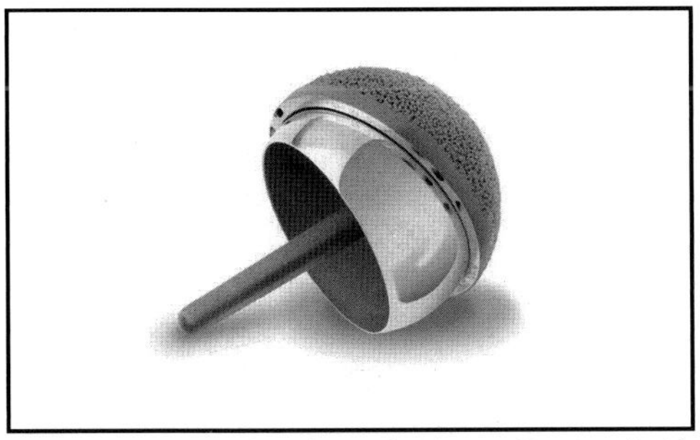

Figure 12-5. Birmingham hip replacement. (Reprinted with permission from Smith and Nephew.)

metal debris and metal ions can cause adverse effects and has received much attention in the media. Although stronger than plastic, metal-on-metal prosthesis still erode and produce debris over time. These free particles have been associated with hypersensitivity reactions and local inflammatory responses, some of which require revision.[19] Similarly, metal ions produced by friction between the 2 metal surfaces can spread throughout the body. Several studies have reported levels of chromium and cobalt in much higher concentrations in the blood and urine of patients with metal-on-metal arthroplasties. There is concern that these elevated levels of metal ions may cause systemic side effects such as cancer. These concerns, however, have not been backed by evidence-based medicine.[20]

Alumina ceramic-on-ceramic bearings were developed as an even stronger surface for articulation. These bearings wear less than their metal counterparts and do not produce metal debris or metal ions. The main issue with these bearings is brittleness and possible fracture within the prosthesis during trauma. Fortunately, new manufacturing techniques to reduce grain size and lower porosity have produced stronger materials. Also, friction between the 2 ceramic surfaces can cause squeaking in a small percentage of patients. Some studies have reported this to be associated with abnormal hip abduction values but often no source is found.[17] It should also be noted that hybrid metal-on-ceramic bearings have been reported to cause higher wear than ceramic alone.[21]

Recently, highly cross-linked polyethylene bearings have emerged as an option for arthroplasty. Unlike its polyethylene cousin, this polymer is chemically reinforced by additional bonds, making it more durable. This material behaves like polyethylene but exhibits slower rates of particulate wear. In this way, it avoids excessive osteolysis while avoiding the adverse effects of both metal and ceramic bearings.[22]

Total Hip Resurfacing

Hip resurfacing is a relatively new procedure designed for younger patients. The acetabulum is prepared in a manner similar to a conventional arthroplasty but the femur is kept intact. Instead of removing the femoral neck and head, a hemispherical cap is placed over the head of the femur and fixed in place by cement. This cap articulates with the acetabular component and spares the pathologic femoral head from irritation. The lack of a femoral stem is theoretically preferred for younger, active patients because osteolysis of the femoral canal due to physical activity is avoided. The procedure also allows for preservation of the proximal femoral bone stock and the option for conversion to THA. Depending on how long the bearing has worn, however, the cup may also need to be revised at revision.

The first hip resurfacing was developed by Charnley in the early 1950s using a Teflon-on-Teflon bearing. Later advances followed as metal-on-metal surfacing and metal-on-polyethylene articulation were introduced. However, the renaissance of hip resurfacing occurred in 1988, with the introduction of carbon-containing, wrought cobalt-chromium (Co-Cr) alloy with excellent wear characteristics. A number of hip resurfacing systems followed with the following properties:

- A bearing made from high carbon-containing Co-Cr alloy
- Cementless fixation of the acetabular component
- Cemented fixation of the femoral component (Figure 12-5)

Short-term results are promising, though concerns remain regarding long-term survival of the system. Long-term results will indicate whether this operation should be used as a bone conservation method before THA or as a reliable operation for durability and permanence.[23]

Despite the popularity of this procedure, little long-term follow-up data are available. Recently, some studies have reported higher than expected failure rates due to femoral neck fracture and collapse of the femoral head. One meta-analysis reported a 1.3% failure rate for THA at an average of 8.4 years follow up while hip resurfacing was twice that at 2.6% over only 3.9 years mean follow-up.[24] Furthermore, several recent studies have shown revision to be higher in patients converted from total hip resurfacing to THA.[25] Even while retaining the proximal femur, revision rates following conversion of a femoral component resurfacing are twice that of revision rates in a primary conventional THA.[26]

Similar to metal-on-metal THA, hypersensitivity and generation metal debris can cause local tissue reactions with metal-on-metal resurfacing. This is of special concern due to the small cup size used in resurfacing. Pseudotumors have been associated with this metal debris characterized by spontaneous dislocation, nerve palsy, and the presence of a palpable mass. Tissue samples of pseudotumors exhibit extensive necrosis, lymphocytic infiltration, and in some cases lymphoreticular spread of metal debris.[27]

New Surgical Approaches

Since Smith-Petersen described his anterior approach to the hip joint, several other approaches have been reported and used. The lateral approach allows a more direct exposure to the hip joint. Some surgeons maintain the posterior approach is technically easier but is associated with a higher rate of dislocation due to release of the short external rotator muscles stabilizing the joint. More recently, minimally invasive approaches have been proposed.

In late 2000, patients began to question the physical burden of undergoing THA. As surgeons grew more skillful, they attempted to minimize the length of their incision. The possibility of performing an arthroplasty with a 4-inch incision rather than an 8- to 12-inch incision excited both patients and surgeons. A study funded by the Orthopaedic Research and Education Foundation revealed the primary concerns of patients to be cosmesis (95%), less violation of the body (93%), and less muscle cutting (89%). Advocates of minimally invasive surgery cite improvements in these fields plus less intraoperative blood loss, less perioperative pain, faster recovery, and a shorter hospital stay as benefits.[28] However, a recent study by Woolson et al observed a significantly high risk of wound complication due to soft tissue injury, a high percentage of acetabular component malposition, and poor fit and fill of uncemented formal components in patients undergoing THA using small incisions.[29] Long-term outcomes of minimally invasive hip replacement surgery are still unknown and more importantly, there are conflicting reports regarding short-term outcomes.[30] Numerous studies indicate that adequate surgical exposure is a pivotal factor in achieving a successful and durable hip arthroplasty. However, as new advances in biotechnology become available and the cumulative experiences of orthopedic surgeons increase, minimally invasive hip replacement has become a priority for researchers and investigations continue.

Recovery Techniques

THA is a major operation that requires substantial postoperative rehabilitation to maximize results and prevent complications. Standard rehabilitation techniques include pain control, early weight bearing, and early mobilization. These interventions have been proven to improve outcomes and reduce complications such as deep vein thrombosis.

New protocols dubbed accelerated intervention have been developed to further reduce duration of hospital stays and improve outcomes. There is contradicting evidence that these protocols have a significant effect. One recent randomized, controlled trial defined its accelerated intervention as informing the patient of discharge goals, pain relief, and mobilization strategies. Also, they sought to achieve 4 hours out of bed on the first postoperative day and 8 hours for each subsequent day. Finally, standard pain, nausea, and constipation control were also implemented. In this study, compared to the control group who received standard rehabilitation protocols, the interventional group enjoyed statistically significant reductions in length of hospital stay. However, accelerating the rehabilitation pathway too much can lead to higher re-admission rates due to dislocation, wound infection, or excessive joint swelling. Care must be taken to find an appropriate balance to optimize outcomes.[31]

Please read Chapter 21 on Controversies in Total Hip Arthroplasty where many of the issues about changes in THA today are discussed.

References

1. Berato J, Dutour O, Williams J, Zakarian H, Acquaviva PC. [Epidemiology of rheumatic diseases in an ancient population. Study of the Necropole du Haut-Empire de Saint-Lambert (Frejus, Var)]. *Rev Rhum Mal Osteoartic.* 1990;57(5):397-400.
2. Peltier LF. A history of hip surgery. In: Callaghan JJ, Rosenberg AG, Rubash HE, eds. *The Adult Hip.* 2nd ed. Philadephia, PA: Lippincott Williams & Wilkins; 2007:3-31.
3. Wiles P. The surgery of the osteoarthritic hip. *Br J Surg.* 1958;45(193):488-497.
4. Steinberg DR, Steinberg ME. The early history of arthroplasty in the United States. *Clin Orthop Relat Res.* 2000;(374):55-89.
5. Sayre LA. Exsection of the head of the femur and removal of the upper rim of the acetabulum for mobus coxarius. *New York J Med.* 1855;(14):70-82.
6. Thompson FR. An essay on the development of arthroplasty of the hip. *Clin Orthop Relat Res.* 1966;44:73-82.

7. Speed K. The unsolved fracture. *Surg Gynecol Obstet.* 1935;(60):341-352.
8. Ufranc OE. Constructive hip surgery with the vitallium mold; a report on 1,000 cases of arthroplasty of the hip over a fifteen-year period. *J Bone Joint Surg Am.* 1957;39-A(2):237-248.
9. Cooper A. *A Treatise on Dislocations and on Fractures of the Joints.* London, England; 1822:114-175.
10. Steele HH. Triple osteotomy of the innominate bone. *Clin Orthop.* 1977;(122):116-127.
11. Gluck T. Die invaginationsmethode der osteo- und arthroplastik. *Berl Klin Wochenscher.* 1890;(28):732-736.
12. McKee GK, Watson-Farrar J. Replacement of arthritic hips by the McKee-Farrar prosthesis. *J Bone Joint Surg Br.* 1966;48(2):245-259.
13. Le Fanu J. Introduction. In: *The Rise and Fall of Modern Medicine.* New York, New York: Basic Books; 2002: XVI.
14. Donald SM. Sir John Charnley (1911-1982): inspiration to future generations of orthopaedic surgeons. *Scott Med J.* 2007;52(2):43-46.
15. Charnley J. The long-term results of low-friction arthroplasty of the hip performed as a primary intervention. *J Bone Joint Surg Br.* 1972;54(1):61-76.
16. Rothman RH, Cohn JC. Cemented versus cementless total hip arthroplasty. A critical review. *Clin Orthop Relat Res.* 1990;(254):153-169.
17. Greene JW, Malkani AL, Kolisek FR, Jessup NM, Baker DL. Ceramic-on-ceramic total hip arthroplasty. *J Arthroplasty.* 2009;24(6 suppl):15-18.
18. Sochart DH. Relationship of acetabular wear to osteolysis and loosening in total hip arthroplasty. *Clin Orthop Relat Res.* 1999;363:135-150.
19. Savarino L, Greco M, Cenni E, et al. Difference in ion release after ceramic-on ceramic and metal-on-metal total hip replacement medium-term follow-up. *J Bone Joint Surg Br.* 2006;88(4):472-476.
20. Dobbs HS, Minski MJ. Metal ion release after total hip replacment. *Biomaterials.* 1980;1:193-198.
21. Affatato S, Spinelli M, Zavalloni M, Trina F, Carmignato S, Toni A. Ceramic-on-metal for total hip replacement: mixing and matching can lead to high wear. *Artif Organs.* 2010;34(4):319-323.
22. McCalden RW, MacDonald SJ, Rorabeck CH, Bourne RB, Chess DG, Charron KD. Wear rate of highly cross-linked polyethylene in total hip arthroplasty. A randomized controlled trial. *J Bone Joint Surg Am.* 2009;91(4):773-782.
23. Grigoris P, Roberts P, Panousis K, Bosch H. The evolution of hip resurfacing arthroplasty. *Orthop Clin North Am.* 2005;36(2):125-134, vii.
24. Springer BD, Connelly SE, Odum SM, et al. Cementless femoral components in young patients: review and meta-analysis of total hip arthroplasty and hip resurfacing. *J Arthroplasty.* 2009;24(6 suppl):2-8.
25. Ollivere B, Darrah C, Barker T, Nolan J, Porteous M J. Early clinical failure of the Birmingham metal-on-metal hip resurfacing is associated with metallo¬sis and soft-tissue necrosis. *J Bone Joint Surg Br.* 2009;91(8):1025-1030.
26. de Steiger RN, Miller LN, Prosser GH, Graves SE, Davidson DC, Stanford TE. Poor outcome of revised resurfacing hip arthroplasty: 397 cases from the Australia Joint Replacement Registry. *Acta Orthopaedica.* 2010;81(1):72-76.
27. Pandit H, Glyn-Jones S, McLardy-Smith P, et al. Pseudotumours associated with metal-on-metal hip resurfacings. *J Bone Joint Surg Br.* 2008;90(7):847-851.
28. Dorr LD, Shahrdar C. The posterior approach for minimally invasive total hip relpacement surgery. In: Callaghan JJ, Rosenberg AG, Rubash HE, eds. *The Adult Hip.* 2nd ed. Philadelphia, PA: Lippincott Williams & Wilkins; 2007:1540-1550.
29. Woolson ST, Mow CS, Syquia JF, Lannin JV, Schurman DJ. Comparison of primary total hip replacements performed with a standard incision or a mini-incision. *J Bone Joint Surg Am.* 2004;86-A(7):1353-1358.
30. Ciminiello M, Parvizi J, Sharkey PF, Eslampour A, Rothman RH. Total hip arthroplasty: is small incision better? *J Arthroplasty.* 2006;21(4):484-488.
31. Larsen K, Sorensen OG, Hansen TB, Thomsen PB, Soballe K. Accelerated perioperative care and rehabilitation intervention for hip and knee replacement is effective: a randomized clinical trial involving 87 patients with 3 months of follow-up. *Acta Orthop.* 2008;79(2):149-159.

13

Indications for Total Hip Arthroplasty and Total Hip Resurfacing

Adam J. Schwartz, MD and Craig J. Della Valle, MD

Total hip arthroplasty (THA) is one of the most successful procedures performed in modern orthopedics.[1,2] The long-term survivorship of contemporary implants is estimated to approach 96% to 99%.[3,4] One consequence of these impressive results is that the prevalence of THA in the United States continues to rise. A recent study estimates that the demand for THA will increase by over 150% during the next 2 decades due in large part to the steadily growing elderly population.[5]

Amidst such growing enthusiasm, it is incumbent upon the orthopedic surgeon to maintain a realistic understanding of the indications and contraindications to this potentially life-changing procedure. In this chapter, the foundations of the patient-surgeon relationship as it pertains to THA are explored and some of the key considerations prior to THA are discussed. The chapter concludes with a brief discussion of the relative indications and contraindications to hip resurfacing.

General Considerations

The decision to undergo any invasive procedure is frequently met with hesitation and anxiety by most patients. A frank, open discussion between patient and surgeon regarding the risks and benefits of THA will provide the foundation for a strong relationship and may alleviate many of the fears harbored by patients with end-stage arthropathy. Ultimately, the selection of THA as the best course of treatment should be made with a clear understanding of the patient's particular goals and the likelihood of complications.

There exists a plethora of literature devoted to the medical decision-making process that is beyond the scope of this chapter. However, it can be quite edifying for the clinician, both from an academic standpoint as well as pragmatically, to review the risks and benefits in detail with the patient, and tabulate the results of this discussion. Such an exercise will clearly define the patient's interest in surgery and will put complication rates into perspective for both patient and clinician. A simple table, such as the one shown in Table 13-1, is a useful tool to help both the patient and surgeon understand one another. On one side of the table, the patient lists the benefits he or she seeks to obtain from the procedure and assigns a score to each benefit with an associated probability. On the opposite side, the clinician lists the complications most likely associated with the procedure, along with the expected probabilities. It may help to enlist the assistance of the patient's medical physician to help determine the risks specific to the particular case. In addition to clearly defining goals and expectations, such a list may also serve useful postoperatively, in the unfortunate instance that a complication does occur, to remind the patient of his or her reasons for accepting that such an event was possible (see Table 13-1).

In practice, it may not be feasible or even desirable to complete the above exercise with each individual patient. In fact, it would be virtually impossible to list every possible benefit or complication associated with THA, or the likelihood that such events could occur. Nonetheless, this mental process can be useful for the surgeon to perform without explicitly reviewing the results with the patient. Such an exercise will prevent the surgeon from approaching

Parvizi J, Klatt BA.
Essentials in Total Hip Arthroplasty (pp 103-113).

Table 13-1

RISK-BENEFIT ANALYSIS FOR CHOOSING TOTAL HIP ARTHROPLASTY IN THE TREATMENT OF END-STAGE HIP ARTHROSIS

BENEFITS	A	B	C
	Benefit (score)	Likelihood (%)	Total (A x B)
1. Decreased pain	10	.95	9.5
2. Improved function	50	.95	47.5
3. Other	##	%	A x B
4. Other	##	%	A x B
Total			**57**
RISKS	A	B	C
	Risk (score)	Likelihood (%)	Total (A x B)
1. Death	100	.2	2
2. Infection	100	.1	1
3. Other	##	%	A x B
4. Other	##	%	A x B
Total			**3**

A simplified risk-benefit analysis can be useful in choosing THA as the best alternative in the treatment of end-stage hip arthrosis. Scores are given based on the patient's desire to achieve the given benefit or avoid the given risk. Risks and benefits may be added depending on the patient's unique conditions. In this case, the benefits (total score = 57) outweigh the risks (total score = 3) and THA is indicated.

patients with rigid algorithms and will reinforce the concept that indications for THA must remain tailored to each individual patient.

Prior to a discussion of specific indications and contraindications, the need for realistic and clear patient expectations cannot be overemphasized. A variety of recent studies have demonstrated that patient expectations are an independent predictor of the outcome of THA. In particular, one recent study cited the patient expectation of complete pain relief as a predictor of improved physical function and pain relief at 6 months following THA.[6] In addition, patients who had expectations of low complication rates had greater postoperative satisfaction than those who did not. Thus, it appears that patient attitudes play a much larger role than previously expected.

INDICATIONS FOR TOTAL HIP ARTHROPLASTY

In general, any patient considered a candidate for THA should have already undergone an earnest attempt at nonoperative management. This typically includes the use of assistive devices, oral nonsteroidal medications, acetaminophen, and activity modifications.[7] It is important to advise patients, however, that nonoperative treatment is not without risk.[8] The chronic use of nonsteroidal anti-inflammatory medications has been shown in numerous studies to cause gastrointestinal, cardiac, renal, and hepatic complications. Patients using oral pain medications for longer than 3 months should undergo routine hepatic and renal screening tests under the supervision of a primary care physician.

The primary indication for THA in a patient with end-stage arthropathy is pain resulting in significant limitation of physical activity. With survivorship of contemporary THA components estimated to approach 20 years, those patients with greater than 20 years life expectancy should be counseled regarding the likelihood of the need for future surgery.[3,9,10] In addition, it is important for the surgeon to remember that the definition of both pain and limitation of physical activity may differ from patient to patient, depending on baseline condition. Important factors to be considered in the decision to recommend or undergo THA are patient age, diagnosis, and medical comorbidities.

Age

The patient and surgeon must recognize that current data describing the longevity of THA are largely drawn from retrospective, nonblinded cohort reviews. It may be gleaned from this limited evidence, however, that excellent long-term pain relief can be obtained in low-demand patients up to 20 years or more.[3,9,10] On the contrary, patients with greater than 20 years' life expectancy can anticipate the high likelihood of a need for future revision surgery. For patients over the age of 65, the need for revision surgery due to wear and aseptic loosening is less likely, and the indication for surgery is typically more straightforward.[11]

The more complex clinical scenario for the surgeon is presented by the patient between 30 to 60 years of age, with a painful hip that limits daily activities. In this group, and in even younger patients, the need for a concerted attempt at nonoperative treatment is essential. It is likely that patients in this age category will require at least one revision procedure in future years, and this should be discussed preoperatively. Additionally, it should be explained that activity modifications, including the avoidance of repetitive high-impact exercises, will protect both the implant fixation and bearing surface after THA. Patients unwilling to modify their activities accordingly are less than ideal candidates.

In the short-term following THA, the main reasons for revision continue to be infection, instability, and aseptic loosening.[12] In the long-term, however, the most common mode of failure is wear of the bearing surface resulting in osteolytic lesions and catastrophic loosening of the implant.[11] As a result, attempts have been made over recent years to improve the wear characteristics of bearing surfaces, particularly for younger, high-demand patients.

Growing data exist to support the contention that newer bearing designs will outlast their older counterparts.[13-22] Again, it must be recognized that these retrospective reviews provide little evidence of implant survivorship beyond 15 years. Additionally, while laboratory data would suggest the absence of clinically significant wear in metal-on-metal, ceramic-on-ceramic, and metal-on-highly-crossed-linked polyethylene bearing surfaces, surgeons have previously witnessed the disastrous results when in vitro data fail to translate in vivo.[23] For these reasons, it is crucial that the surgeon remains realistic with younger, higher-demand patients, and explains the limitations in accurately predicting implant survivorship (Figure 13-1).

Aside from the above limitations, many authors have demonstrated excellent long-term results from THA even in extremely young patients. In a retrospective review of THAs in patients with early-onset juvenile rheumatoid arthritis (mean age 17.8 years), Kitsoulis et al demonstrated excellent long-term results. With over 20-year follow-up, only one acetabular component was revised due to aseptic loosening. The authors advised that surgery in this age population is technically more difficult and should be performed in specialized centers.[24] It is encouraging, however, that such results may be obtained when other treatment modalities fail in this patient population.

Diagnosis

The most common diagnosis for which THA is indicated is osteoarthritis.[5] The results of THA in patients with radiographic signs of severe degenerative joint disease coupled with anterior thigh or groin pain are quite reliable. Less commonly, the surgeon will encounter patients with radiographic findings of severe hip degeneration and the absence of characteristic hip pain, or patients with pain out of proportion to the radiographic findings. In either scenario, it is important to search for other sources of pain, and if the pain has been present for more than 3 to 6 weeks, it would be prudent to obtain further imaging, typically with magnetic resonance imaging.

It must be remembered that in patients with osteoarthritis of the hip other joints are typically affected as well, in addition to long-standing gait and posture disorders. Specifically, concomitant lumbosacral spine arthropathy is quite common among these patients, and pain radiating below the knee to the foot is more likely to be attributable to disease within the spine than the hip. Such patients should be advised that THA will not likely relieve pain radiating from the spine, and while the patient's gait may improve postoperatively, there is a possibility of worsening pain from other joints due to increased mobility.

Patients with end-stage arthrosis secondary to inflammatory arthropathy are also excellent candidates for THA. Preoperative evaluation of patients with rheumatoid arthritis should include radiographs of the cervical spine to rule out pre-existing C1-C2 subluxation. In addition, large erosions and severe bone deficiencies are typical of this patient population, and preoperative templating should alert the surgeon to the need for special implants. Results in this group are encouraging, even in those with early-onset or juvenile rheumatoid arthritis. Various studies have shown a decreased incidence of implant loosening, and the highest rate of implant survivorship for this group.[25,26] Sochart et al reviewed the results of 226 Charley low-friction arthroplasties at a mean of 20 years and found the lowest incidence of implant failure in the 63 patients with rheumatoid arthritis compared to those with congenital hip dislocation or

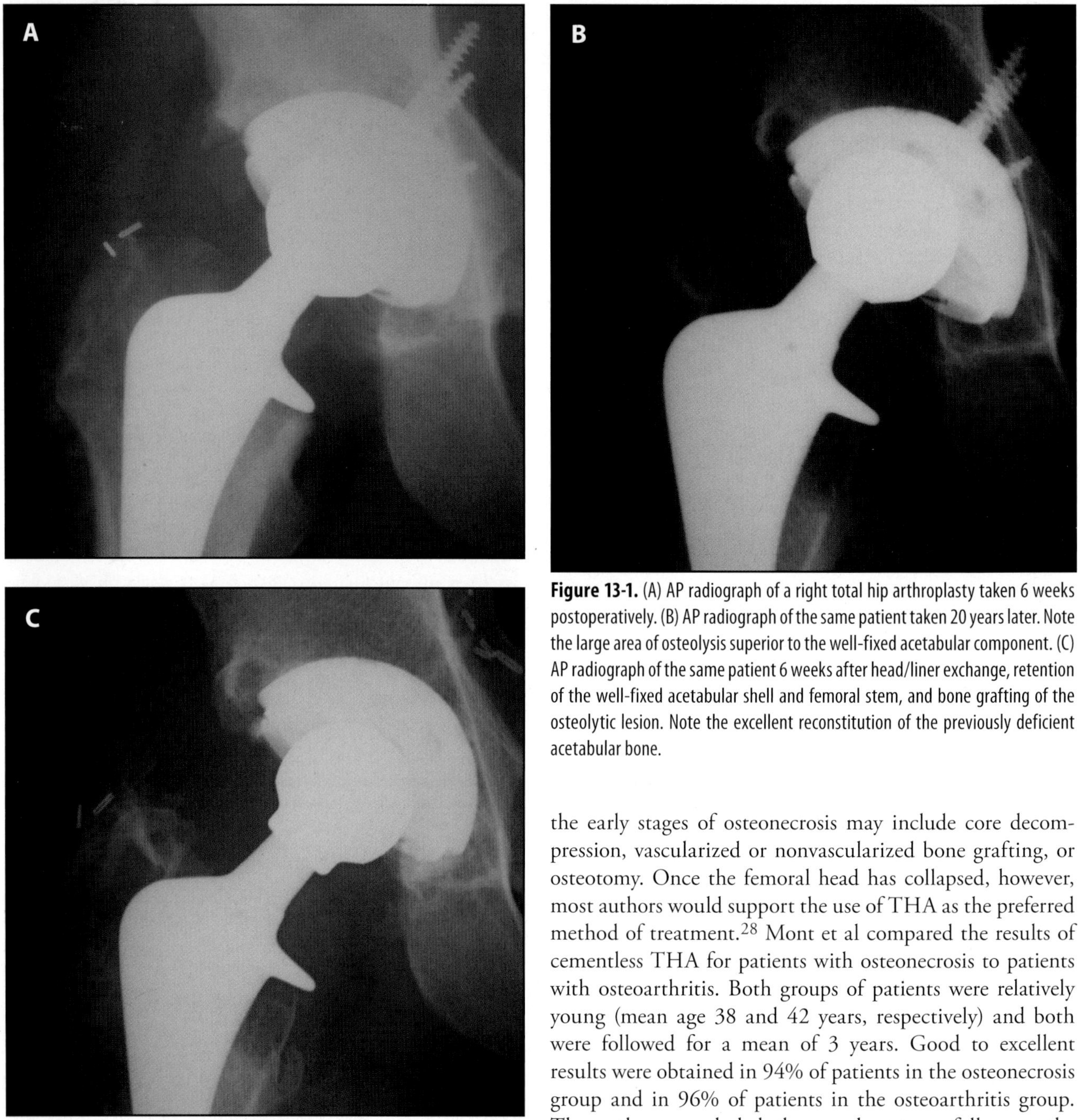

Figure 13-1. (A) AP radiograph of a right total hip arthroplasty taken 6 weeks postoperatively. (B) AP radiograph of the same patient taken 20 years later. Note the large area of osteolysis superior to the well-fixed acetabular component. (C) AP radiograph of the same patient 6 weeks after head/liner exchange, retention of the well-fixed acetabular shell and femoral stem, and bone grafting of the osteolytic lesion. Note the excellent reconstitution of the previously deficient acetabular bone.

osteoarthritis. This increased longevity is likely due to the lower level of activity typical of patients with severe rheumatoid arthritis.[26]

Osteonecrosis of the hip is a common cause of end-stage arthropathy. The etiology of osteonecrosis is simplified to include direct and indirect causes.[27] The most common direct cause is trauma resulting in decreased blood supply to the femoral head, while atraumatic osteonecrosis is most likely due to corticosteroid use or alcoholism. Treatment of the early stages of osteonecrosis may include core decompression, vascularized or nonvascularized bone grafting, or osteotomy. Once the femoral head has collapsed, however, most authors would support the use of THA as the preferred method of treatment.[28] Mont et al compared the results of cementless THA for patients with osteonecrosis to patients with osteoarthritis. Both groups of patients were relatively young (mean age 38 and 42 years, respectively) and both were followed for a mean of 3 years. Good to excellent results were obtained in 94% of patients in the osteonecrosis group and in 96% of patients in the osteoarthritis group. The authors concluded that at short-term follow-up the results appear equivalent.[27]

The debate regarding the role of THA in patients with an acute femoral neck fracture continues to evolve.[29,30] The 2 most important predictors of outcome in this group of patients seem to be physiologic age and fracture displacement. For younger patients with nondisplaced fractures, internal fixation and joint salvage remains the gold standard treatment. For elderly patients with a displaced femoral neck fracture, prosthetic replacement seems to be both cost-effective and associated with improved pain and

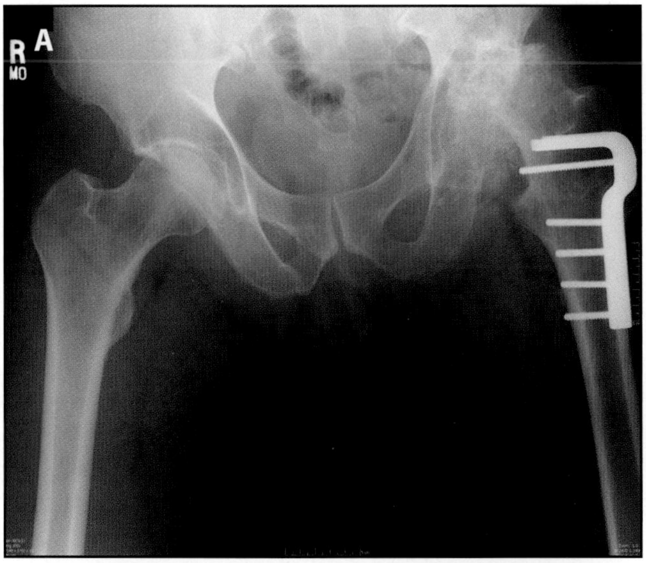

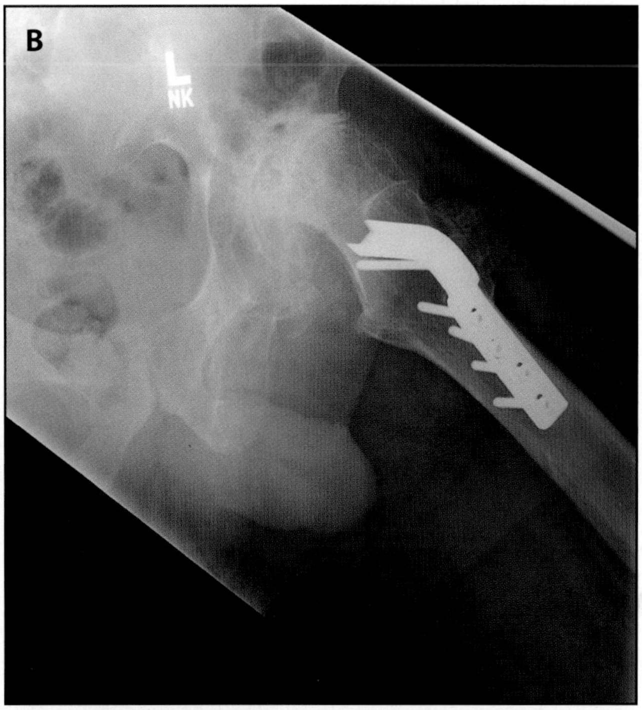

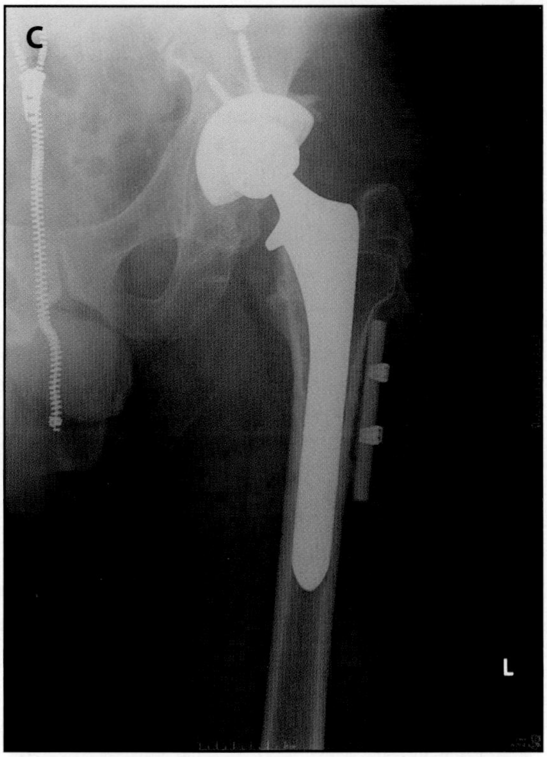

Figure 13-2. (A) AP radiograph of a 62-year-old male with a history of previous proximal femoral osteotomy. (B) Lateral radiograph of the same patient. (C) Postoperative AP radiograph of the left hip after conversion to THA and supplemental fixation with a cortical allograft strut and cerclage cables.

function scores in multiple long-term studies. The literature would support the use of THA in this patient population as the most durable, cost-effective treatment alternative.[31,32] Hemiarthroplasty is useful in patients without evidence of acetabular wear, but concerns exist regarding the early development of groin pain.[33] There does not appear to be any difference between the use of bipolar and unipolar hemiarthroplasty in this group.[32,34-36]

THA in patients with a previous history of trauma or surgery can be technically challenging (Figure 13-2). As discussed previously, the patient's anatomy is typically abnormal. Preoperative templating and planning is particularly useful in this scenario to alert the surgeon to potential intraoperative problems, and the need for special instruments to remove previously placed hardware. For patients with a history of multiple previous surgeries, or even multiple previous attempts at total joint arthroplasty, the Charnley "pseudarthrosis" test is helpful to decide whether to proceed with a repeated attempt at salvage. The essence of the pseudarthrosis test is to proceed with an attempt at THA if the patient would be no worse off with a resection arthroplasty than the present condition.[37] Previous hip fracture and prior hip surgery certainly confers a higher risk of perioperative complications, including dislocation and fracture.[38-40] Because it can be difficult in such cases to obtain a good repair of the deficient posterior soft tissues, some authors have advocated the use of an anterior approach in these patients to reduce dislocation rates. Despite these limitations, the longevity of implants after failed internal fixation is excellent, with one study demonstrating 100% survivorship at 7-year follow-up, and 87.5% survivorship at 10-year follow-up.[38]

The results of THA for severe developmental dysplasia are mixed, with some series showing excellent long-term survivorship and others reporting a greater than 25% revision rate.[41-44] Many patients with long-standing congenital

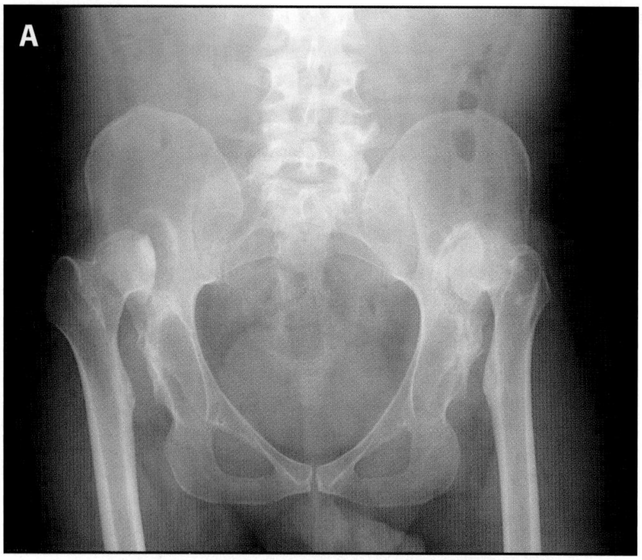

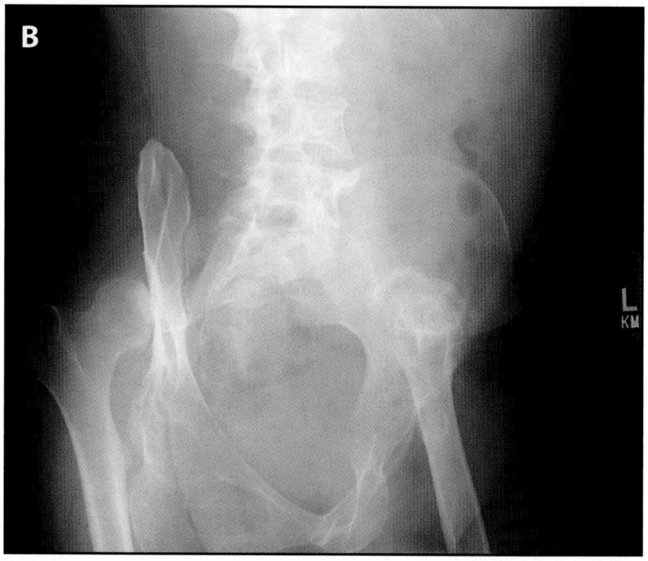

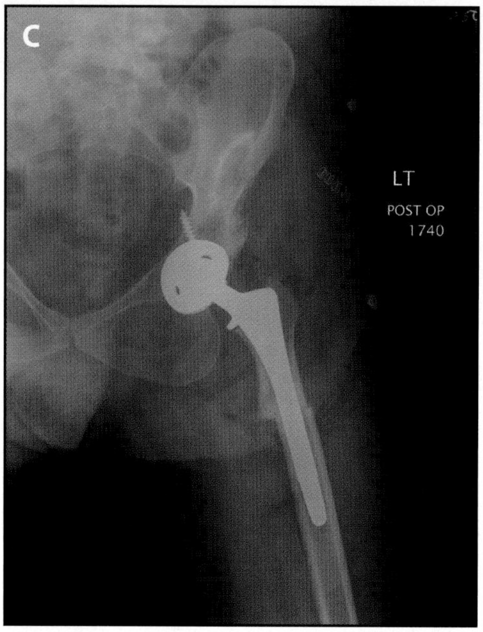

Figure 13-3. (A) AP pelvis radiograph of an otherwise healthy 46-year-old male with a history of bilateral developmental hip dysplasia. Note the location of the acetabular tear-drop, indicating the native location of the hip center of rotation. (B) Lateral radiograph demonstrating excessive superior migration of the femoral head. (C) Postoperative radiograph following THA and femoral shortening osteotomy. The hip center of rotation has been restored.

hip dislocation are surprisingly functional and have very little pain. It is not uncommon for patients to accommodate to this hip deformity into their fifth and sixth decades. The major indication for joint replacement in this population is significant pain leading to a progressive deterioration of function. The surgeon should have an open discussion with the patient prior to surgery regarding the particular risks involved with THA for severe dysplasia. Specifically, it should be explained that restoring the hip center of rotation may involve significant lengthening of the limb, placing the neurovascular structures at risk of injury. For patients with Crowe IV deformity, when the expected limb-lengthening will exceed 3 cm, a subtrochanteric shortening osteotomy is indicated (Figure 13-3).

Medical Comorbidities

THA is designed to improve patient quality of life, and as such, it should be presented to the patient as an elective procedure. In rare instances, the need for THA becomes more urgent, such as in cases of rapidly progressing acetabular bone loss, which could compromise the outcome of future surgery (Figure 13-4). More typically, however, the decision to undergo THA should be made in a controlled manner as described above, allowing for a discussion of the particular risks and benefits to each particular patient.

The existence of significant pre-existing medical comorbidities certainly places the patient at greater risk for perioperative and postoperative complications after any elective procedure, and THA is no exception.[45] In a retrospective review of over 30,000 patients who underwent THA over a period of 30 years, Parvizi et al reported 90 deaths (0.29%) within 30 days of surgery.[46] Mortality rates were statistically higher for patients with pre-existing cardiovascular disease and those greater than 70 years of age. Interestingly, during the last decade of the study period, there was a statistically significant decline in mortality rates (0.29% to 0.15%). Similarly, Dearborn et al reviewed the results of 2736 primary and revision THAs performed over the same time period.[47] Eight deaths (0.3%) occurred within the first 90 days after surgery. The authors attributed half of this mortality rate to pre-existing severe cardiovascular or hepatorenal disease.

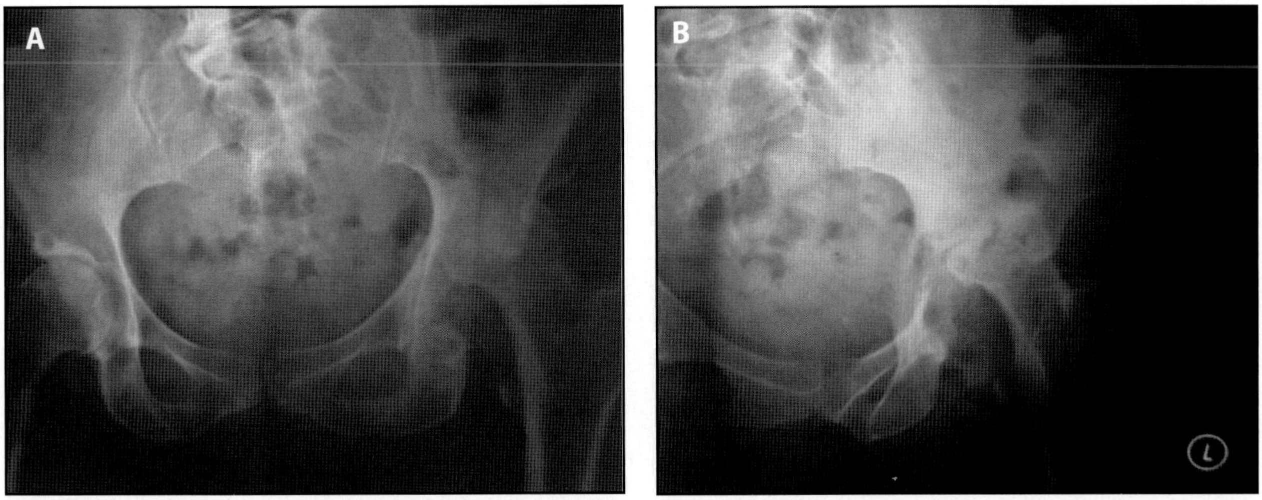

Figure 13-4. (A) AP pelvis radiograph of a 46-year-old female with a history of severe left hip pain. Note the superior migration of the femoral head and resultant leg length discrepancy. (B) AP hip radiograph of the same patient demonstrating severe acetabular bone loss in this native hip.

Preoperative evaluation should include a thorough history and physical examination by a medical physician to determine the existence of significant medical comorbidities. A team approach to patient care will provide a more clear understanding of the patient's particular risks and aid in the immediate perioperative management.

Contraindications to Total Hip Arthroplasty

The main contraindication to THA is active local or systemic infection.[48] Patients with a history of previous hip infection should undergo thorough preoperative evaluation, including erythrocyte sedimentation rate, C-reactive protein, complete blood count, and joint aspiration. If all these tests are negative, the likelihood of infection is low; however, the patient should be counseled that intra-operative findings may dictate the need for resection arthroplasty and antibiotic spacer placement. Intra-operative biopsy in such patients may help to confirm the absence of a subacute infection. Excellent clinical results have been demonstrated in patients with a history of joint infection greater than 10 years prior to THA.[49] Active acquired immunodeficiency syndrome (AIDS) may also be considered a contraindication as the risks of infection and other medical complications may outweigh the risks of surgery.

While not considered a firm contraindication to THA, morbid obesity has been shown in numerous studies to result in higher perioperative complication rates.[50,51] In a review of 1071 THAs, Namba et al found that 36% of patients were classified as morbidly obese, with a higher proportion being female. The odds ratio for infection was 4.2 times higher in obese patients (BMI >35) than nonobese patients.[51] Similarly, Lubekke et al reviewed a cohort of 93 patients, of whom 31 were classified as being obese (BMI >35). Obese patients had a higher dislocation rate and higher risk of revision.[50] Other studies repudiate these claims, citing technical error as the reason for higher complication rates among morbidly obese patients, but the issue remains controversial.

Hip Resurfacing

Two devices are presently FDA approved for use in the United States for metal-on-metal total hip resurfacing; the Birmingham Hip Resurfacing (Smith and Nephew, Memphis, TN) and the Cormet 2000 (Stryker, Mahwah, NJ). The putative benefits of hip resurfacing when compared to conventional THA are conservation of femoral bone stock, relative ease of femoral revision, wear resistance, increased range of motion, and a decreased risk of dislocation.[52,53] In addition, the available literature would support a higher likelihood of patients with hip resurfacing returning to running and heavy manual labor.[54-56]

A discussion regarding the indications for hip resurfacing is essentially a discussion of the history of the procedure and the previous failures encountered with its use. Early designs introduced in the 1960s were fraught with fixation and wear issues. The poor tolerance of the metal-on-metal manufacturing process resulted in high rates of wear and osteolysis. Due to the success of other designs at the time, interest in metal-on-metal as a bearing surface quickly waned.[57]

Contemporary manufacturing techniques confer much greater precision, and several studies have demonstrated superior wear characteristics of newer metal-on-metal bearings in the realm of THA.[15,17,20,21] Similarly, the early results of metal-on-metal resurfacing arthroplasty have demonstrated excellent clinical results at 10 years.[55,56] Concerns regarding metal hypersensitivity and increased blood ion levels have tempered some enthusiasm over the metal-on-metal bearing surfaces. While no long-term data suggest adverse outcomes from increased blood ion levels, the threat of systemic complications has caused a general hesitance to use this type of bearing surface in women of child-bearing years or the very young.

More recently, locally aggressive lesions that have been described as "pseudotumors" have been described and have further made surgeons more cautious regarding hip resurfacing and metal-on-metal bearings in general.[58] These local soft tissue reactions are thought to be related to edge loading of the bearing surface, which causes high wear and a subsequent local inflammatory response that can lead to pain, swelling (hence the name *pseudotumor*), and if neglected soft tissue and even bony damage. Risk factors for this complication include component malposition (typically vertical acetabular components), small component size, and female sex.[59] It is thought that the relationship with female sex may be related to increased femoral and acetabular anteversion, particularly seen in younger female patients with hip dysplasia, which similarly causes edge loading of the bearing surface.

The main concern following hip resurfacing arthroplasty, however, continues to be postoperative femoral neck fracture.[60] Several studies have attempted to define the various factors that confer an increased risk of femoral neck fracture. Excessive varus or valgus positioning (greater than 10 degrees) has been shown to be associated with notching of the femoral neck and reduced load to fracture.[61] In addition, female gender, poor bone quality, and femoral head cysts greater than 1 cm in diameter were all associated with a higher likelihood of postoperative femoral neck fracture.[52,60-62] Although not absolute contraindications to hip resurfacing, the above factors need to be carefully considered preoperatively and discussed with the patient. In a series of 3500 hip resurfacing arthroplasties performed by 89 surgeons, the rate of femoral neck fracture in women was nearly double that seen among men (1.9% versus 0.98%, relative risk 1.95, $p < 0.01$) When compared with conventional THA, the risk of early revision for any reason was increased in women over the age of 60, and not significantly different for men under the age of 55 who carried a diagnosis of osteoarthritis.[54]

The role of hip resurfacing in patients with osteonecrosis of the femoral head continues to be defined. Some authors have expressed concern regarding the ability of the diseased subchondral bone to support the resurfacing component. Two recent studies demonstrated similar short-to-medium term results following hip resurfacing in this patient population. Mont et al reported excellent results in 93% of patients with osteonecrosis of the femoral head, compared to 98% of patients with a diagnosis of osteoarthritis.[63] Similarly, Revell et al demonstrated 93% good to excellent results at a mean of 6 years postoperatively.[64] Such results certainly indicate that hip resurfacing can be effective for the treatment of osteonecrosis, but patients who carry this diagnosis should be advised of these slightly inferior results.

The lack of modularity is also a consideration for patients with greater pre-existing deformity. Hip resurfacing arthroplasty is a technically demanding procedure that does not allow the surgeon the intra-operative flexibility to tailor leg lengths or offset and thus patients with symptomatic leg length discrepancy are better handled with conventional THA. Furthermore, abnormal acetabular anatomy, as seen in cases of moderate to severe dysplasia, may be problematic as most resurfacing systems do not allow for the use of adjunctive screw fixation. This may limit the surgeon's ability to reconstruct a shallow or otherwise deficient acetabulum.

In general, the absolute contraindications to hip resurfacing are the same as those previously discussed in the section on conventional THA. Currently available resurfacing implants require the use of a metal-on-metal bearing surface, which has been shown in numerous studies to elevate blood metal ion levels. The surgeon must recognize that while the clinical significance of this side effect has not been firmly established, the potential for future complications cannot be dismissed. This is particularly true for women of child-bearing age as metal ions have been shown to freely cross the placenta, leading to elevated fetal ion levels. Additionally, patients with chronic renal failure who cannot metabolize these ions and patients with a known diagnosis of metal allergy should be discouraged from undergoing prosthetic joint replacement with a metal-on-metal bearing surface.

Based on a review of the available literature, patients with the lowest risk of early revision appear to be males with osteoarthritis who are less than 55 years of age. As this same patient population is at higher risk for revision with conventional THA, hip resurfacing seems a reasonable alternative.

Summary

THA is a potentially life-altering procedure that offers the advantages of reliable pain relief, improved function, and increased independence. The primary indication for THA is pain and limited activity due to end-stage arthropathy refractory to nonoperative treatment. The definitions of pain and limited activity may vary widely from patient to patient, and as a result, it is the surgeon's duty to convey his or her knowledge and experience in a manner that allows the patient to make an informed decision. Such a decision should be founded upon a clear understanding of the particular risks involved, the likely benefits to be obtained, and the various treatment alternatives. With current techniques and the proper indications, the vast majority of patients who choose to undergo THA will experience years of lasting pain relief and improved function.

References

1. Jones CA, Voaklander DC, Johnson DW, et al. Health related quality of life outcomes after total hip and knee arthroplasties in a community based population. *J Rheumatol.* 2000;27;1745-1752.
2. Laupacis A, Bourne R, Rorabeck C, et al. The effect of elective total hip replacement on health related quality of life. *J Bone Joint Surg Am.* 1993;75:1619-1626.
3. Velyvis JH, Rubash HE, Callaghan JJ. Primary total hip arthroplasty: cementless and cemented. In: Barrack RL, Booth RE, Lonner JH, McCarthy JC, Mont MA, Rubash HE, eds. *Orthopaedic Knowledge Update: Hip and Knee Reconstruction 3.* Rosemont, IL: AAOS; 2006.
4. Archibeck MJ, Berger RA, Jacobs JJ, et al. Second-generation cementless total hip arthroplasty. Eight to eleven-year results. *J Bone Joint Surg Am.* 2001;83-A(11):1666-1673.
5. Kurtz, S, Ong, K, Lau, E, Mowat, F, Halpern M. Projections of primary and revision hip and knee arthroplasty in the United States from 2005 to 2030. *J Bone Joint Surg Am.* 2007;89(4):780-785.
6. Mahomed NN, Liang MH, Cook EF, et al. The importance of patient expectations in predicting functional outcomes after total joint arthroplasty. *J Rhematol.* 2003;30(7):1656-1657.
7. Brand RA, Crowninshield RD. The effect of cane use on hip contact force. *Clin Orthop Relat Res.* 1980;147:181-184.
8. Fries JF, Bruce B. Rates of serious gastrointestinal events from low dose use of acetylsalicylic acid, acetaminophen, and ibuprofen in patients with osteoarthritis and rheumatoid arthritis. *J Rhematol.* 2003;30(10):2226-2233.
9. Callaghan JJ, Albright JC, Goetz DD, et al. Charnley total hip arthroplasty with cement: minimum twenty-five year followup. *J Bone Joint Surg Am.* 2000;82:487-497.
10. Della Valle CJ, Berger RA, Shott S, et al. Primary total hip arthroplasty with a porous coated acetabular component: a concise follow-up of a previous report. *J Bone Joint Surg Am.* 2004;86;1217-1222.
11. Ulrich SD, Seyler TM, Bennett D, et al. Total hip arthroplasties: what are the reasons for revision? *Int Orthop.* 2008;32(5):597-604.
12. Dobzyniak M, Fehring TK, Odum S. Early failure in total hip arthroplasty. *Clin Orthop Relat Res.* 2006;447:76-78.
13. D'Antonio J, Capello W, Manley M, Naughton M, Sutton K. Alumina ceramic bearings for total hip arthroplasty: five-year results of a prospective randomized study. *Clin Orthop Relat Res.* 2005;(436):164-171.
14. Digas G, Kärrholm J, Thanner J, Malchau H, Herberts P. The Otto Aufranc Award. Highly cross-linked polyethylene in total hip arthroplasty: randomized evaluation of penetration rate in cemented and uncemented sockets using radiostereometric analysis. *Clin Orthop Relat Res.* 2004;(429):6-16.
15. Dorr LD, Wan Z, Longjohn DB, Dubois B, Murken R. Total hip arthroplasty with use of the Metasul metal-on-metal articulation. Four to seven-year results. *J Bone Joint Surg Am.* 2001;83-A(5):783-785.
16. Geerdink CH, Grimm B, Ramakrishnan R, Rondhuis J, Verburg AJ, Tonino AJ. Crosslinked polyethylene compared to conventional polyethylene in total hip replacement: pre-clinical evaluation, in-vitro testing and prospective clinical follow-up study. *Acta Orthop.* 2006;77(5):719-725.
17. Grubl A, Marker M, Brodner W, et al. Long-term follow-up of metal-on-metal total hip replacement. *J Orthop Res.* 2007;25(7):841-848.
18. Kim SY, Kim DH, Oh CW, Kim PT, Ihn JC, Kim SY. Total hip arthroplasty with the use of nonmodular cementless acetabular component. *J Arthroplasty.* 2005;20(5):632-638.
19. Leung SB, Egawa H, Stepniewski A, Beykirch S, Engh CA Jr, Engh CA Sr. Incidence and volume of pelvic osteolyisis at early follow-up with highly cross-linked and noncross-linked polyethylene. *J Arthroplasty.* 2007;22(6 suppl 2):134-139.
20. MacDonald SJ, McCalden RW, Chess DG, et al. Metal-on-metal versus polyethylene in hip arthroplasty: a randomized clinical trial. *Clin Orthop Relat Res.* 2003;(406):282-296.
21. Saito S, Ryu J, Watanabe M, Ishii T, Saigo K. Midterm results of Metasul metal-on-metal total hip arthroplasty. *J Arthroplasty.* 2006;21(8):1105-1110.
22. Seyler TM, Bonutti PM, Shen J, Naughton M, Kester M. Use of alumina-on-alumina bearing system in total hip arthroplasty for osteonecrosis of the hip. *J Bone Joint Surg Am.* 2006;88(suppl 3):116-125.
23. Livingston, BJ, Chmell MJ, Spector M, Poss R. Complications of total hip arthroplasty associated with the use of an acetabular component with a Hylamer liner. *J Bone Joint Surg Am.* 1997;79(10):1529-1538.
24. Kitsoulis PB, Siamopoulou A, Beris AE, Xenakis TA. Total hip and knee arthroplasty for juvenile rheumatoid arthritis. *Folia Med (Plovdiv).* 2006;48(3-4):42-49.

25. Katsimihas M, Taylor AH, Lee MB, et al. Cementless acetabular replacement in patients with rheumatoid arthritis: A 6 to 14 year prospective study. *J Arthroplasty.* 2003;18(1):16-22.
26. Sochart DH, Porter ML. The long-term results of Charnley low-friction arthroplasty in young patients who have congenital dislocation, degenerative osteoarthrosis, or rheumatoid arthritis. *J Bone Joint Surg Am.* 1997;79(11):1599-1617.
27. Mont MA, Seyler TM, Plate JF, Delanois RE, Parvizi J. Uncemented total hip arthroplasty in young adults with osteonecrosis of the femoral head: a comparative study. *J Bone Joint Surg Am.* 2006;88(suppl 3):104-109.
28. Mont MA, Lonner JH, Ragland PS. Osteonecrosis of the hip. In: Barrack, RL, Booth, RE, Lonner JH, McCarthy JC, Mont MA, Rubash HE, eds. *Orthopaedic Knowledge Update: Hip and Knee Reconstruction 3.* Rosemont, IL: AAOS; 2006.
29. Bhandari M, Devereaux PJ, Tornetta P III, et al. Operative management of displaced femoral neck fractures in elderly patients. An international survey. *J Bone Joint Surg Am.* 2005;87(9):2122-2130.
30. Iorio R, Schwartz B, Macaulay W, Teeney SM, Healy WL, York S. Surgical treatment of displaced femoral neck fractures in the elderly: a survey of the American Association of Hip and Knee Surgeons. *J Arthroplasty.* 2006;21(8):1124-1133.
31. Blomfeldt R, Törnkvist H, Eriksson K, Söderqvist A, Ponzer S, Tidermark J. A randomised controlled trial comparing bipolar hemiarthroplasty with total hip replacement for displaced intracapsular fractures of the femoral neck in elderly patients. *J Bone Joint Surg Br.* 2007;89(2):160-165.
32. Narayan KK, George T. Functional outcome of fracture neck of femur treated with total hip replacement versus bipolar arthroplasty in a South Asian population. *Arch Orthop Trauma Surg.* 2006;126(8):545-548.
33. Macaulay W, Pagnotto MR, Iorio R, Mont MA, Saleh KJ. Displaced femoral neck fractures in the elderly: hemiarthroplasty versus total hip arthroplasty. *J Am Acad Orthop Surg.* 2006;14(5):287-293.
34. Ong BC, Maurer SG, Aharonoff GB, Zuckerman JD, Koval KJ. Unipolar versus bipolar hemiarthroplasty: functional outcome after femoral neck fracture at a minimum of thirty-six months of follow-up. *J Orthop Trauma.* 2002;16(5):317-322.
35. Raia FJ, Chapman CB, Herrera MF, Schweppe MW, Michelsen CB, Rosenwasser MP. Unipolar or bipolar hemiarthroplasty for femoral neck fractures in the elderly? *Clin Orthop Relat Res.* 2003;(414):259-265.
36. Wathne RA, Koval KJ, Aharonoff GB, Zuckerman JD, Jones DA. Modular unipolar versus bipolar prosthesis: a prospective evaluation of functional outcome after femoral neck fracture. *J Orthop Trauma.* 1995;9(4):298-302.
37. Charnley J. *Low Friction Arthroplasty of the Hip: Theory and Practice.* New York, NY: Springer Verlag; 1979.
38. Haidukewych GJ, Berry DJ. Hip arthroplasty for salvage of failed treatment of intertrochanteric hip fractures. *J Bone Joint Surg Am.* 2003;85-A(5):899-904.
39. Sierra RJ, Cabanela ME. Conversion of failed hip hemiarthroplasties after femoral neck fractures. *Clin Orthop.* 2002;399:129-139.
40. Jacobs JJ, Kull LT, Frey GA, et al. Early failure of acetabular components inserted without cement after previous pelvic irradiation. *J Bone Joint Surg Am.* 1995;77;1829-1835.
41. Cabanela ME. Total hip arthroplasty for developmental dysplasia of the hip. *Orthopedics.* 2001:24(9):865-866.
42. Cameron HU, Lee OB, Chou H. Total hip arthroplasty in patients with deficient bone stock and small femoral canals. *J Arthroplasty.* 2003;18(1):35-40.
43. DiFazio F, Shon WY, Salvati EA, Wilson PD. Long-term results of total hip arthroplasty with a cemented custom designed swan neck femoral component for congenital dislocation or severe dysplasia: a follow-up note. *J Bone Joint Surg Am.* 2002;84-A(2):204-207.
44. Ito H, Matsuno T, Minami A, Aoki Y. Intermediate-term results after hybrid total hip arthroplasty for the treatment of dyplastic hips. *J Bone Joint Surg Am.* 2003;85-A(9):1725-1732.
45. Sakalkale DP, Hozak WJ, Rothman RH. Total hip arthroplasty in patients on long-term renal dialysis. *J Arthroplasty.* 1999;14:571-575.
46. Parvizi J, Johnson BG, Rowland C, Ereth MH, Lewallen DG. Thirty-day mortality after elective total hip arthroplasty. *J Bone Joint Surg Am.* 2001;83-A(10):1524-1528.
47. Dearborn JT, Harris WH. Postoperative mortality after total hip arthroplasty. An analysis of deaths after two thousand seven hundred and thirty-six procedures. *J Bone Joint Surg Am.* 1998;80(9):1291-1294.
48. Della Valle CJ, Rosenberg AG. Primary total hip arthroplasty: indications and contraindications. In: Callaghan JJ, Rosenberg AG, Rubash HE, eds. *The Adult Hip.* Lippincott Williams & Wilkins; 2007.
49. Robbins GM, Masri BA, Garbuz DS, et al. Primary total hip arthroplasty after infection. Instr Course Lect. 2001;50:317-333.
50. Lübbeke A, Stern R, Garavaglia G, Zurcher L, Hoffmeyer P. Differences in outcomes of obese women and men undergoing primary total hip arthroplasty. *Arthritis Rheum.* 2007;57(2):327-334.
51. Namba RS, Paxton L, Fithian DC, Stone ML. Obesity and perioperative morbidity in total hip and total knee arthroplasty patients. *J Arthroplasty.* 2005;20(7 suppl 3):46-50.
52. Amstutz HC, Ball ST, Le Duff MJ, Dorey FJ. Resurfacing THA for patients younger than 50 years: results of 2- to 9-year followup. *Clin Orthop Relat Res.* 2007;460:159-164.
53. Amstutz HC, Campbell P, Le Duff MJ. Metal-on-metal hip resurfacing: what have we learned? *Instr Course Lect.* 2007;56:149-161.
54. Buergi M, Walter W. Hip resurfacing arthroplasty: the Australian experience. *J Arthroplasty.* 2007:22(7):61-65.
55. Daniel J, Pynsent PB, McMinn DJ. Metal-on-metal resurfacing of the hip in patients under the age of 55 years with osteoarthritis. *J Bone Joint Surg Br.* 2004;86(2):177-184.
56. Pollard TC, Baker RP, Eastaugh-Waring SJ, Bannister GC. Treatment of the young active patient with osteoarthritis of the hip. A five- to seven-year comparison of hybrid total hip arthroplasty and metal-on-metal resurfacing. *J Bone Joint Surg Br.* 2006;88(5):592-600.

57. Mont MA, Ragland PA, Etienne G, et al. Hip resurfacing arthroplasty. *J Am Acad of Orthop Surg.* 2006;14(8):454-463.

58. Pandit H, Glyn-Jones S, McLardy-Smith P, et al. Pseudotumours associated with metal-on-metal hip resurfacings. *J Bone Joint Surg Br.* 2008;90(7):847-851.

59. Glyn-Jones S, Pandit H, Kwon YM, Doll H, Gill HS, Murray DW. Risk factors for inflammatory pseudotumour formation following hip resurfacing. *J Bone Joint Surg Br.* 2009;91(12):1566-1574.

60. Shimmin AJ, Back D. Femoral neck fractures following Birmingham hip resurfacing: a national review of 50 cases. *J Bone Joint Surg Br.* 2005;87(4):463-464.

61. Anglin C, Masri BA, Tonetti J, Hodgson AJ, Greidanus NV. Hip resurfacing femoral neck fracture influenced by valgus placement. *Clin Orthop Relat Res.* 2007;465:71-79.

62. Marker DR, Seyler TM, Jinnah RH, Delanois RE, Ulrich SD, Mont MA. Femoral neck fractures after metal-on-metal total hip resurfacing: a prospective cohort study. *J Arthroplasty.* 2007;22(7 suppl 3):66-71.

63. Mont MA, Seyler TM, Marker DR, Marulanda GA, Delanois RE. Use of metal-on-metal total hip resurfacing for the treatment of osteonecrosis of the femoral head. *J Bone Joint Surg Am.* 2006;88(suppl 3):90-97.

64. Revell MP, McBryde CW, Bhatnagar S, Pynsent PB, Treacy R. Metal on metal hip resurfacing in osteonecrosis of the femoral head. *J Bone Joint Surg Am.* 2006;88(suppl 3): 98-103.

14

Preoperative Templating

Ravi K. Bashyal, MD; Benjamin Bender, MD; and Robert L. Barrack, MD

The re-establishment of appropriate hip biomechanics is an objective of paramount importance in total hip arthroplasty (THA).[1-4] Numerous texts have discussed the value of preoperative x-ray review and measurement to help achieve this goal. Early techniques that utilized cement on both the femoral and acetabular side allowed the surgeon to adjust the position of either component within the cement mantle and more easily compensate to achieve proper hip biomechanics. The increased popularity of cementless implants beginning in the 1980s forced a change in this practice.[5] With cementless implants, the placement of the components was most significantly determined by the patient's native anatomy. Thus, the surgeon's ability to dictate and customize component position within the cement mantle became limited. This change made preoperative templating an even more crucial step in the planning of a cementless THA and refined the preoperative planning process. Engh et al published enhanced radiographic techniques and templating principles that addressed these developments.[6,7] With the advent of digital x-rays, some templating is now being done with computer software. This chapter will focus on the use of the printed radiograph, and the principles of digital templating are the same. Overall, the common goals of hip reconstruction are to recreate the anatomic biomechanical axis as accurately as possible by focusing on restoring the anatomic center of rotation and femoral offset while attempting to equalize limb length.

Acetabular Templating

In standard THA, intraoperative acetabular preparation is completed prior to addressing the femur. Templating appropriately begins with the acetabular side as well. Typically the acetabular template is positioned just lateral to the lateral edge of the teardrop at a 40- to 45-degree angle. Ideally, the cup is covered completely by bone and should span the distance between the teardrop and the superolateral margin of the acetabulum. If the acetabulum is shallow and the hip dysplastic, complete coverage will not be possible without either excessive medialization or vertical cup orientation. In this scenario, a portion of the acetabular component should be left uncovered. Screw fixation as well as the use of an enhanced porous metal surface is often elected in this scenario for increased mechanical stability. The amount of uncovered acetabular shell in millimeters should be noted during templating so it can be used as an intraoperative check for appropriate component orientation.

Component-specific templates are used to size and select the component that best accomplishes this with minimal removal of subchondral bone. Cemented sockets require that a uniform 2- to 3-mm space be reserved for cement. The center of rotation is then marked through the template. Evaluation of the center of rotation is most easily achieved if the component's medial edge is just lateral to the teardrop. In this situation, the horizontal and vertical distances from

Parvizi J, Klatt BA.
Essentials in Total Hip Arthroplasty (pp 115-123).

the teardrop should closely approximate those of the contralateral normal hip. If a limb length discrepancy is present with the affected side shorter (most common), the center of rotation planning point is moved superiorly above the templating point the number or millimeters of the planned correction, and this point is utilized for subsequent templating. Normally only a portion of the discrepancy is corrected (one-half to two-thirds) since the appropriate side often feels longer to the patient and full correction may also lead to excessive tissue tension and contracture.

Lateralized Acetabulum

Lateralization of the hip center is a common phenomena noted in many cases of degenerative osteoarthritis of the hip. In these cases, hypertrophic osteophytes in the acetabulum cause lateralization of the hip's center of rotation. This condition occurs most frequently in men with hypertrophic osteoarthritis. During templating, the presence of a lateralized hip center becomes apparent when 1 or 2 cm of reaming is found to be necessary in order to place the acetabular component in its appropriate position just lateral to the teardrop. If this crucial finding is not recognized, the acetabular component is at risk for being placed in an inappropriately lateralized position. This may result in incomplete bony coverage and subsequent suboptimal stability, especially in cases where a press-fit noncemented acetabular component is implanted without screws. In press-fit components, complete peripheral rim contact is desired in order to obtain immediate stability. Complete bony coverage is desirable for cemented sockets as well. Sarmiento et al demonstrated lower rates of acetabular component loosening were associated with higher degrees of cemented acetabular component coverage.[8] Karachalios et al found that increased horizontal distance from the teardrop was the most significant factor predictive of an unfavorable radiographic appearance of a cemented acetabular component.[9]

Identifying the true anatomic location of the hip joint in these cases can be challenging and often requires careful intraoperative examination. The most reliable landmark is the transverse acetabular ligament that marks the inferior border of the true acetabulum and the location of the teardrop.[10] The cotyloid notch ("horseshoe"), which is often used can be difficult to visualize as is it often completely overgrown with cartilage and osteophytes. In these situations, careful straight medial reaming with smaller reamers to the desired depth followed by progressively larger reamers to enlarge the periphery in the desired orientation can be used to avoid excessive superior placement of the acetabular component. However, it is not necessarily desirable to ream all the way to the unicortical plate in all cases with lateralized acetabuli. As described by Charnley, overreaming can result in an increased risk of impingement, instability, and restricted motion.[2] An additional potential benefit from this slight lateralization of the cup is that this position relatively increases offset and therefore the abductor moment arm.

Superolateral Migration

Another common pattern of hip deformity is superolateral migration, which is more common in women, especially those with some degree of hip dysplasia. In these cases, the shallow nature of the acetabulum and incomplete coverage of the femoral head result in a concentration of forces on the superolateral joint surface. This can cause a progressive flattening and erosion of the joint with subsequent superior migration of the hip and associated shortening of the limb. During the templating process, this set of conditions becomes most apparent when the acetabular template is placed just adjacent to the teardrop and a significant portion of the lateral margin of the cup remains uncovered. A wide variety of surgical options can be considered during the templating phase of these cases.

If there is a well-established pseudoacetabulum, some surgeons advocate a smaller component placed at a high hip center.[11,12] However, there are a number of potential disadvantages to this approach. Often, the amount of supporting bone in this location is relatively small in dimension and may be inadequate to provide proper coverage and support of the implant. In addition, this approach usually requires the use of smaller components and smaller head sizes in order to accommodate for an appropriately sized polyethylene liner. This exacerbates the tendency for instability resulting from impingement on the anterior column and anterior-inferior iliac spine with flexion and internal rotation, as well as on the ischium in extension and external rotation. Superior and lateral placement of the acetabular component disrupts the native, nondiseased biomechanics of the hip and increases joint reaction forces. These increased forces carry an increased risk of accelerated polyethylene wear and component loosening. In less severe cases of dysplasia where there is some degree of superolateral migration but no clear pseudoacetabulum, there is often inadequate bone stock present to ream in the superolateral margin and anatomic cup placement is preferred.[13,14,4]

Templating in these cases is of critical importance for proper preoperative planning. When planning, the surgeon must understand that greater than 10% to 20% lateral uncoverage of the acetabular component is suboptimal. There are numerous techniques available to try and achieve at least 80% to 90% coverage of the cup in these cases.

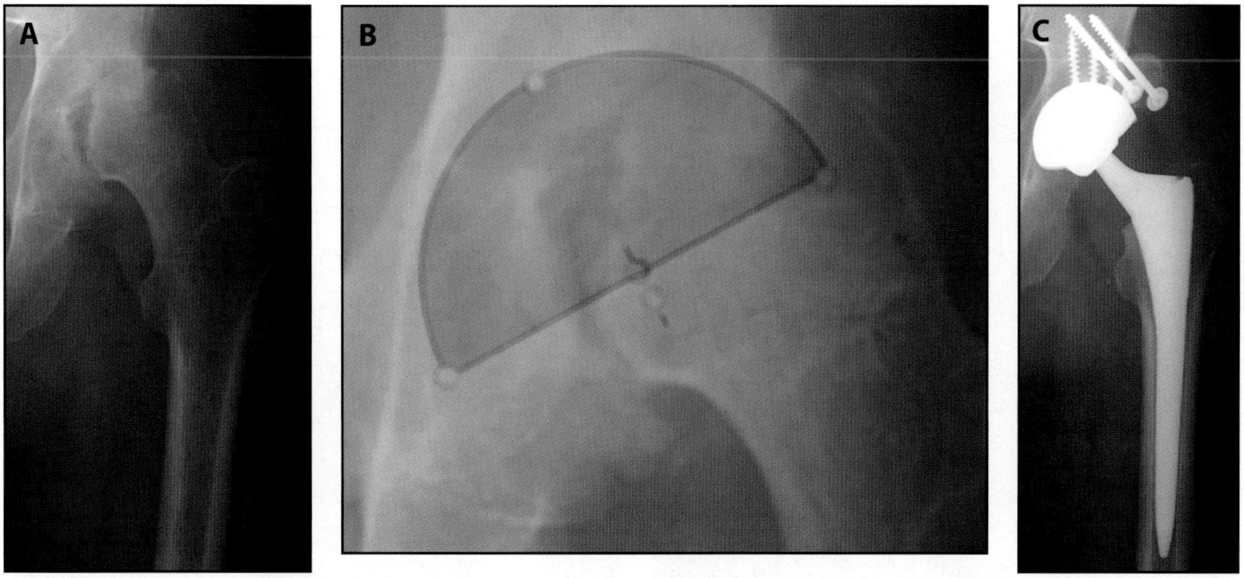

Figure 14-1. (A) AP radiograph of patient with a history of prior hip fracture dislocation with post-traumatic osteoarthritis and hip subluxation. (B) Preoperative templating demonstrated that greater than 20% to 30% of the acetabular shell would most likely remain uncovered after appropriate placement. This was confirmed following intraoperative reaming and trial insertion. (C) The acetabular component was subsequently augmented with structural femoral head autograft.

Medial reaming to the subchondral plate and use of a low profile component is one strategy to achieve an appropriate level of coverage. In addition, screws can be used to augment the fixation of cementless components as they will likely not have the benefits of circumferential peripheral contact in these situations. Another technique is to fix the acetabular component in a slightly less abducted position than usual, and use an offset liner in the superior position to compensate for this. However, an acetabular inclination angle of greater than 50 degrees should be avoided to prevent increased edge wear and decreased stability, and this technique should be altogether avoided in hard-hard bearing surfaces. If the acetabular component still remains 20% to 30% uncovered, structural graft fixed to the pelvis can be considered (Figure 14-1). It is crucial to recognize this possibility during the templating phase as a significant amount of additional equipment may be required intraoperatively. Various studies have described the use of structural femoral head autograft in these cases and have discussed the need for additional equipment in order to properly complete the procedure.[13,14] In cemented components, cement augmentation of the superolateral deficiency has been described without deleterious effects on component fixation in the 5- to 10-year follow-up range.[15] A more contemporary option is the use of metal augments.[16]

In many of these cases, especially those requiring structural grafting, significant lengthening will occur through the acetabular component. This may subsequently require a lower neck cut and shorter neck length to avoid over-lengthening. It has been demonstrated that in cases where significant length changes are anticipated, an intraoperative measurement device (most commonly utilizing a pin fixed to the superior ileum and a fixed point on the lateral femur) is particularly indicated for use.[17,18] In addition, if the anticipated lengthening is to be 2 cm or more, the use of somatosensory evoked potentials (SSEPs) should be considered in order to minimize the risk of a postoperative nerve palsy.[17,19]

When templating a dysplastic hip, particular attention should be paid to the patient's degree of femoral anteversion. Excessive femoral anteversion is a common coexisting condition in patients with hip dysplasia.[20] If a cemented stem is chosen, a smaller, straighter stem that allows for rotation within the cement column to correct for excessive anteversion prior to hardening may be required. In addition, the greater trochanter is often posteriorly rotated in these patients and close monitoring of the abductor moment arm is necessary. A greater trochanter osteotomy with subsequent reattachment more anteriorly and laterally may be required if the direction of pull of the abductors is inappropriate, especially if this is present in conjunction with impingement of the trochanter with extension and external rotation. If a press fit stem is chosen, a variety of options are available, including use of a modular stem or an anteverted stem made for the contralateral hip. In cases of abnormal femoral version, the surgeon may elect to prepare the femur first and adjust the acetabular version accordingly. Generally, a

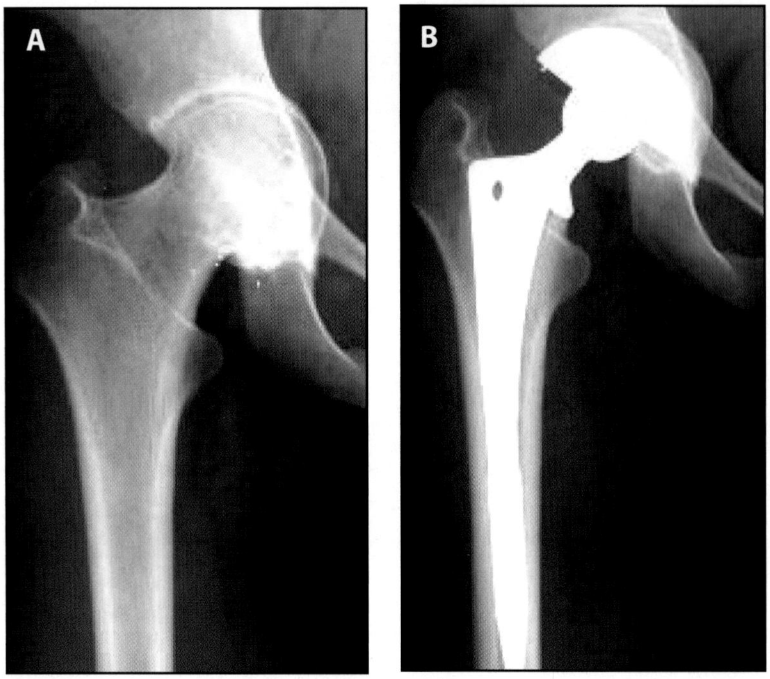

Figure 14-2. Protrusio is noted on the preoperative x-rays. During the procedure, impaction grafting of reamed femoral head autograft was used to augment the medial wall, and a trabecular metal acetabular component with peripheral rim fit was utilized.

combined femoral and acetabular version of approximately 30 degrees is the goal. When femoral version dictates placing the stem beyond 10 degrees of anteversion, a corresponding decrease in acetabular anteversion should be considered.

Regardless of the system and techniques used, there are significant surgical implications in patients with superolateral acetabular migration and possible increased femoral anteversion. It is essential that these abnormalities, if present, be recognized preoperatively and that these details are incorporated during the templating phase in order to come up with the most efficient and effective operative plan.

Protrusio Acetabuli

Protrusio acetabuli is a condition present in a significant portion of patients undergoing THA. It is especially prevalent in patients with a history of rheumatoid arthritis, ankylosing spondylitis, Paget's disease, or any metabolic bone disease that results in the weakening of subchondral bone.[21] In these cases, it is important to recognize the lack of bone stock during preoperative x-ray review and templating in order to avoid medialization of the hip center. Medialized acetabular components often lack ideal bony structural support from the pelvis. Restoring medial bone stock is an essential step in achieving success in these cases. Morselization of the femoral head is a common technique used to create medial graft. However, in some cases, a larger amount of bone may be required to achieve adequate lateralization of the hip center and augmentation with allograft is sometimes necessary. In addition to more accurately recreating the native biomechanics of the hip, lateralization of the hip center in protrusio cases also has the added benefit of increasing femoral offset and decreasing the tendency for impingement (Figure 14-2).

Though lateralization affords the benefits described above, it is essential to recognize and address the structural limitations present in these cases. Because the cup is contacting only bone graft medially rather than structurally supportive subchondral bone, a large component with excellent peripheral rim fit is necessary. Failure to achieve a tight rim fit peripherally risks potential complications including medial wall fracture during component insertion, as well as progressive medial component migration and subsequent recurrence of protrusio acetabuli over time.

Another consequence of acetabular component lateralization in protrusio cases is limb lengthening. This lengthening can be a desirable effect as the affected limb is often shortened in unilateral protrusio acetabuli. However, the condition commonly affects both hips. In these cases, both limbs have progressively shortened and may not have a great deal of disparity between each other. These patients should be advised that there may be a significant degree of lengthening of the first hip to be operated on, but that there will be an opportunity for correction when the contralateral hip replacement is performed. In addition to these concerns, cases of longstanding protrusio are often associated with ankylosis of the hip and associated joint capsule and soft tissue contracture. When lengthening occurs by lateralizing the acetabular component, it is critical to understand that these issues may limit the amount of further lengthening. As a result, a lower neck cut and shorter neck segment may need to be utilized in these cases.

Femoral Templating

Following appropriate acetabular templating and marking of the hip center of rotation, attention should be turned to the femoral side. The first step is determining whether a cemented or cementless stem is to be used. Although in practice most surgeons tend to implant the same type of stem for most of their cases, it is prudent to template for both a cemented and noncemented stem, especially in cases where any anatomic abnormality is identified. Cementless components require immediate stable fixation at the time of implantation. If there is intraoperative difficulty encountered in reaming or broaching, or if immediate stability is not achieved, it is advisable to implant a cemented stem in some cases.

The size of the femoral component is judged from the anteroposterior (AP) radiograph of the hip. Thus, it is essential that femoral templating be performed using an image that was taken with appropriate positioning. Fifteen to 20 degrees of internal rotation has been found to most accurately predict stem size, neck length, offset, and neck resection level. If the operative leg has a fixed external rotation contracture and the contralateral side is normal, templating of the acetabulum can be performed on the operative side. Once the center of rotation is determined on this side, the horizontal and vertical distances from the teardrop to this point should be recorded. Using these measurements, this point is then transposed to the AP hip radiograph of the normal side (with the leg in suitable 15 to 20 degrees of internal rotation). Femoral templating can then take place using this appropriate x-ray.[7]

For proximally coated noncemented stems, emphasis should be placed on proximal fit and fill. For more fully coated cementless stems, fixation is obtained distally and the goal is to obtain a tight isthmus fit. Contact of the stem medially and laterally with the endosteal sidewalls over 4 to 6 cm is recommended.[6,7] When templating for a cemented stem, it is important to keep in mind that a 2- to 3-mm circumferential cement mantle is required for optimal fit.

Regardless of the stem type utilized, it is important to keep the template centered over the neutral axis of the femur and to avoid any varus or valgus inclination. With this in mind, the femoral template is moved vertically along the neutral axis of the femur until the center of the femoral head template is at the same vertical height as the planned center of rotation. If the center of rotation of the femoral head directly overlaps the planned center of rotation of the hip based on the acetabular templating, then the length and offset will be restored. The neck resection level is marked through the template and the distance above the lesser trochanter can be measured with an appropriately scaled ruler so that appropriate neck resection level can be reproduced during surgery. Ideally, femoral bone stock should be maintained and neck cuts should be planned 1 to 2 cm above the lesser trochanter.

If the center of the femoral head template lies medial to the planned center of hip rotation determined during acetabular templating, stem insertion to this level will increase femoral offset. This is generally advantageous, especially if it is increased by 3 to 4 mm, due to the increased abductor moment arm created. However, excessive increase in offset can cause trochanteric prominence and an increased risk for development of trochanteric bursitis and muscle tightness and contracture.

If the center of the femoral head lies lateral to the planned center of hip rotation, stem insertion in this position will decrease femoral offset. Decreasing the femoral offset has a number of deleterious effects. One of the cornerstones of Charnley's early work on restoring hip biomechanics was the restoration or improvement of the abductor moment arm.[2] McGrory et al demonstrated less strength in isokinetic testing in hips with lower offset.[22] Rothman et al showed a higher incidence of limp with low-offset hip replacements.[23] Decreasing the abductor moment arm increases joint reaction forces, which in turn could lead to higher rates of loosening and polyethylene wear. Robinson et al were able to demonstrate a correlation between low offset and higher rate of polyethylene wear.[24] The abductor laxity caused by decreased offset could also lead to a higher incidence of instability.

Numerous options exist to avoid performing a reconstruction that decreases offset. Small decreases in offset can be corrected by seating the component lower, using a longer (lower) neck cut, and using a larger head. More recent innovations have included use of the dual offset total hip. This allows the same stem and neck resection level to be utilized with 2 different base offsets. Neck resection should be planned to ideally utilize a neck length without a "skirt" or thickened extension of the head as this tends to restrict

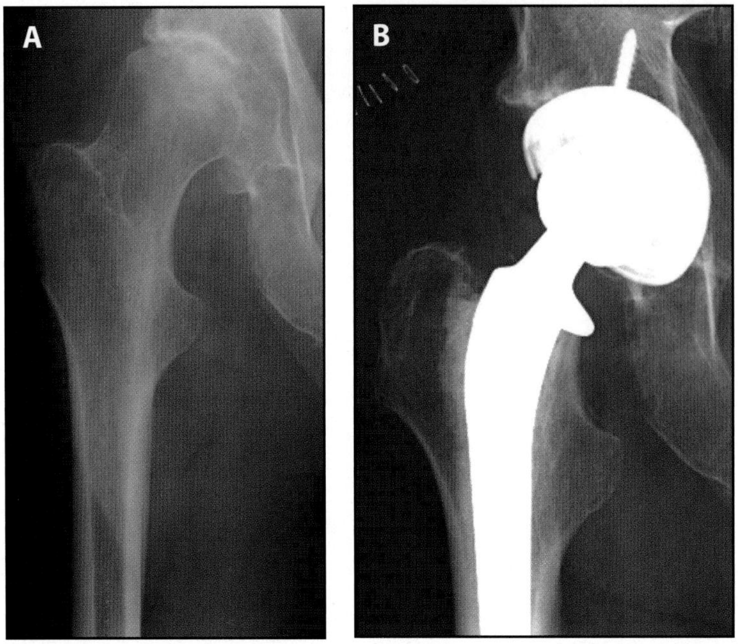

Figure 14-3. (A) AP radiograph of a patient with significant coxa valga. A high (>20 mm) neck cut and short neck component were utilized in order to maintain offset and length. (B) A high (>20 mm) neck cut and short neck component were utilized in order to maintain anatomic offset and length.

motion and cause impingement at extremes of motion.[25] Most implant systems offer 4 or 5 head choices of which the first 2 or 3 do not have a skirt or an extension. In general, reconstruction should be planned around a short (but not shortest) component neck (high femoral neck cut). Calcar planing and further countersinking of the component can be used and the neck can always be recut if need be. This is preferable to too low of a resection level, which may force the surgeon to use a long or extra-long prosthetic neck, which typically come with a skirt.

After templating to determine femoral component size and neck resection level, the lateral radiographs must be templated in order to assure that fit can be achieved with the planned stem diameter and length. If stem impingement is predicted, options include varying the entry point in the AP plane, switching to an anatomically bowed stem, or implanting a cemented stem.

The planned component size and distal canal diameter should be measured and recorded from the AP radiograph so that this information can be used as an intraoperative reference. If there is difficulty in seating reamers and broaches below the planned size, intraoperative reassessment of entry point should be undertaken. The most frequent error in these circumstances is an entry point that is too medial and reaming/broaching being completed in a varus orientation. An intraoperative radiograph with a reamer or broach in place is often helpful to confirm the source of the problem. Alternatively, if reaming/broaching is proceeding easily past the planned size, it may also be useful to obtain an intraoperative radiograph to ensure that significant cortical bone is not being reamed away. If cortical bone is being reamed without significant resistance, conversion to a cemented stem should be considered. In these cases, awareness of the measured isthmus diameter is useful in order to select and appropriately size the cement restrictor plug.

Femoral Neck Abnormalities

The average anatomic neck-shaft angle is approximately 125 degrees. Values significantly lower than this represent coxa vara and values significantly above represent coxa valga. Patients with coxa vara have a higher than usual femoral offset. This can be compensated for by utilizing a component with a lower neck-shaft angle, or by making a lower neck cut and utilizing a longer neck. The opposite situation exists when the patient's neck-shaft angle significantly exceeds that of the prosthesis. There is relatively low offset and more length. To compensate for this, it is necessary to utilize a higher neck cut and use a shorter neck length to maintain length and offset (Figure 14-3).

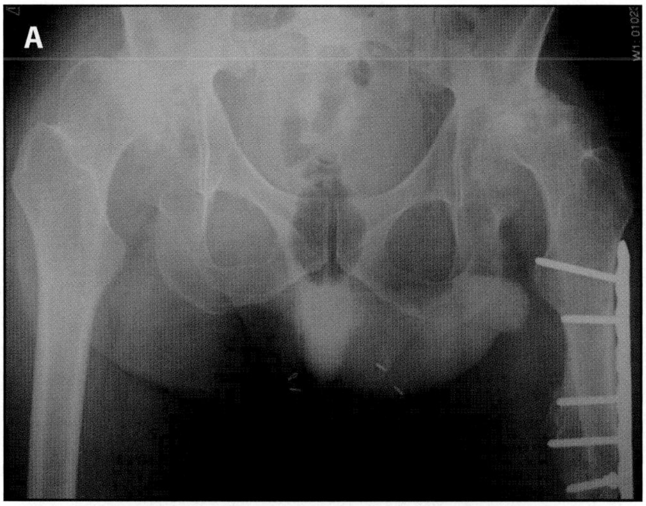

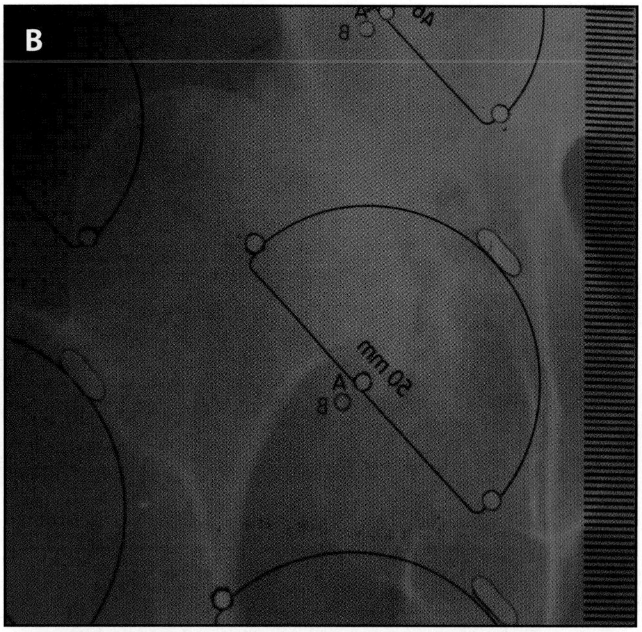

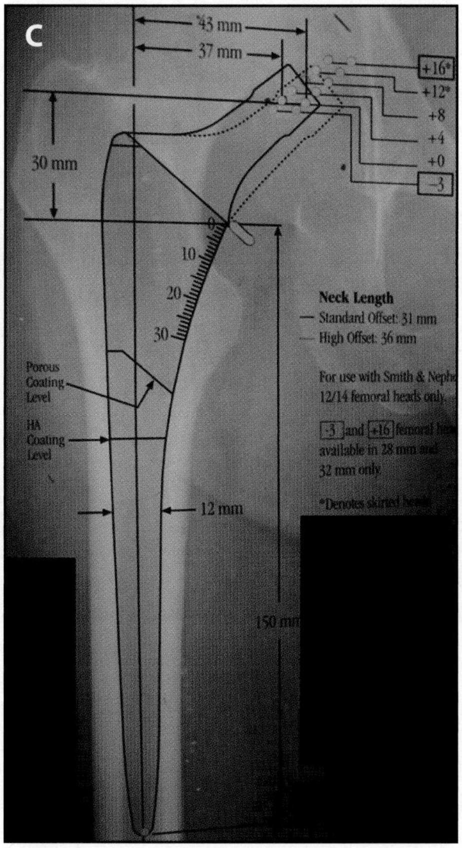

Figure 14-4. (A) An AP radiograph demonstrating a patient with a history of bilateral hip dysplasia with secondary osteoarthritis as well as a left femur fracture treated with plate and screws. (B) Acetabular templating on the more symptomatic right side demonstrates a lowering of the hip center, and anticipated amount of cup uncoverage. (C) Femoral templating demonstrating predicted stem size as well as addition of offset as indicated by the position of the neck center of rotation medial to the center of rotation from the previously templated acetabular component (outlined by black dots and dash).

Patients with a history of Perthes disease or other childhood history of hip avascular necrosis have a higher incidence of abnormally shortened femoral necks (coxa breva). In these patients, length and offset are generally increased when using a standard acetabular component. To avoid overlengthening, a low neck cut and short neck may need to be utilized.

Summary

Carter et al demonstrated that an experienced surgeon can accurately predict component size during preoperative templating in approximately 95% of cases.[26] When proper planning and templating is combined with intraoperative limb-length measurement, the incidence of overlengthening significantly decreases.[4,27,28] Clearly, preoperative planning is crucial to the success of primary THA. Data gathered from the history, review of systems, physical examination, review of radiographs, and templating are synthesized into an organized plan to approach each case. This includes selection of the proper type and size of components to be used in the procedure as well as consideration of possible alternatives. An organized approach insures that the need for appropriate implants, instruments, and graft materials can be anticipated well in advance and intraoperative surprises can be minimized. This type of preparation is most likely to lead to consistent, reproducible results while making the most efficient use of available resources (Figure 14-4).

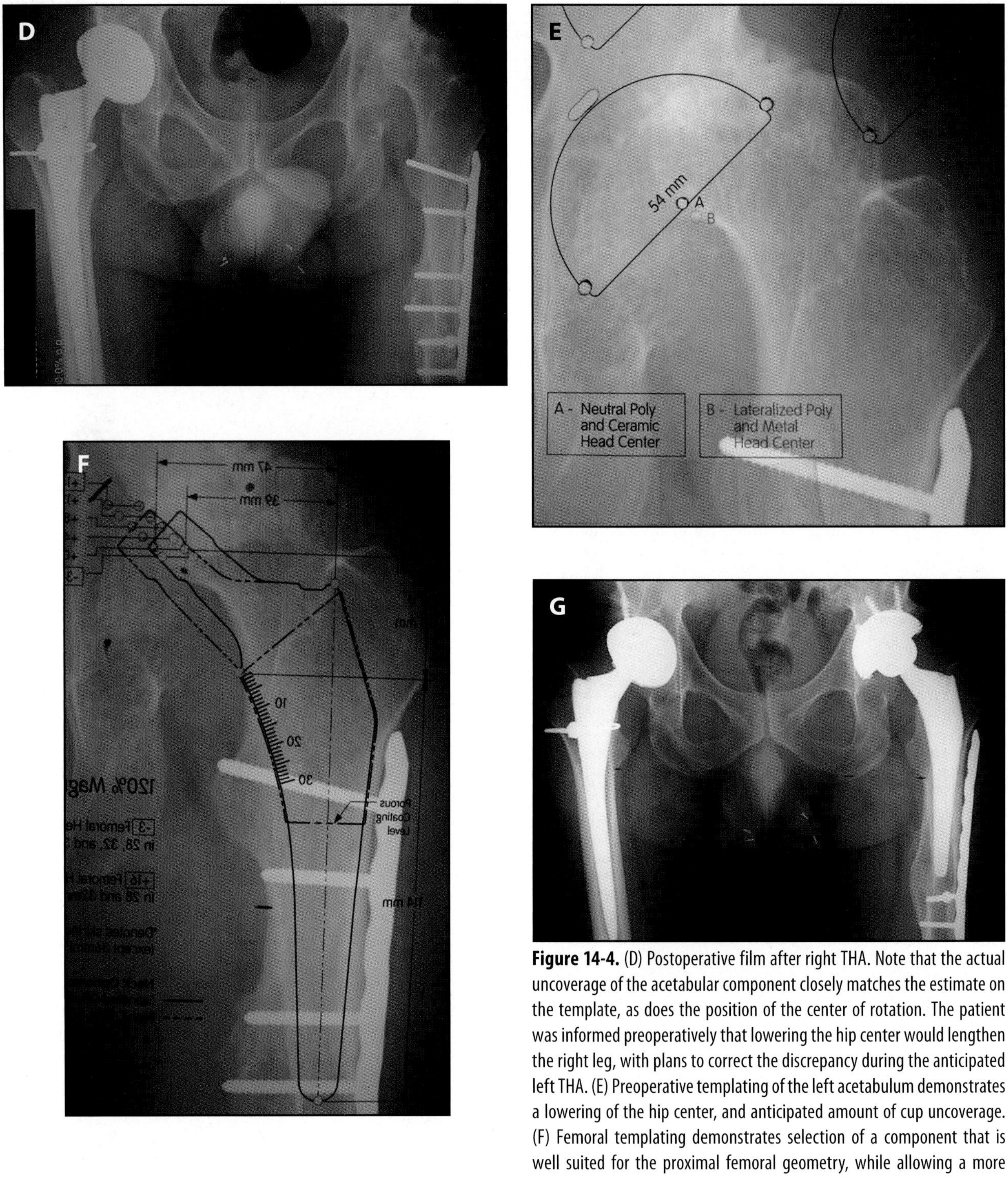

Figure 14-4. (D) Postoperative film after right THA. Note that the actual uncoverage of the acetabular component closely matches the estimate on the template, as does the position of the center of rotation. The patient was informed preoperatively that lowering the hip center would lengthen the right leg, with plans to correct the discrepancy during the anticipated left THA. (E) Preoperative templating of the left acetabulum demonstrates a lowering of the hip center, and anticipated amount of cup uncoverage. (F) Femoral templating demonstrates selection of a component that is well suited for the proximal femoral geometry, while allowing a more limited removal of hardware as compared to a longer stem design. Also note to position of the femoral center of rotation superior to the center of rotation of the acetabular component (again marked with black dots and a dash) indicating plans to slightly lengthen the leg to correct leg length discrepancy. (G) Final postoperative images demonstrating predicted acetabular uncoverage on the left side as well as restoration of equal leg lengths.

References

1. Capello WN. Preoperative planning of total hip arthroplasty. *Instr Course Lect.* 1986;35:249-257.
2. Charnley J. *Low Friction Arthroplasty of the Hip.* New York, NY: Springer-Verlag; 1979.
3. Dorr LD. Optimizing results of total joint arthroplasty. *Instr Course Lect.* 1985;34:401-404.
4. Barrack RL. Preoperative planning. In: Callaghan JJ, editor. *The Adult Hip.* Lippincott Williams & Wilkins: Philadelphia, PA; 1998:925-950.
5. Harris, WH and CB Sledge, Total hip and total knee replacement (1). *N Engl J Med.* 1990;323(11):725-731.
6. Engh C. *Biological Fixation in Total Hip Arthroplasty.* Engh C, Bobyn JD, eds. Thorofare, NJ: SLACK, Inc; 1985.
7. Engh C. Recent advances in cementless total hip arthroplasty using the AML prosthesis. *Techniques Orthop.* 1991;6(3):59-72.
8. Sarmiento A, Ebramzadeh E, Gogan WJ, McKellop HA. Cup containment and orientation in cemented total hip arthroplasties. *J Bone Joint Surg Br.* 1990;72(6):996-1002.
9. Karachalios T, Hartofilakidis G, Zacharakis N, Tsekoura M. A 12- to 18-year radiographic follow-up study of Charnley low-friction arthroplasty. The role of the center of rotation. *Clin Orthop Relat Res.* 1993;(296):140-147.
10. Dore DD, Rubash HE. Primary total hip arthroplasty in the older patient: optimizing the results. *Instr Course Lect.* 1994;43:347-357.
11. Russotti GM, Harris WH. Proximal placement of the acetabular component in total hip arthroplasty. A long-term follow-up study. *J Bone Joint Surg Am.* 1991;73(4):587-592.
12. Schutzer SF, Harris WH. High placement of porous-coated acetabular components in complex total hip arthroplasty. *J Arthroplasty.* 1994;9(4):359-367.
13. Barrack RL, Newland CC. Uncemented total hip arthroplasty with superior acetabular deficiency. Femoral head autograft technique and early clinical results. *J Arthroplasty.* 1990;5(2):159-167.
14. Barrack RL, Newland CC. A technique of acetabular reconstruction for uncemented total hip replacement. *Orthop Rev.* 1990;19(9):807-817.
15. McQueary FG, Johnston RC. Coxarthrosis after congenital dysplasia. Treatment by total hip arthroplasty without acetabular bone-grafting. *J Bone Joint Surg Am.* 1988;70(8):1140-1144.
16. Sporer SM, Paprosky WG. The use of a trabecular metal acetabular component and trabecular metal augment for severe acetabular defects. *J Arthroplasty.* 2006;21(6 suppl 2):83-86.
17. Williamson JA , Reckling FW. Limb length discrepancy and related problems following total hip joint replacement. *Clin Orthop Relat Res.* 1978;(134):135-138.
18. Woolson ST, Harris WH. A method of intraoperative limb length measurement in total hip arthroplasty. *Clin Orthop Relat Res.* 1985;(194):207-210.
19. Wasielewski RC, Crossett LS, Rubash HE. Neural and vascular injury in total hip arthroplasty. *Orthop Clin North Am.* 1992;23(2):219-235.
20. Ruby L, Mital MA, O'Connor J, Patel U. Anteversion of the femoral neck. *J Bone Joint Surg Am.* 1979;61(1):46-51.
21. Kaplan FS, Singer FR. Paget's disease of bone: pathophysiology, diagnosis, and management. *J Am Acad Orthop Surg.* 1995;3(6):336-344.
22. McGrory BJ, Morrey BF, Cahalan TD, An KN, Cabanela ME. Effect of femoral offset on range of motion and abductor muscle strength after total hip arthroplasty. *J Bone Joint Surg Br.* 1995;77(6):865-869.
23. Rothman R. The effect of varying offset on component fixation in cemented total hip arthroplasty. Presented at the 60th annual meeting of the American Academy of Orthpaedic Surgeons. San Francisco, CA; 1993.
24. Robinson E. Effect of implant position on polyethylene wear in total hip arthroplasty. Presented at the 62nd annual meeting of the American Academy of Orthpaedic Surgeons. Orlando, FL; 1995.
25. Krushell RJ, Burke DW, Harris WH. Range of motion in contemporary total hip arthroplasty. The impact of modular head-neck components. *J Arthroplasty.* 1991;6(2):97-101.
26. Carter LW, Stovall DO, Young TR. Determination of accuracy of preoperative templating of noncemented femoral prostheses. *J Arthroplasty.* 1995;10(4):507-513.
27. Abraham WD, Dimon JH III. Leg length discrepancy in total hip arthroplasty. *Orthop Clin North Am.* 1992;23(2):201-209.
28. Woolson ST. Leg length equalization during total hip replacement. *Orthopedics.* 1990;13(1):17-21.

15

Surgical Approaches in Total Hip Arthroplasty

Elie Ghanem, MD and Matt Austin, MD

Background

Total hip arthroplasty (THA) is the preferred surgical procedure for patients suffering from the pain and dysfunction associated with degenerative hip osteoarthritis.[1] There are 4 basic approaches that can be used for performing THA: anterior, anterolateral, direct lateral, and posterior. These approaches take advantage of the muscular intervals that surround the hip joint.

Bony Landmarks

There are some bony landmarks of the pelvis and femur that offer direction to performing the various approaches of the hip during THA (Figure 15-1). The anterior-superior iliac spine (ASIS) is the most anterior limit of the iliac spine and serves as an attachment to the sartorius muscles and inguinal ligament. The iliac crest curves posteriorly and ends at the posterior-superior iliac spine (PSIS). The greater trochanter with its prominent tubercle located in the posterior-superior area is the site of the gluteus medius tendon attachment. The rectus femoris tendon originates from the anterior-inferior iliac spine (AIIS) and passes underneath the inguinal ligament close to the ASIS.

Muscular Layout

The anterior thigh muscle group consists of the tensor fascia lata, sartorius, and quadriceps (rectus femoris, vastus medius, vastus intermedius, and vastus lateralis) (Figure 15-2). The rectus femoris consists of 2 heads that originate from the AIIS and the superior acetabular labrum and/or hip capsule. The lateral abductors consist of the gluteus medius and gluteus minimus that lies underneath it (Figure 15-3). The medius arises from the external surface of the ilium and the underbelly of the tensor fascia and plays the major role of abduction and internal rotation of the hip. Posteriorly, the gluteus maximus arises from the posterior gluteal line, iliac crest, sacrum, and coccyx; its tendon merges with the fascia lata to form the iliotibial tract. The piriformis muscle exits through the sciatic foramen and attaches to the piriformis fossa of the greater trochanter. The sciatic nerve runs within the nearby fat pad and deep to the piriformis. The obturator internus tendon located nearby also exits the sciatic notch and inserts caudally on the greater trochanter. The smaller gamelli lie superior and inferior to the obturator internus.

Anterior Approach

The anterior approach is known as the Smith-Peterson approach and utilizes the internervous intervals between the sartorius and tensor fascia lata in the superficial plane and the rectus femoris muscle and gluteus medius and minimus in the deep plane[2] (Figure 15-4). The sartorius and rectus femoris are supplied by the femoral nerve, while the tensor fascia lata and glutei receive innervations from the superior gluteal nerve.

Parvizi J, Klatt BA.
Essentials in Total Hip Arthroplasty (pp 125-131).

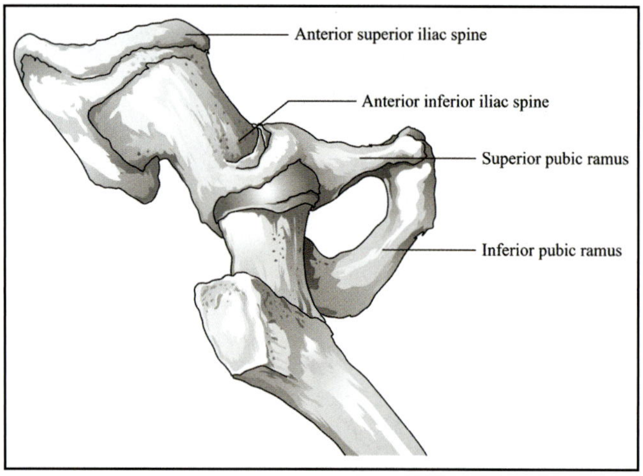

Figure 15-1. Bony landmarks of the pelvis.

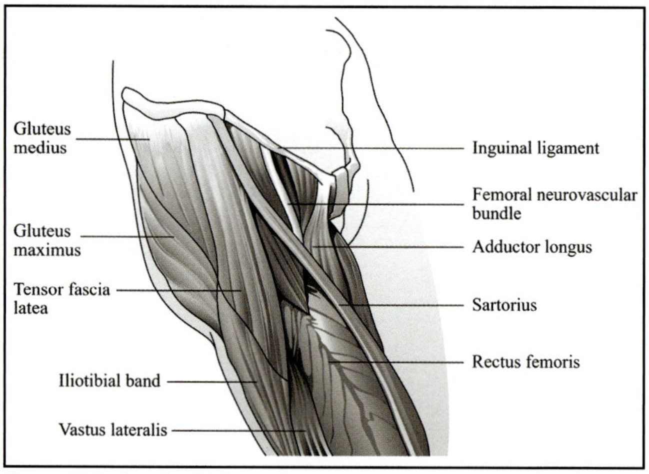

Figure 15-2. Anterior thigh muscle group.

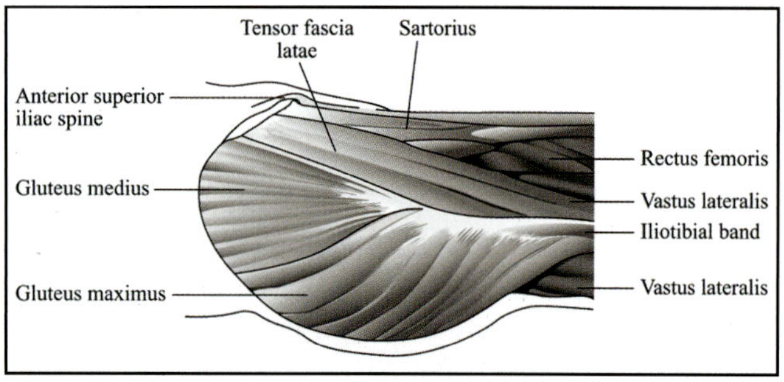

Figure 15-3. Abductors and gluteus maximus viewed laterally.

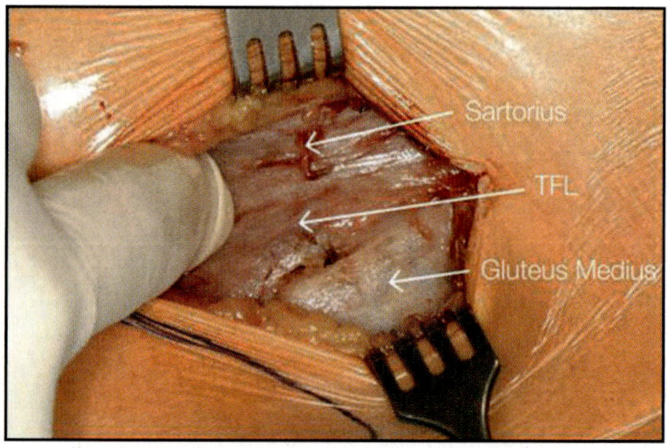

Figure 15-4. Superficial surgical plane of the anterior approach.

Patient Positioning

The patient is placed in the supine position with a bump under the affected side to allow the posterior soft tissues to fall posteriorly.

Surgical Dissection

The skin incision runs 2 to 3 cm lateral to the iliac crest border until it approaches the ASIS where it runs distally along the anterior border of the thigh for 8 to 10 cm (Figure 15-5).

Superficial Exposure

1. External rotation of the leg stretches the sartorius and develops the gap between the sartorius and tensor fascia lata.
2. The fascia encompassing the tensor fascia muscle can be opened laterally and dissected anteriorly to protect the lateral femoral cutaneous nerve, which penetrates the sartorial fascia 2 to 3 cm below the ASIS.
3. Retract the anterior and posterior fascial flaps and the underlying tensor and sartorius muscles. The rectus femoris and gluteus medius found in the deeper plane underneath are then exposed. The tensor muscle is then released from the lateral iliac wing for better exposure of the gluteus.

Deep Exposure

1. The major ascending branch of the lateral circumflex artery is located between the rectus femoris and gluteus medius; hemostasis and ligation of the artery are crucial.
2. The direct and reflected heads of the rectus muscle may be divided and retracted medially to expose the anterior hip capsule (Figure 15-6). Proper placement of the retractors can obviate the need for muscular detachment.
3. Adduct and externally rotate the leg to stretch the capsule.

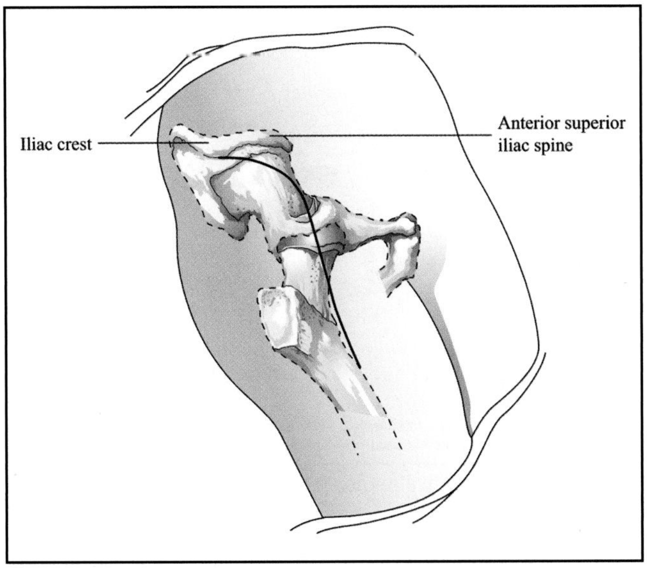

Figure 15-5. Skin incision for the anterior using bony landmarks.

4. Use a T-shaped or longitudinal capsulotomy to expose the femoral head and neck.
5. Following capsulectomy or capsulotomy, dislocation of the hip can be achieved by external rotation, adduction, and flexion of the femur, or a double cut can be made to the femoral neck in situ. This allows for removal of a small segment of the neck and then the head can be removed with a corkscrew.

Improving the Exposure

1. Detach the origins of the tensor fascia and sartorius from the anterior iliac wing for better visualization of the abductors.
2. The acetabular exposure in the anterior approach is limited compared to other approaches; hence, the abductors can be stripped off the ileum.
3. Lengthen the incision proximally along the iliac crest or distally down the anterolateral aspect of the thigh in the interval between the vastus lateralis and rectus femoris to expose the femoral shaft.
4. The inguinal ligament and sartorius can be released from their origin at the ASIS for optimal visualization of the medial acetabulum and quadrangular space.

Pitfalls

1. Dissection medial to the sartorius muscle will lead to lateral femoral cutaneous nerve damage, which may cause paresthesias along the lateral thigh or a painful neuroma.
2. Beware of the ascending branch of the lateral femoral circumflex that crosses the deep internervous plane. Hemostasis must be obtained.
3. Do not stray far out of the plane of dissection, especially medial to the rectus. The femoral nerve is the most lateral element of the femoral sheath.

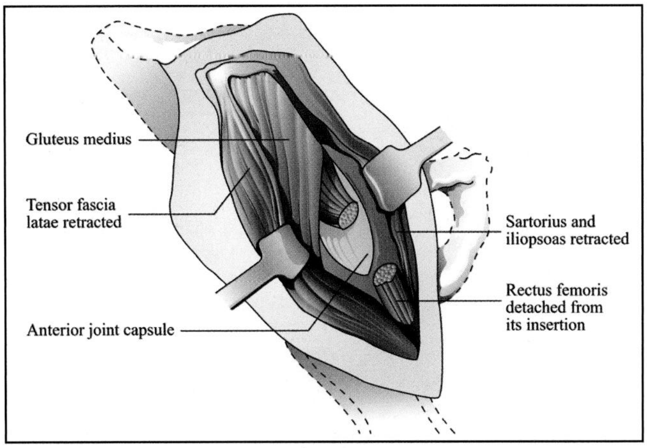

Figure 15-6. Deep surgical plane of the anterior approach.

Anterolateral Approach

The anterolateral approach was popularized by Watson-Jones early on for hip fracture fixation.[3] The anterolateral approach utilizes the plane between the gluteus medius and tensor fascia muscle that are both innervated by the superior gluteal nerve. Although the anterolateral approach does not permit extensive exposure of the anterior column as the anterior approach, it allows good acetabular exposure with safe femoral reaming. There is also less dissection of the abductors as compared to the Smith-Petersen approach.[2]

Patient Positioning

The patient is positioned commonly in the supine position with a bump below the midline to allow for the posterior tissues to fall posteriorly.

Surgical Dissection

A curved skin incision is made with the apex directed posteriorly over the tip of the greater trochanter, which can then be extended along the length of the femoral shaft (Figure 15-7).

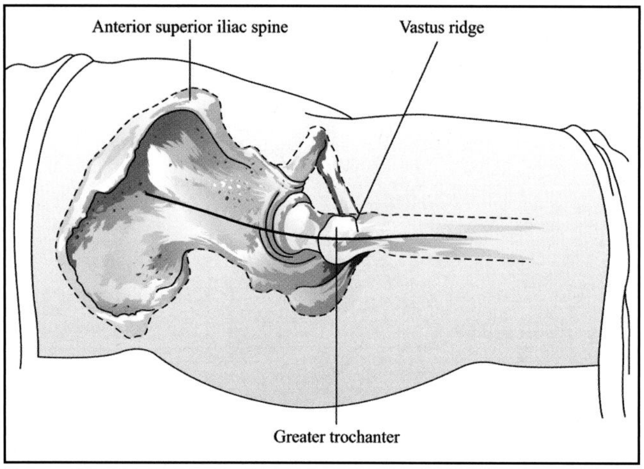

Figure 15-7. Skin incision for the anterolateral approach.

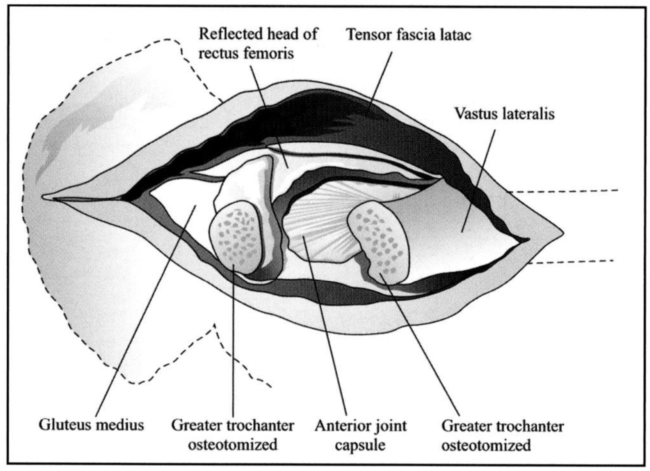

Figure 15-8. Deep surgical dissection of the anterolateral approach.

Superficial Exposure

1. The fascia is divided parallel to the skin incision and along the posterior margin of the greater trochanter proximally and distally.
2. Use forceps to elevate the fascial flap and retract it anteriorly. The tensor fascia muscle will elevate with the fascia.
3. Ligate the vessels in the interval between the tensor fascia and gluteus medius muscle.
4. Retract the abductors laterally and externally rotate the femur to expose the hip capsule.
5. The vastus lateralis can be partially released for capsular exposure.

Deep Exposure

1. The vastus ridge, where the greater trochanter merges with the femoral shaft, is identified and a trochanteric osteotomy is performed using a Gigli saw or an oscillating saw at the base of the ridge (Figure 15-8).
2. The anterior capsule can also be exposed by partial release of the gluteus from the anterior greater trochanter.
3. Retractors are placed under the rectus tendon and above the anterior column.
4. Use an H-shaped capsulotomy and retract the capsular flaps.
5. Following capsulectomy or capsulotomy, dislocation of the hip can be achieved by external rotation and adduction of the femur.

Improving the Exposure

1. The posterior thigh can be relaxed by incising the posterior fascia lata, which will allow for greater leverage.
2. Exposure of the femoral neck can be improved with elevation of the vastus muscle from the proximal femur using a periosteal elevator.
3. The rectus tendon can be released and later reattached for better exposure of the anterior capsule.
4. A partial release of the vastus lateralis origin from the vastus ridge uncovers the femoral neck and shaft.

Pitfalls

1. Compression neuropraxia can occur. The retractors should be placed over the anterior column and gentle traction implemented.
2. The superior gluteal neurovascular bundle is encountered when dissecting the gluteus medius too superiorly.
3. The lateral femoral circumflex artery may be encountered during inferomedial dissection on the anterior column and below the level of the femoral head.
4. Spiral fractures of the femoral shaft may occur while the hip is being dislocated.

Direct Lateral Approach

The direct lateral approach was popularized by Harding for performing THA.[4] It can provide excellent exposure to

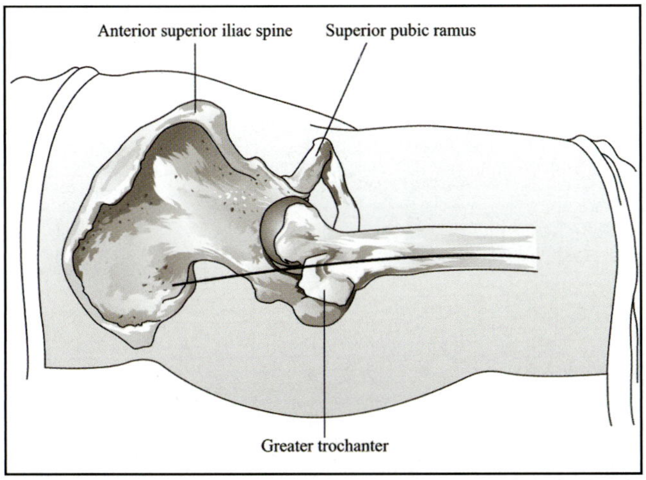

Figure 15-9. Skin incision for the direct lateral approach using bony landmarks

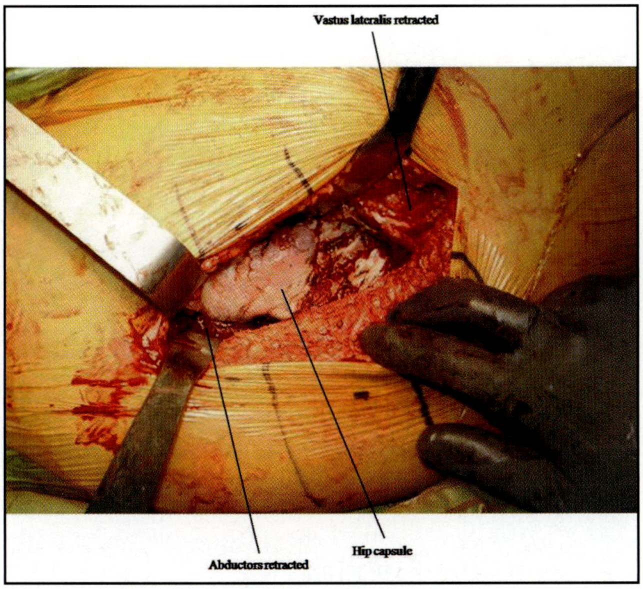

Figure 15-11. Joint capsule is completely exposed.

both the anterior hip and upper femur without the need for trochanteric osteotomy. At the same time, the posterior hip soft tissue structures are preserved, which decreases the risk of postoperative dislocation.[5]

Patient Positioning

The patient can be placed in either the supine or lateral position.

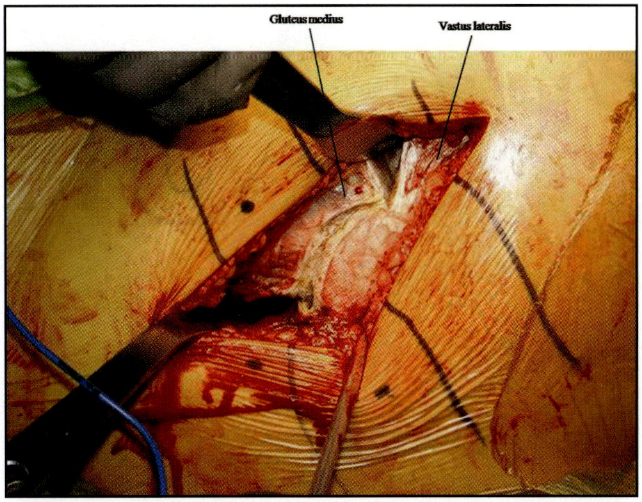

Figure 15-10. Anterior and posterior flaps of the gluteus medius and vastus lateralis are created.

Surgical Dissection

The skin incision is made directly over the center of the greater trochanter and runs parallel to the femoral shaft. The proximal incision ends at the level of the ASIS (Figure 15-9).

Superficial Exposure

1. The fascia lata is divided over the center of the greater trochanter and parallel to the skin incision superiorly/inferiorly.
2. Retract the anterior and posterior fascial flaps which expose the gluteus medius and vastus lateralis (Figure 15-10).

Deep Exposure

1. Incise the gluteus medius over the center of the trochanter and extend superiorly.
2. The vastus lateralis is also split at its insertion at the greater trochanter and carried distally.
3. Develop an anterior flap of muscle including both the gluteus medius and vastus lateralis during medial dissection and retract it anteriorly. Split the gluteus medius muscle to reveal the underlying joint capsule (Figure 15-11).
4. Use T-shaped capsulotomy and then osteotomize the femoral neck and extract the head.

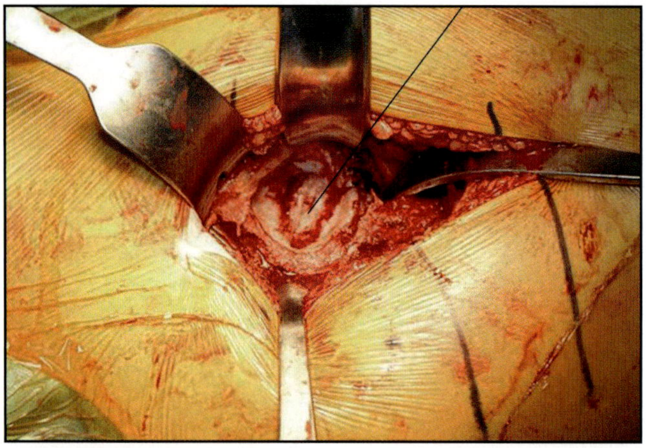

Figure 15-12. Line points to the center of the acetabulum that is exposed with properly placed retractors.

5. Properly place acetabular retractors around the acetabulum (Figure 15-12).

Improving the Exposure

1. Extend the distal incision along the vastus lateralis to expose the femur. The proximal incision cannot be extended due to the superior gluteal nerve innervations of the gluteus medius.

Pitfalls

1. Beware of the superior gluteal nerve that innervates the gluteus medius and minimus 5 cm above the tip of the trochanter. The superior gluteal nerve is at risk if the gluteus medius dissection is carried too superiorly above the acetabulum.
2. Do not infringe upon the psoas and the neurovascular structures. Properly placed acetabular retractors can obviate neurovascular damage.

Posterior/Posterolateral Approach

The posterior approach was originally described by Austin Moore and utilized for exposure of the posterior capsule and acetabular wall by splitting the gluteus maximus.[6] It permits excellent exposure of the proximal femoral shaft. One advantage over the other approaches is the preservation of the abductor mechanism.

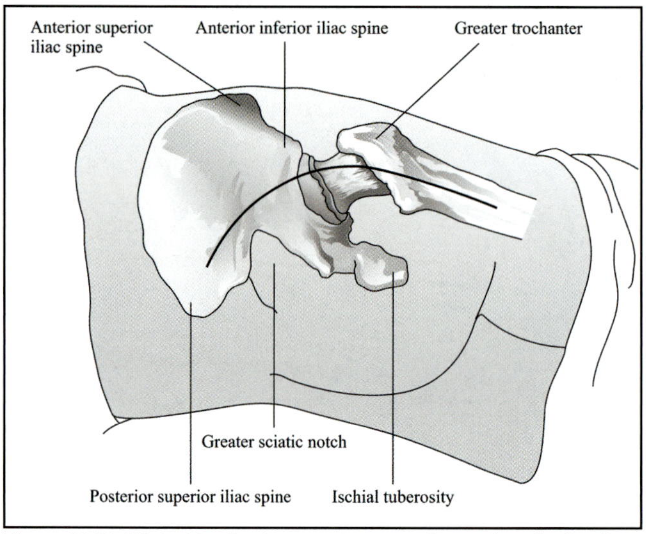

Figure 15-13. Skin incision for the posterior approach using bony landmarks.

Patient Positioning

The patient can be positioned in the lateral decubitus position for arthroplasty cases. The bony prominences must be padded under the lateral malleolus and a pillow placed between the knees.

Surgical Dissection

The skin incision starts at the level of the PSIS, 5 to 8 cm cephalad to the posterior aspect of the greater trochanter (Figure 15-13). The incision curves anteriorly 10 to 12 cm along the posterior border of the femoral shaft. The posterolateral approach differs slightly in that the distal incision is located more anterior to the greater trochanter.

Superficial Exposure

1. Incise the fascia lata in the direction of the skin incision.
2. The anterior and posterior fascial flaps are then retracted.
3. Split the fibers of the gluteus maximus.
4. The gluteus maximus tendon insertion into the femur can be safely released to relieve tension.

Deep Exposure

1. The hip is extended to relax the gluteus maximus and internally rotated to improve exposure of the external rotators (Figure 15-14).

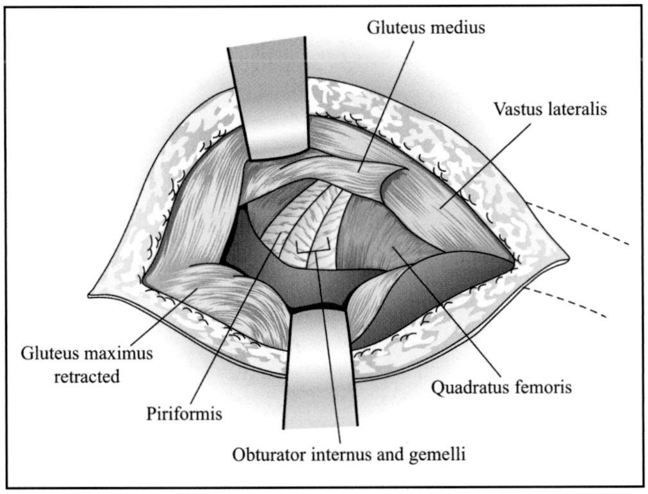

Figure 15-14. Deep surgical dissection of the posterior approach.

2. Properly placed superior and inferior retractors can improve visualization of the capsule. Place the retractors within the substance of the gluteus maximus and away from the soft tissues that encase the sciatic nerve.
3. The short rotators can be detached at their femoral insertion and reflected backward to protect the sciatic nerve while exposing the hip capsule.
4. A longitudinal or T-shaped capsulotomy is performed to preserve a portion of the capsule for later reconstitution.
5. The femoral head and neck are exposed by dislocating the hip posteriorly in flexion, adduction, and internal rotation.
6. The femoral head and neck can be osteotomized in situ if dislocation is difficult.
7. The femur can be retracted anteriorly and properly placed acetabular retractors allow adequate acetabular exposure.

Improving the Exposure

1. A trochanteric osteotomy can be performed in cases of a poorly visualized acetabulum.
2. Detach the quadratus or the insertion of the gluteus maximus from the femur to expose the shaft and neck better.

Pitfalls

1. Place the acetabular retractors over the anterior acetabulum in neutral to rostral direction; this decreases the risk of damaging the femoral neurovascular bundle.
2. Keep the retractors on the cut surfaces of the rotators to help protect the sciatic nerve.
3. Beware of early bifurcation of the sciatic nerve.
4. The gluteus maximus is supplied by the superior and inferior gluteal arteries and has an extensive venous network. Hence, hemostasis during gentle splitting of the gluteus maximus is essential.

References

1. Ng CY, Ballantyne JA, Brenkel IJ. Quality of life and functional outcome after primary total hip replacement. A five-year follow-up. *J Bone Joint Surg Br.* 2007;89(7):868-873.
2. Smith-Peterson MN. Approach to and exposure of the hip joint for mold arthroplasty. *J Bone Joint Surg Am.* 1949;31A(1):40-46.
3. Watson-Jones R. The classic: "Fractures and Joint Injuries" by Sir Reginald Watson-Jones, taken from "Fractures and Joint Injuries," by R. Watson-Jones, Vol. II, 4th ed. Baltimore, MD: Williams & Wilkins; 1955. *Clin Orthop Relat Res.* 1974;(105):4-10.
4. Hardinge K. The direct lateral approach to the hip. *J Bone Joint Surg Br.* 1982;64(1):17-19.
5. Kwon MS, Kuskowski M, Mulhall KJ, Macaulay W, Brown TE, Saleh KJ. Does surgical approach affect total hip arthroplasty dislocation rates? *Clin Orthop Relat Res.* 2006;447:34-38.
6. Moore AT. Metal hip joint; a new self-locking vitallium prosthesis. *South Med J.* 1952;45(11):1015-1019.

16

Operating Room Setup

Eric Levicoff, MD; Manny Porat, MD; and Brian A. Klatt, MD

Since Sir John Charnley ushered in the modern era of joint replacement in the 1960s, total hip arthroplasty (THA) has become a useful and reliable treatment for end-stage pathology of the hip joint.[1] Careful attention to detail with respect to patient selection, preoperative planning, operative technique, and postoperative care are all essential in achieving the goal of a successful operation.

Preoperative preparation, including proper use and arrangement of equipment, and meticulous patient preparation can greatly increase the probability of an excellent outcome. The purpose of this chapter is to discuss some of the options available to the surgeon in terms of the setup of the operating room (OR) prior to THA, and to highlight the importance of both operating room and patient preparation.

Equipment

Prior to bringing a patient into the OR, the surgeon should develop a system to ensure that proper equipment is present and functional. X-rays of the patient, including anteroposterior (AP) and lateral views of the hip and an AP view of the pelvis, should be clearly visible in addition to a preoperative template of the proposed implant. The template should include a brief summary of important data, including relevant past medical history, medications, allergies, and key components of the physical exam. The OR table should be assessed to make sure it functions properly and has a level surface. The horizontal plane is an important landmark for component insertion and improper tilting of the OR table can result in significant component malalignment.[2] For this reason, it can be helpful to use a leveler to ensure proper table position prior to patient transfer. Properly functioning suction and electrocautery systems should also be readily available.

Before beginning an arthroplasty procedure, the surgeon must also make sure that all necessary instruments have been properly sterilized and made available. In addition to the instrument packs, it is critical that a range of arthroplasty components are on hand. While preoperative templating will provide an intraoperative guide to the types and sizes of the components, intraoperative variations are common.[3] It is wise for the surgeon to make known to both the hospital staff as well as any necessary company representatives exactly what items might be needed and to make sure that these components are on hand prior to the start of the case (Table 16-1).

Asepsis

Providing an aseptic environment during joint arthroplasty procedures is crucial in achieving consistent, successful outcomes. The relative immunodeficiency of the joint space combines with the large surface area of the components to create a significant risk of infection that is difficult to eradicate. Though the incidence of infection following THA has decreased since Charnley's original cases,[4,5] deep sepsis following THA often results in severe consequences and can ultimately prove catastrophic.[6,7]

Parvizi J, Klatt BA.
Essentials in Total Hip Arthroplasty (pp 133-138).

Table 16-1

CHECKLIST OF ESSENTIAL EQUIPMENT AND MATERIALS FOR TOTAL HIP ARTHROPLASTY

- Radiographs (AP pelvis, AP, and lateral hip)
- Template
- Level OR table
- Functioning suction/electrocautery
- Implant selection
- Specialty items (ie, navigation systems, novel implants)
- Preoperative antibiotics

Antibiotic prophylaxis has become a mainstay in infection prevention for almost all orthopedic procedures and THA is no exception. As numerous studies have reported, there is no doubt as to the benefit of preoperative antibiotics.[8-10] Particularly when given within 30 to 60 minutes prior to skin incision, infection rates are decidedly lower in those patients receiving a dose of antibiotics preoperatively.[11] Furthermore, including antibiosis as a part of a system for preoperative setup has been shown to increase compliance rates.[12]

In addition to preoperative antibiosis, there is an emerging trend toward the preoperative treatment of community-acquired methicillin-resistant *Staphylococcus aureus* (MRSA). The incidence of MRSA in the community is growing and studies have shown an increased risk of MRSA infection postoperatively in patients known to be colonized.[13] Given the potentially disastrous consequences of MRSA infection following total joint arthroplasty, some centers have instituted routine preoperative testing for MRSA colonization, treating those patients with positive cultures prior to surgery. Treatment strategies vary but typically include the application of intranasal mupirocin over a 5-day period with or without the use of a total body wash with an anti-MRSA agent.[14] Though there is currently no definitive evidence of the cost-effectiveness of this practice, several studies have reported a decreased number of MRSA infections following orthopedic procedures with such a regimen.[15]

While the best methods used to limit the bacterial count in the OR have not been clearly established, no discussion of OR setup is complete without addressing different equipment and strategies that may enhance the aseptic environment. Air flow and filtration has become a central issue in maintaining a sterile environment in the OR, and to this end, laminar flow systems and exhaust suits have become popular tools utilized in arthroplasty procedures. It has been shown that infection following total joint arthroplasty correlates directly with OR contamination and that laminar flow systems significantly reduce the number of bacterial colony-forming units in the OR.[16,17] Exhaust suits reduce the shed of bacteria from the surgeon onto his or her surgical gown. In their initial studies, Charnley and Eftekhar demonstrated lower rates of infection using laminar flow rooms and filtered exhaust helmets.[18] Despite the fact that a statistically significant decrease in infections with the use of laminar flow and exhaust suits has yet to be clearly established,[19] both the Centers for Disease Control and Prevention and the National Institutes of Health have supported the use of both strategies to control OR contamination.[20,21] In addition, the traffic into and out of the OR should be kept to a minimum. Many surgeons will allow access to the OR through only one door and post signs outside the OR doors indicating that a total joint replacement procedure is in progress. Finally, all tables and equipment should be placed away from OR entry and exit points to avoid accidental contamination during the procedure.

In addition to clothing, the gloving technique has also been cited as a way to decrease bacterial contamination during surgical procedures. Common gloving techniques include single-gloving, standard double-gloving, and double-gloving with the use of indicator gloves. Though no studies show a statistically significant decrease in surgical site infections using any of the gloving techniques, frequency of inner glove perforations is clearly decreased with the use of a double-gloving technique, and use of indicator gloves definitively increases the recognition of outer glove tears.[22]

PATIENT POSITIONING

Once the room has been prepared and the choice of equipment has been made, it is time for the patient to be brought into the OR. Positioning of the patient on the table should be done in a systematic manner with a mental checklist of the steps necessary to achieve a safe and successful procedure (Table 16-2). When performing a THA, the surgeon can opt to place the patient in a supine or lateral position (Figure 16-1). For the most part, positioning the patient in the lateral or supine position is a matter of surgeon training, preference, and comfort (Table 16-3). In either case, it is of the utmost importance to make sure that all bony prominences are well padded and pressure is taken off of neurovascular structures at risk. It is important to remember that neurovascular structures are more susceptible to injury

Table 16-2

Positioning Checklist

- Placement of positioning device (ie, bean bag, peg board) on OR table
- Foley catheter
- Padding of neurovascular structures at risk (ie, peroneal nerve, sacral pad, axillary roll)
- Secure patient once positioned
- Electrocautery pad placed away from internal metal and devices (ie, pacemakers)
- Pneumatic compression devices on nonoperative limb
- Free access to nonoperative limb landmarks (ie, knee, malleoli, heel)
- Unobstructed movement of operative limb

Table 16-3

Advantages of Lateral Versus Supine Positioning

Lateral Position	Supine Position
• Gravity-assisted soft tissue retraction • Improved diaphragmatic excursion • Fewer required assistants	• Fewer problems with pelvic obliquity • Greater anesthesia access to airway • More facile evaluation of limb length • More efficient for bilateral procedures

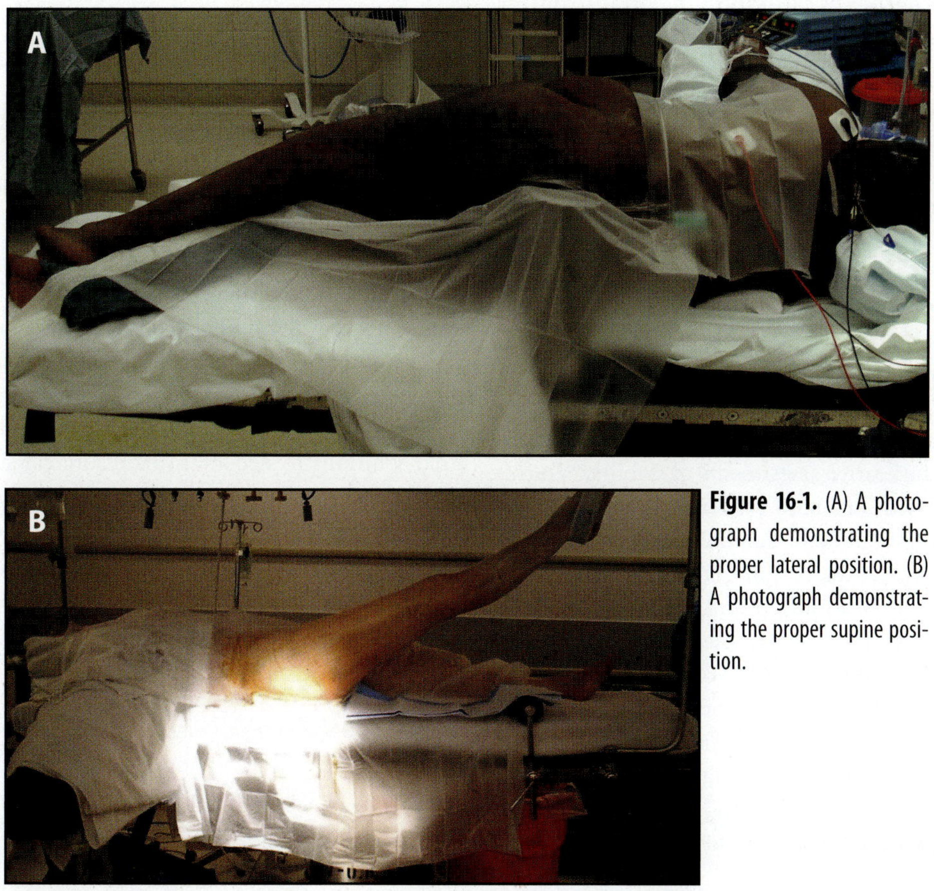

Figure 16-1. (A) A photograph demonstrating the proper lateral position. (B) A photograph demonstrating the proper supine position.

during the use of muscle relaxant medications. Particularly in the lateral decubitus position, special attention must be paid to the contralateral peroneal nerve and lateral leg compartment, as these structures are at risk for the development of iatrogenic injuries including neuropraxia and compartment syndrome.[23]

Neurologic injuries to the upper extremities have also been reported following THA, presumably from inadequate patient positioning.[24] Positioning injuries to the upper extremity appear to be significantly more common in patients with inflammatory arthritis, perhaps due to an underlying pre-existing neuropathy, and include most commonly the ulnar nerve and brachial plexus.[25] To limit such complications, an axillary roll is positioned on the chest wall and slightly inferior to the axilla such that enough space is present to allow a hand to easily slide in and out of the axilla, keeping pressure off of the neurovascular structures as they pass through this vulnerable region.

Once all potentially vulnerable neurovascular structures are protected, further issues specific to THA are addressed. The issue of limb length is of the utmost importance during total hip replacement surgery, and the nonoperative lower extremity should be placed in a position of access to allow for limb length estimation. Several different methods are used to assess limb length during the trial phase of the procedure, including intraoperative radiographs, knee height, malleolar symmetry, and heel height. In order to properly assess length, access to the nonoperative limb must be uninhibited save for the presence of sterile drapes. Pillows, towels, tape, and other positioning aids must be strategically placed prior to draping to allow for adequate intraoperative comparisons of limb length to avoid significant inequalities. In addition, the operative limb must be free to be taken through a large range of motion to allow for surgical dislocation as well as intraoperative assessments of stability. To this end, positioning boards or suction-deflated bean bags must be placed in a manner allowing for uninhibited motion of the operative extremity. Again, anterior or posterior listing of the patient must be minimized and pelvic tilt must be accounted for prior to draping as these factors can significantly impact component placement. Foley catheters, placed prior to final patient positioning, should be placed with the tubing facing away from the surgical site. Grounding pads for electrocautery should be placed away from any internal or external magnetic objects including metallic hardware, internal pacemakers or defibrillators, or other such devices, typically safe with placement on the contralateral thigh, flank, or abdomen. Finally, some surgeons choose to implement pneumatic compression devices on the nonoperative leg in an attempt to decrease the risk of intraoperative and postoperative deep vein thromboses.[26]

Hand Scrubbing, Patient Preparation, and Draping

The topics of hand scrubbing, patient preparation, and draping also deserve mention in a discussion of OR setup. While a detailed account of the various methods and materials used in these processes is beyond the scope of this chapter, some general points are worth noting. First, though the products and techniques of hand sanitation vary widely, consistent use of hand washing protocols has been shown to significantly reduce the number of bacterial colonies on a surgeon's hands.[27] Traditional methods involve the use of aqueous scrubs for various durations typically lasting between 2 and 5 minutes. Scrubs utilizing chlorhexidine gluconate have been shown to be more effective than povidine-iodine scrubs in decreasing the bacterial counts on surgeons' hands, but superiority with regard to surgical site infections has not been shown.[28] More recently alcohol-based hand rubs have been marketed to surgeons as an alternative to traditional aqueous scrubs. Typically a routine hand wash with antibacterial soap and water is followed with the application of a hand rub prior to gloving. While again there is no evidence that surgical site infections are any more or less common following the use of a sanitizing rub, there is evidence that rubs may help to maintain their antiseptic properties for a longer period of time than aqueous scrubbing.[29]

Historically, preparation of the operative extremity included scrubs with various bactericidal solutions lasting approximately 5 minutes, followed by a paint that would remain in the patient throughout the procedure. More recently, however, studies have shown equivalent result utilizing paint-only technique with no scrub.[30] Commonly used solutions to decontaminate surgical sites include tincture of iodine, povidine-iodine, and various other alcohol-based disinfectants. Particularly when using tincture of iodine, one must be careful not to allow excess solution to drip beneath the patient or to pool in any skin creases or folds, as this renders the patient at risk for chemical burns and other skin complications. Recently, hospitals have routinely begun providing fast-drying, one-step, alcohol-based preparation solutions to be used in place of traditional scrub-and-paint techniques. Though these solutions are relatively new, there is evidence that they are at least as effective as traditional solutions, and may also be less expensive and more helpful with regard to drape adhesion.[31] Bactericidal solutions should be applied over a surface area reasonably larger than the intended skin exposure to allow for adequate space for draping. Sponges or other solution applicators should start over the anticipated area of incision and work outward, and to avoid contamination they should not be brought back into the field after preparation of the peroneal and foot regions. Though the order of surgical scrubbing, patient preparation, and the opening of instruments in the room has not been standardized, preparation of the patient by a gowned and gloved member of the surgical team has been shown to significantly decrease bacterial air counts and therefore may be beneficial to complete prior to the opening of sterile instruments.[32]

The final step of the setup of the OR is the sterile draping of the patient. Ideally, the draping of the patient should be undertaken by an experienced member of the surgical staff, if not the attending surgeon. Again there are many different methods employed by surgeons to successfully create a sterile field, and while there is no standard, there are some general points worth remembering to decrease the risk of complications. Foundation layer drapes should be placed at least 3 to 5 cm inside the outer edge of the sterilely prepared skin.[33] U-drapes are often used to properly seal off the perineum and gluteal areas while allowing maximum possible exposure, and top drapes should be waterproof to avoid soaking contamination during the operation. If patients are placed in the lateral position, top drapes should be arranged to allow for a sterile pocket in which to place the leg following dislocation. In addition, many surgeons have also begun to routinely employ the use of iodophor-impregnated adhesive drapes to further seal off the operative area. Theoretically, these drapes help to isolate the incision site and they provide another barrier to fluid leakage and drape liftoff. While there is little evidence to demonstrate a decrease in surgical site infections while using adhesive drapes, there have been reports of decreased wound contamination with their use in hip surgery.[34] Finally, due to the risk of glove contamination during the draping process, it is advisable to change the top pair of gloves prior to making an incision as gloves used exclusively for draping have been shown to be frequently contaminated prior to hip arthroplasty procedures.[35]

Summary

THA has become one of the most common and most successful procedures in orthopedic surgery. Demographic studies project a tremendous increase in the demand for hip arthroplasty over the next 20 years.[36] In order to increase the efficiency of total hip replacement surgery and optimize patient outcomes, the development of an efficient, reliable, and reproducible preoperative routine is essential. The setup of the OR is a critical component of this preoperative plan, and the surgeon must pay great attention to detail during the process to limit chances of failure. Diligent preparation of the OR and the patient will not only improve the efficiency of the procedure, but will also greatly enhance sterility and decrease the likelihood of both intraoperative and postoperative complications.

References

1. Ethgen O, Bruyère O, Richy F, Dardennes C, Reginster JY. Health-related quality of life in total hip and total knee arthroplasty: a qualitative and systematic review of the literature. *J Bone Joint Surg Am.* 2004;86-A(5):963-974.
2. DiGioa A, Jaramaz B, Blackwell M, et al. The Otto Aufranc Award. Image guided navigation system to measure intraoperatively acetabular implant alignment. *Clin Orthop Relat Res.* 1998;(355):8-22.
3. Della Valle AG, Padgett DE, Salvati EA. Preoperative planning for primary total hip arthroplasty. *J Am Acad Ortho Surg.* 2005;13:455-462.
4. Blom A, Taylor AH, Pattison G, Whitehouse S, Bannister GC. Infection after total hip arthroplasty. The Avon experience. *J Bone Joint Surg Br.* 2003;85(7):956-959.
5. Fitzgerald R. Infected total hip arthroplasty: diagnosis and treatment. *J Am Acad Ortho Surg.* 1995;3:249-262.
6. Whitehouse J, Friedman ND, Kirkland KB, Richardson WJ, Sexton DJ. The impact of surgical-site infections following orthopedic surgery at a community hospital and a university hospital: adverse quality of life, excess length of stay, and extra cost. *Infect Control Hosp Epidemiol.* 2002;23:183–189.
7. Manniën J, Wille JC, Snoeren RL, van den Hof S. Impact of postdischarge surveillance on surgical site infection rates for several surgical procedures: results from the nosocomial surveillance network in The Netherlands. *Infect Control Hosp Epidemiol.* 2006;27:809–816.
8. Fitzgerald R. Total hip arthroplasty sepsis. Prevention and diagnosis. *Orthop Clin North Am.* 1992;23(2):259-264.
9. Bratzler D, Houck PM, Richards C, et al. Use of antimicrobial prophylaxis for major surgery: baseline results from the National Surgical Infection Prevention Project. *Arch Surg.* 2005;140:174-82.
10. Sia IG, Berbari EF, Karchmer AW. Prosthetic joint infections. *Infect Dis Clin North Am.* 2005;19:885-914.
11. Hanssen A, Osmon D. The use of prophylactic antimicrobial agents during and after hip arthroplasty. *Clin Orthop Relat Res.* 1999;369:124-138.
12. Rosenberg AD. Ensuring appropriate timing of antimicrobial prophylaxis. *J Bone Joint Surg Am.* 2008;90(2):226-32.
13. Davis K, Stewart JJ, Crouch HK, Florez CE, Hospenthal DR. Methicillin-resistant Staphylococcus aureus (MRSA) nares colonization at hospital admission and its effect on subsequent MRSA infection. *Clin Infect Dis.* 2004;15;39(6):776-782.
14. Rohr U, Mueller C, Wilhelm M, Muhr G, Gatermann S. Methicillin-resistant Staphylococcus aureus whole-body decolonization among hospitalized patients with variable site colonization by using mupirocin in combination with octenidine dihydrochloride. *J Hosp Infect.* 2003;54(4):305-309.

15. Wilcox M, Hall J, Pike H, et al. Use of perioperative mupirocin to prevent methicillin-resistant Staphylococcus aureus (MRSA) orthopaedic surgical site infections. *J Hosp Infect.* 2003;54(3):196-201.
16. Lidwell O, Lowbury EJ, Whyte W, Blowers R, Stanley SJ, Lowe D. Airborne contamination of wounds in joint replacement operations: the relationship to sepsis rates. *J Hosp Infect.* 1983;4:111-131.
17. Nelson J, Glassburn AR Jr, Talbott RD, McElhinney JP. The effect of previous surgery, operating room environment, and preventive antibiotics on post-operative infection following total hip arthroplasty. *Clin Orthop Relat Res.* 1980;147:167-169.
18. Charnley J, Eftekhar N. Postoperative infection in total prosthetic replacement arthroplasty of the hip-joint. With special reference to the bacterial content of the air of the operating room. *Br J Surg.* 1969;56(9):641-649.
19. Shaw J, Bordner MA, Hamory BH. Efficacy of the steri-shield filtered exhaust helmet in limiting bacterial counts in the operating room during total joint arthroplasty. *J Arthroplasty.* 1996;11(4): 469-473.
20. Hospital Infections Program, Centers for Disease Control and Prevention. Guideline for prevention of surgical site infection. *Infect Control Hosp Epidemiol.* 1999;20(4):247-278.
21. Memarzadeh F, Manning A. Reducing risks of surgery. *ASHRAE Journal.* 2002;108:1-13.
22. Tanner J, Parkinson H. Double-gloving to reduce surgical cross-infection. *Cochrane Database Syst Rev.* 2006 19;3:CD003087.
23. Guss D, Bhattacharyya T. Perioperative management of the obese orthopaedic patient. *J Am Acad Orthop Surg.* 2006;14(7):425-432.
24. Nercessian OA, Macaulay W, Stinchfield FE. Peripheral neuropathies following total hip arthroplasty. *J Arthroplasty.* 1994;9(6):645-651.
25. Posta AG Jr, Allen AA, Nercessian OA. Neurologic injury in the upper extremity after total hip arthroplasty. *Clin Orthop Relat Res.* 1997;(345):181-186.
26. Woolston ST, Watt JM. Intermittent pneumatic compression to prevent proximal deep venous thrombosis during and after total hip replacement. A prospective, randomized study of compression alone, compression and aspirin, and compression and low-dose warfarin. *J Bone Joint Surg Am.* 1991;73(4):507-512.
27. Morton HE. Alcohols. In: Block SS, ed. *Disinfection, Sterilization and Preservation.* Philadelphia, PA: Lea and Febiger; 1983:225–239.
28. Tanner J, Swarbrook S, Stuart J. Surgical hand antisepsis to reduce surgical site infection. *Cochrane Database Syst Rev.* 2008;(1):CD004288.
29. Carro C, Camilleri L, Traore O, et al. An in-use microbiological comparison of two surgical hand disinfection techniques in cardiothoracic surgery: hand rubbing versus hand scrubbing. *J Hosp Infect.* 2007;67(1):62-66.
30. Gilliam DL, Nelson CL. Comparison of a one-step iodophor skin preparation versus traditional preparation in total joint surgery. *Clin Orthop Relat Res.* 1990;(250):258-260.
31. Jacobson C, Osmon DR, Hanssen A, et al. Prevention of wound contamination using DuraPrep solution plus Ioban 2 drapes. *Clin Orthop Relat Res.* 2005;439:323-327.
32. Brown AR, Taylor GJS, Gregg PJ. Air contamination during skin preparation and draping in joint replacement surgery. *J Bone Joint Surg Br.* 1996;78(1):92-94.
33. Crenshaw AH Jr. Surgical Techniques and Approaches. In: Canale ST, ed. *Campbell's Operative Orthopaedics.* 10th ed. Philadelphia, PA: Mosby; 2003:9-10.
34. Fairclough JA, Johnson D, Mackie I. The prevention of wound contamination by skin organisms by the pre-operative application of an iodophor impregnated plastic adhesive drape. *J Int Med Res.* 1986;14(2):105-109.
35. McCue SF, Berg EW, Saunders EA. Efficacy of double-gloving as a barrier to microbial contamination during total joint arthroplasty. *J Bone Joint Surg Am.* 1981;63(5):811-813.
36. Kurtz S, Ong K, Lau E, Mowat F, Halpern M. Projections of primary and revision hip and knee arthroplasty in the United States from 2005 to 2030. *J Bone Joint Surg Am.* 2007;89(4):780-785.

17

Implants

Elie Ghanem, MD; Javad Parvizi, MD, FRCS; and Brian A. Klatt, MD

The implants we use to replace a hip are far more complex than they seem at first glance. The variances are numerous and this topic can take some time to master. Even when describing one general class of implant there are differences in materials, sizes, and insertion techniques. The designs of these implants vary in effort to optimize fixation, biomechanical function, and long-term survival. A good knowledge of the various implants on the market is essential to aid the surgeon in choosing the proper implant for each patient. In this chapter, the goal will be to provide a basic overview of implant types and some differences. It will require further time and study for the surgeon to master this topic. As you see surgeons use various implants, be sure to ask questions about why the implant was chosen and how the technique to insert the implant differs.

Femoral Component

A basic division between stem types is the fixation method. Today there are 2 main techniques to fix the stem to the femoral bone. The first great successes in total hip arthroplasty (THA) came with "cemented" fixation. In attempts to overcome issues related to cemented fixation, press-fit stems were developed, which allow bone ingrowth or ongrowth for fixation. Within both the cemented and press-fit stems there are also many variances.

Common Variances in Both Cemented and Press-Fit Stems

Only a few stem designs will be discussed in this section. These stems are used as examples only. There are numerous other stems that are not discussed here. The reader can take the examples here and read the relevant company literature to determine how other stems compare in these common variances.

Neck Angle

The neck angle varies between implants. This is an important consideration to explore when trying to replicate the native biomechanics for your patient. If the patient has a varus neck angle, options can be explored to match this angle. For example, the original Taperloc stem (Biomet, Warsaw, IN) had a 138-degree neck-shaft angle (Figure 17-1A). This high neck angle contrasts that of the Accolade stem (Stryker, Mahwah, NJ), which offers 132- and 127-degree neck-shaft angle options (Figure 17-1B). While at first evaluation this difference may seem of minimal consequence, it can be very helpful. Using a longer head adds more to offset with a lower neck-shaft angle than with a higher neck-shaft angle. Stability can be achieved with offset rather than

Parvizi J, Klatt BA.
Essentials in Total Hip Arthroplasty (pp 139-146).

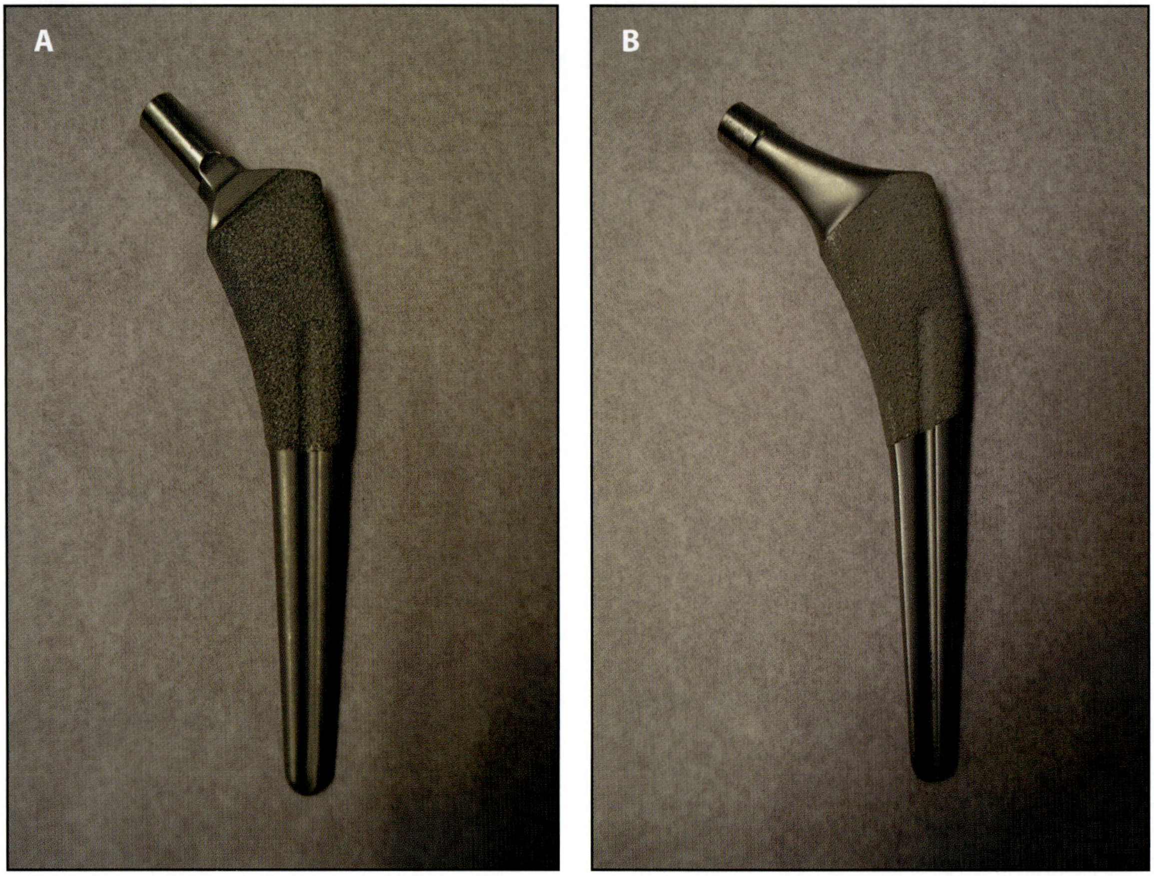

Figure 17-1. Two examples of tapered wedge, proximal ingrowth stems. (A) Taperloc stem with 138-degree neck angle. (B) Accolade stem with 132-degree neck angle.

increasing leg length. The new Taperloc Complete stem (Biomet) now offers a 133-degree neck-shaft angle. It is important for the surgeon to think about what the consequences of the neck-shaft angle are and plan for the proper stem to recreate the biomechanics of the hip.

Offset Options

Instead of having a neck-shaft angle change like the Accolade, other systems offer 2 offset options in the same neck angle. This provides for an increase in offset without changing the stem size or leg length. Some prefer this to the angle change that is available in the Accolade stem. The offset option in the Taperloc system is 7-mm greater with the high offset option. There may be variances in the amount of offset available with each system.

Anatomic Versus Straight Stems

Anatomic stems may offer a built-in version within the neck of the femoral component to replicate the native 15 degrees of femoral anteversion. The Prodigy stem (DePuy, Warsaw, IN) is one such stem.

Cemented Stems

Studies have shown that the cemented Charnley prosthesis provides excellent long-term results, but there have been multiple reports that have shown less favorable results in young patients.[1] There is evidence to support the use of either cemented or press-fit stems, so the choice is really up to the surgeon. In the elderly patient with poor bone stock, the cemented stem is often the best choice. When choosing a cemented implant, there are variances that one needs to be aware of to make an educated choice.

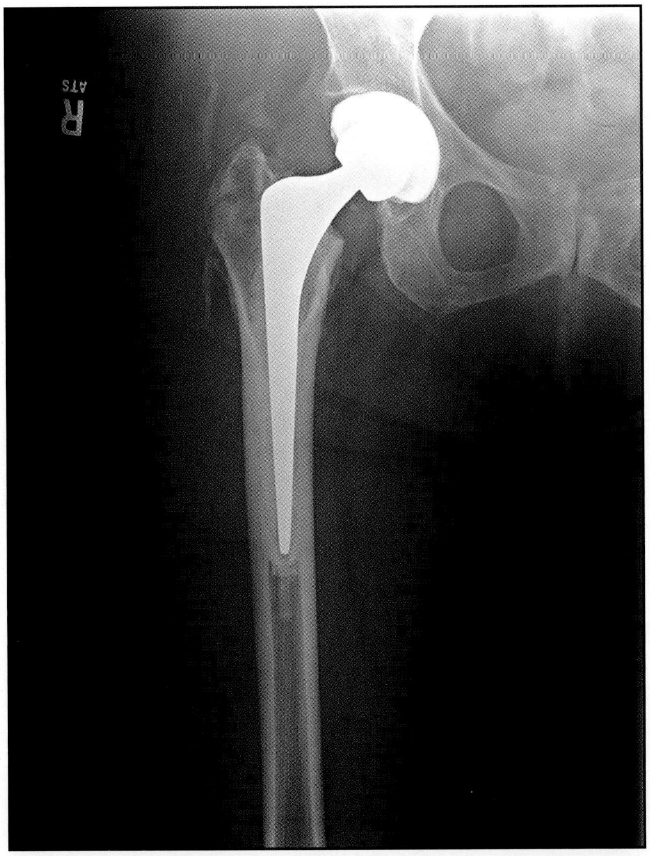

Figure 17-2. AP radiograph of a left THA with an Exeter cemented stem. Stem is a smooth, polished stem with no collar.

Design Differences in Cemented Stems

Collar

There are proposed benefits to the use of a collar but there are also proposed disadvantages. The collar aids the surgeon in the placement of the stem. It is far easier to control the depth and varus-valgus position with the collar. Also, the collar potentially allows for greater load transfer to the proximal femur, preventing stress shielding, decreasing proximal stem stresses, diminishing micromotion, and decreasing strain on the proximal cement mantle. Opponents of the collar believe that the collar is not in contact in all cases and can generate wear debris at this contact point. Most of the opponents are also in favor of the use of a smooth, collarless, tapered stem, which allows controlled subsidence in the cement mantle. Adding a collar to a smooth, tapered stem would not make sense for controlled subsidence philosophy. A great example of a collarless, tapered, polished stem is the Exeter stem (Stryker) (Figure 17-2). The collar is usually added to an implant that maintains stability by being contained within the cement mantle. A good example of a stem with a collar is the Omnifit EON (Stryker) (Figure 17-3).

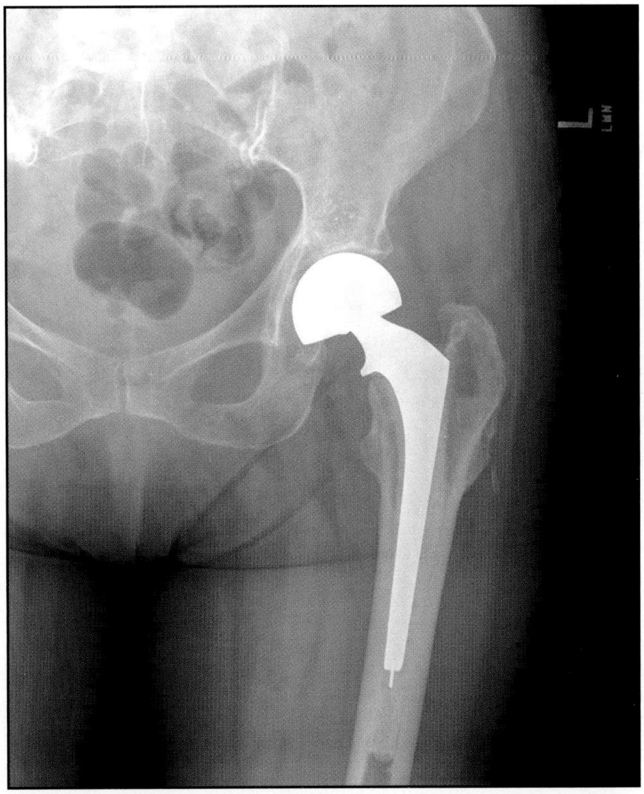

Figure 17-3. AP radiograph of a right hip hemiarthroplasty (bipolar) with an Omnifit EON stem. The stem has a collar.

Material

The original stems were stainless steel, but the most commonly used materials now are cobalt-chrome (Co-Cr) and titanium. The stiffer stems made from Co-Cr are able to reduce cement stresses. The less stiff titanium stem may be prone to micromotion and this may lead to debonding. The Exeter and Omnifit EON are both made of Co-Cr.

Surface Texturing

The texturing of the cemented component is a controversial subject. Studies are available to support or refute the use of this technique. Historically, the polished smooth stem has done extremely well. Stems of this design include the Exeter. The stem is smooth and this allows for controlled subsidence within the cement mantle. Other implants have been tried with enhanced surfaces of various types, such as macrotexturing, microtexturing, and precoating. These surface treatments seek to improve the bond between implant and cement. The concern is for cases of debonding. If the textured stem debonds from the cement, this interface can generate a large amount of debris.

Cementless Femoral Components

The earliest of the cementless femoral components achieved stability through bone growth into large fenestrations in the implants. An example of this type of ingrowth is the Austin Moore prosthesis (DePuy). Newer implants have evolved with grit-blasted titanium, plasma sprayed titanium, and porous metals that achieve ongrowth or ingrowth to the metal itself. The Harris-Galante Porous I stem (Zimmer, Warsaw, IN) was introduced to overcome the failure rate of the cemented prosthesis. Long-term results were disappointing with a survivorship of 82% at 15 years follow-up.[2] This stem was not circumferentially coated with ingrowth surface, and this allowed wear debris a passage around the stem. Distal osteolysis was a concern. Proximal porous coated stems have a survival rate of over 90% at 10 years and good to excellent clinical results.[3] All current stem designs involve circumferential coating of the proximal portion of the stem. There are many versions of this type of stem that now have proven results with long-term follow-up.

The designs can be loosely classified into several categories to simplify the discussion: tapered stems, extensively coated stems, and modular components.

When the ingrowth stems were first being discussed, the classification was anatomic or straight stems. Currently, this is really not an easy way to classify stems. Most of the stems on the market are straight but some anatomic features have been included in the designs. Historically, anatomic stems were designed to fill the canal of the femur anatomically and the straight stems were designed to either wedge into the metaphysis for stability or gain fill of the diaphysis for initial scratch fit.

The anatomic stems have a slight proximal posterior bow at the metaphysis and a distal anterior bow to fit the anatomy of the femoral canal.[4] The femoral neck is anteverted to compensate for the predetermined rotational alignment.[5] Porous-coated anatomic stems have good long-term survivorship and functional outcome in young, active patients.[6]

The straight stems can be tapered and fill the proximal portion of the femur or parallel side and achieve less proximal fill of the metaphysic.[7] Cylindrical stems allow for close contact between the cortical bone of the proximal diaphysis for initial stability.[8] Wedge-shaped stems achieve contact with metaphyseal bone but lack contact with the proximal diaphysis.[9] Stems with a wide proximal body and a rectangular shape in the horizontal cross-section allow for excellent rotational and torsional stability.[7]

Coatings can be added to the stem to enhance the ingrowth of bone. Hydroxyapatite (HA) coating was first introduced in 1985 to facilitate the formation of a biological bond between the host bone and implant.[10] Several studies have reported encouraging results with HA-coated stems in young, active patients, with a survivorship of 90% to 100% at 10 to 12 years.[11]

Tapered Stems

The tapered stem is a straight stem that encompasses several basic designs, such as the tapered wedge stem with proximal ingrowth, the Zweymuller stems (Sulzer, Switzerland), and the ream and broach stems.

The tapered wedge stem with proximal ingrowth includes stems such as the Tri-Lock (DePuy), the Taperloc, and the Accolade stems (see Figure 17-1). These stems are inserted with a technique that involves a canal finder only and then a broach-only technique. Porous coating is only present on the proximal portion of the stem. Any of the tapered stems can result in a femoral fracture, but this becomes a rare event with experience.

The Zweymuller stem is a straight, tapered wedge that is long enough to gain press-fit fixation in the upper diaphysis. The entire surface of this implant is roughened by corundum blasting to promote bone apposition. There are a number of companies that offer similar stems.

The ream and broach stems mostly rely on a proximal tapered body. This stem is the best of the tapered stems for dealing with the Dorr A type femur. Both the tapered wedge stem and the Zweymuller type stems can become potted distally in a narrow femur and thus not get a proper tapered fit in the metaphysis. With the ream and broach stems, the canal can be reamed so this does not happen. Stems that would be considered in this class are the Summit (DePuy) and the Secur-Fit (Stryker).

Extensively Coated Stems

Extensively coated stems are usually straight stems. Extensive porous-coated stems that achieve purchase more distally have shown a 96% rate of good to excellent clinical results at long-term follow-up.[12] The first stem to demonstrate this success was the Anatomical Medullary Locking stem (AML) (DePuy). Many companies offer an implant of this type now. The ingrowth and long-term survival is good. The concerns with the implant type are stress shielding of proximal bone and the difficulty of removing the stem if revision is needed. Again, there are differences in the stems and the surgeon needs to understand these factors as discussed for the proximal ingrowth stems. An anatomic neck with built-in 10 degrees anteversion was added to the Prodigy (DePuy).

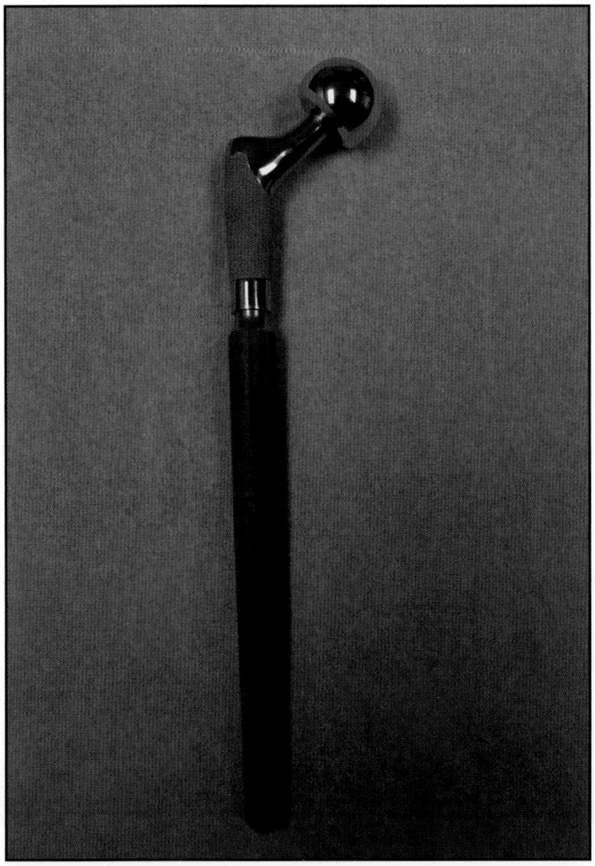

Figure 17-4. Restoration Modular System. The revision stem is shown with a cobalt-chromium head, cone body, and conical stem.

Modular Components

One of the first modular components introduced was the S-ROM stem (DePuy). The S-ROM stem was first introduced in 1984 to facilitate the management of difficult and complex THA, especially in patients with juvenile rheumatoid arthritis and developmental dysplasia of the hip (DDH) or in patients following fracture or corrective osteotomy.[13] The S-ROM is a unique system that allows 360 degrees of rotation of the femoral neck with relation to the stem and sleeve. The modularity of this implant allows for a wide variety of options to match native bone.

Excellent midterm follow-up (average, 5.3 years) of the S-ROM stem with 98% stable bone ingrowth and 7% bone lysis restricted to above the sleeve has been reported.[14] Some surgeons use this implant for all cases while others restrict its use to the complex cases that require its flexibility.

Recently, a new class of modular implants was brought to the market. These implants had a modular neck in proximally tapered stems. There were issues with fretting, corrosion, and breakage at this modular junction. The promise of the modularity is attractive to achieve balance and stability of the hip, but the downside of this additional junction seems to outweigh that benefit. Most of the stems are no longer on the market and those that are should be used with caution.

A new generation of modular implants continues to evolve for use in revision THA. To address the complexities of revision in the femoral component, these implants offer a wide variety of distal stem types and proximal bodies. A good example of this versatile revision stem is the Restoration Modular System (Stryker) (Figure 17-4). Distal stem options include a conical stem, a plasma stem, and a fluted stem. Proximal bodies have 5 options: broached, calcar, milled, cone, and MT3.

When using a modular implant, it is important to remember that the junctions are always potential sites for wear debris generation or implant fatigue. The history of this class has shown multiple fatigue failures and at the junctions. The most recent generation of modular implants has been introduced with "beefed up" junctional metal but unless the forces are kept below the endurance limit, a fracture could occur in time. The surgeon needs to prepare the bone in such a manner as to prevent this occurrence by achieving ingrowth on both sides of the junction.

ACETABULAR COMPONENTS

Originally, the acetabular component consisted of a cemented all-polyethylene (PE) cup.[15] The cemented all-PE cup performed well in elderly and low-demand patients. Most studies have shown that this design is plagued by a high rate of loosening in young patients.[16] The cemented cup still serves a role in the tumor patient with highly irradiated bone or in situations where ingrowth is unlikely to occur. To provide for longer survival in young patients, cementless acetabular components were introduced in an attempt to improve fixation and osseointegration. Long-term stability is determined by the osseous ingrowth and depends on the acetabular coating.[17]

Early designs included threaded cups designed to cut through the bone for the initial fixation and primary stability. However, long-term results (>10 years) proved to be disappointing with the smooth-threaded and roughened acetabular component because of poor biologic fixation of the smooth surface and lack of osteointegration.[18] Other early designs included tri-spiked sockets. This cup design was found to decrease micromotion of the acetabular component in the ischial and pubic regions.[19] The porous-coated acetabular component (Harris-Galante) has shown excellent survivorship in the elderly at 10 years follow-up and reproducible midterm to long-term survivorship in the younger population.[20] Polywear, liner problems, and osteolysis were the major problems with first-generation cementless acetabular components.[21] Improvements in the liner material have resolved many of these issues.

Most modern designs are hemispherical shells with screw holes in the shell to improve initial stability as needed. These cups have grit-blasted or plasma-sprayed rough surfaces that can be either porous-coated or have HA coating for additional bone ingrowth. HA-coated acetabular components have not consistently shown successful results as the HA-coated femoral components.[22] HA-coated cups have better radiographic results and midterm survivorship as compared with a similar, non-HA-coated cup.[23] The surface of the cup can be smooth (microstructured) using grit blasting or roughened (macrostructured) with the metal coating arc deposited. Newer materials such as porous titanium and tantalum shells promise a surface more conductive to bony ingrowth. Screws can be added through holes in the shell to improve acetabular fixation as needed. Two screws are usually adequate if added in a primary hip replacement.

Choice of Bearing Surfaces

Metal-on-PE bearing surfaces remain the most widely used combination in THA. Although ultra-high molecular weight polyethylene (UHMWPE) has low friction and dampening properties,[24] it is marred by adhesive and abrasive wear. The UHMWPE particles produced from cyclical loading are thought to play a major role in particle-induced osteolysis and secondary implant failure and loosening.[25] There are many new alternatives to conventional PE, including highly cross-linked PE and hard-on-hard surfaces like alumina-on-alumina and metal-on-metal.

Highly Cross-Linked Polyethylene

The cross-linking process involves irradiation of the PE followed by heating to a temperature less than the melting point (annealing) or higher than the melting point (remelting). Remelting clears the original material of any free radicals.[26] Remelting does alter the mechanical properties of the PE, and this may lead to a higher risk of implant fracture than in the conventional or annealed liners. The annual linear wear for highly cross-linked PE has been reported to be 45% that of the conventional liner at 5 years after implantation.[27] Long-term results (10 to 20 years) of highly cross-linked PE support that the low wear rates reported approach that of metal-on-metal and ceramic-on-ceramic bearings.[28]

Ceramic-on-Ceramic

Ceramic-on-ceramic surfaces include alumina and zirconia oxides. Ceramics are hard and strong but brittle. Ceramics are resistant to mechanical and chemical corrosion as well as oxidation.[29] Although alumina is relatively brittle, the risk of fracture has been reported to be 0.02%.[30] Newer ceramics such as BIOLOX delta ceramic (CeramTec AG, Plochingen, Germany) is a zirconia-toughened, platelet-reinforced alumina ceramic designed to incorporate the wear properties and stability of alumina with vastly improved material strength and toughness. As the quality of ceramic materials has improved, the incidence of ceramic fracture has decreased. Alumina ceramics have been shown to have a lower wear rate than PE-on-metal and metal-on-metal combinations resulting from a greater resistance to wear and a lower coefficient of friction. Favorable results in terms of decreased wear rate and limited osteolysis have been reported in young and active patients with a survival rate of 85.6% in patients with cementless acetabular components.[31] However, ceramic-on-ceramic bearings have been associated with some setbacks, such as implant loosening, component fracture, and impingement between the cup and stem neck. Also, ceramic-on-ceramic components can at times emit an audible squeaking sound in as high as 7% of hips done with this bearing surface. This sound can be audible and troubling and it has lead to many revisions for squeaking joints. A sandwich design of ceramic-PE liner is 30 times less stiff than a ceramic-only liner and has shown encouraging short-term (5 years) results in terms of radiographic and clinical outcome.[32] However, a recent study reported a 17% failure rate due to alumina liner fracture and component dissociation.[33]

Metal-on-Metal

At this time, the metal-on-metal hip replacement has fallen out of favor due to issues with metallosis causing local and systemic damage. Although the troubles have been largely associated with several implants, there has been a drastic reduction in the use of the metal-on-metal bearings.

Metal-on-metal bearings lost favor in the 1950s because of poor outcomes with the McKee-Farrar design and the introduction of the Charnley low-friction metal-on-PE prosthesis.[34] Second-generation metal-on-metal components included certain improvements in metallurgy and design. Metal-on-metal designs can produce metallosis when impingement occurs and produce third-body effect in the articulating surface.[35] Cobalt levels must be measured to assess wear of a metal-on-metal bearing because

Table 17-1

Examples of Various Stems From Four Different Implant Manufacturers

	Biomet	DePuy	Stryker	Zimmer
Collared cemented stem	Echo	Summit Cemented	Omnifit EON	Versys Advocate
Polished, tapered, collarless cemented stem	Gen 4 (has a collar)	C-Stem AMT	Exeter	CPT
Tapered stem	Taperloc	Tri-lock	Accolade	M/L Taper
Fit and fill	Bimetric	Summit	Secur-Fit	Fibermetal Taper (FMT)
Long porous coated	Reach	Prodigy/AML	Restoration HA	VerSys Epoch
Modular primary stems		S-ROM		
Modular revision stems	Arcos	ReClaim	Restoration Modular	ZMR

conventional radiographic methods are not helpful. Hypersensitivity reactions have been described in hip capsules.[28] The dislocation rate was 4 times lower in the metal-on-metal bearing group versus the alumina-on-alumina group.[28] Osteolysis is rarely present in metal-on-metal components that are well fixed. The 5-year survival rate of metal-on-metal articulation in young patients was reported to be slightly higher than that of their control group in terms of age and gender when using ceramic-on-PE bearings (97%).[36] Metal-on-metal articulation had less aseptic loosening and excellent patient satisfaction rating of the acetabular and femoral components compared to the metal-on-PE articulation.[37]

Recommendations for Young Patients

Cementless THA using proximally coated stems and an alternative bearing surface is currently preferred in North America. Due to the issues with metal-on-metal and ceramic-on-ceramic, the pendulum has swung back to PE. The newer PE liners are performing well with low wear rates.

Summary

This chapter has only scratched the surface of a rather large topic. Each company offers multiple stems and cups, and the variances in the implants can be confusing (Table 17-1). A good arthroplasty surgeon needs to understand the implants to choose the ones that offer the best outcomes for his or her patients. Good luck!

References

1. Devitt A, O'Sullivan T, Quinlan W. 16- to 25-year follow-up study of cemented arthroplasty of the hip in patients aged 50 years or younger. *J Arthroplasty.* 1997;12(5):479-489.
2. Parvizi J, Sullivan T, Duffy G, Cabanela ME. Fifteen-year clinical survivorship of Harris-Galante total hip arthroplasty. *J Arthroplasty.* 2004;19(6):672-677.
3. Eskelinen A, Paavolainen P, Helenius I, Pulkkinen P, Remes V. Total hip arthroplasty for rheumatoid arthritis in younger patients: 2,557 replacements in the Finnish Arthroplasty Register followed for 0-24 years. *Acta Orthop.* 2006;77(6):853-865.
4. Herrera A, Canales V, Anderson J, Garcia-Araujo C, Murcia-Mazon A, Tonino AJ. Seven to 10 years followup of an anatomic hip prosthesis: an international study. *Clin Orthop Relat Res.* 2004;(423):129-137.
5. Kim YH. Titanium and cobalt-chrome cementless femoral stems of identical shape produce equal results. *Clin Orthop Relat Res.* 2004;(427):148-156.
6. Butler JB, Lansky D, Duwelius PJ. Prospective evaluation of total hip arthroplasty with a cementless, anatomically designed, porous-coated femoral implant: mean 11-year follow-up. *J Arthroplasty.* 2005;20(6):709-716.
7. Pospischill M, Knahr K. Cementless total hip arthroplasty using a threaded cup and a rectangular tapered stem. Follow-up for ten to 17 years. *J Bone Joint Surg Br.* 2005;87(9):1210-1215.

8. Bobyn JD, Pilliar RM, Cameron HU, Weatherly GC. The optimum pore size for the fixation of porous-surfaced metal implants by the ingrowth of bone. *Clin Orthop Relat Res.* 1980;(150):263-270.
9. Engh CA, Bobyn JD, Glassman AH. Porous-coated hip replacement. The factors governing bone ingrowth, stress shielding, and clinical results. *J Bone Joint Surg Br.* 1987;69(1):45-55.
10. Singh S, Trikha SP, Edge AJ. Hydroxyapatite ceramic-coated femoral stems in young patients. A prospective ten-year study. *J Bone Joint Surg Br.* 2004;86(8):1118-1123.
11. Capello WN, D'Antonio JA, Feinberg JR, Manley MT. Ten-year results with hydroxyapatite-coated total hip femoral components in patients less than fifty years old. A concise follow-up of a previous report. *J Bone Joint Surg Am.* 2003;85-A(5):885-889.
12. la Valle CJ, Paprosky WG. The middle-aged patient with hip arthritis: the case for extensively coated stems. *Clin Orthop Relat Res.* 2002;(405):101-107.
13. Buly R. The S-ROM stem: versatility of stem/sleeve combinations and head options. *Orthopedics.* 2005;28(9 suppl):s1025-s1032.
14. Tanzer M, Chan S, Brooks CE, Bobyn JD. Primary cementless total hip arthroplasty using a modular femoral component: a minimum 6-year follow-up. *J Arthroplasty.* 2001;16(8 suppl 1):64-70.
15. Kavanagh BF, Dewitz MA, Ilstrup DM, Stauffer RN, Coventry MB. Charnley total hip arthroplasty with cement. Fifteen-year results. *J Bone Joint Surg Am.* 1989;71(10):1496-1503.
16. Mulroy WF, Estok DM, Harris WH. Total hip arthroplasty with use of so-called second-generation cementing techniques. A fifteen-year-average follow-up study. *J Bone Joint Surg Am.* 1995;77(12):1845-1852.
17. Cheung KW, Yung SH, Wong KC, Chiu KH. Early failure of smooth hydroxyapatite-coated press-fit acetabular cup--7 years of follow-up. *J Arthroplasty.* 2005;20(5):627-631.
18. Pupparo F, Engh CA. Comparison of porous-threaded and smooth-threaded acetabular components of identical design. Two- to four-year results. *Clin Orthop Relat Res.* 1991;(271):201-206.
19. Perona PG, Lawrence J, Paprosky WG, Patwardhan AG, Sartori M. Acetabular micromotion as a measure of initial implant stability in primary hip arthroplasty. An in vitro comparison of different methods of initial acetabular component fixation. *J Arthroplasty.* 1992;7(4):537-547.
20. Lachiewicz PF, Messick P. Precoated femoral component in primary hybrid total hip arthroplasty: results at a mean 10-year follow-up. *J Arthroplasty.* 2003;18(1):1-5.
21. Harris WH. Results of uncemented cups: a critical appraisal at 15 years. *Clin Orthop Relat Res.* 2003;(417):121-125.
22. Hermida JC, D'Lima DD, Steklov N, Colwell CW Jr. Outcome of an acetabular design with hydroxyapatite coating on a rough substrate. *Clin Orthop Relat Res.* 2005;441:298-304.
23. D'Antonio JA, Capello WN, Manley MT, Naughton M, Sutton K. A titanium-encased alumina ceramic bearing for total hip arthroplasty: 3- to 5-year results. *Clin Orthop Relat Res.* 2005;441:151-158.
24. Eschbach L. Nonresorbable polymers in bone surgery. *Injury.* 2000;31(suppl 4):22-27.
25. Schmalzried TP, Jasty M, Harris WH. Periprosthetic bone loss in total hip arthroplasty. Polyethylene wear debris and the concept of the effective joint space. *J Bone Joint Surg Am.* 1992;74(6):849-863.
26. Collier JP, Currier BH, Kennedy FE et al. Comparison of cross-linked polyethylene materials for orthopaedic applications. *Clin Orthop Relat Res.* 2003;(414):289-304.
27. Dorr LD, Wan Z, Shahrdar C, Sirianni L, Boutary M, Yun A. Clinical performance of a Durasul highly cross-linked polyethylene acetabular liner for total hip arthroplasty at five years. *J Bone Joint Surg Am.* 2005;87(8):1816-1821.
28. Delaunay CP. Metal-on-metal bearings in cementless primary total hip arthroplasty. *J Arthroplasty.* 2004;19(8 suppl 3):35-40.
29. Konttinen YT, Zhao D, Beklen A, et al. The microenvironment around total hip replacement prostheses. *Clin Orthop Relat Res.* 2005;(430):28-38.
30. Willmann G. Ceramics for total hip replacement--what a surgeon should know. *Orthopedics.* 1998;21(2):173-177.
31. Sedel L, Nizard RS, Kerboull L, Witvoet J. Alumina-alumina hip replacement in patients younger than 50 years old. *Clin Orthop Relat Res.* 1994;(298):1751-83.
32. Ravasi F, Sansone V. Five-year follow-up with a ceramic sandwich cup in total hip replacement. *Arch Orthop Trauma Surg.* 2002;122(6):350-353.
33. Hasegawa M, Sudo A, Uchida A. Alumina ceramic-on-ceramic total hip replacement with a layered acetabular component. *J Bone Joint Surg Br.* 2006;88(7):877-882.
34. McKee GK, Chen SC. The statistics of the McKee-Farrar method of total hip replacement. *Clin Orthop Relat Res.* 1973;(95):26-33.
35. Harris WH. Highly cross-linked, electron-beam-irradiated, melted polyethylene: some pros. *Clin Orthop Relat Res.* 2004;(429):63-67.
36. Migaud H, Jobin A, Chantelot C, Giraud F, Laffargue P, Duquennoy A. Cementless metal-on-metal hip arthroplasty in patients less than 50 years of age: comparison with a matched control group using ceramic-on-polyethylene after a minimum 5-year follow-up. *J Arthroplasty.* 2004;19(8 suppl 3):23-28.
37. Naudie D, Roeder CP, Parvizi J, Berry DJ, Eggli S, Busato A. Metal-on-metal versus metal-on-polyethylene bearings in total hip arthroplasty: a matched case-control study. *J Arthroplasty.* 2004;19(7 suppl 2):35-41.
38. Won CH, Hearn TC, Tile M. Micromotion of cementless hemispherical acetabular components. Does press-fit need adjunctive screw fixation? *J Bone Joint Surg Br.* 1995;77(3):484-489.

18

Surgical Principles of Total Hip Arthroplasty

Luis Pulido, MD and William J. Hozack, MD

Total hip arthroplasty (THA) is one of the greatest advances in orthopedic surgery. Since Sir John Charnley's revolution with the development of the low friction hip arthroplasty, THA has been ruled as the gold standard treatment for end-stage hip disease with excellent long-term clinical results.[1,2] Patients' improvement of function and pain relief are commonly achieved goals after a successful THA. An adequate operative exposure is crucial for optimal component fixation, soft tissue balancing, and successful clinical results.

The advances in modern hip arthroplasty have reduced the failure rate while accommodating to the higher activity and longevity profile of our patients. The evolution in cementation techniques and uncemented fixation has shown excellent long-term outcomes using both methods. Cemented femoral fixation is the most popular method worldwide. Recognized disadvantages of cemented fixation include the presence of 2 separate interfaces with the lack of bone remodeling. Cementless fixation is more commonly used in the United States. This biological method of fixation allows bone remodeling in the metal-bone interface.[3]

Soft tissue balancing and adequate implant positioning are the key surgical principles of total hip replacement. Charnley addressed the importance of soft tissue balancing to increase the abductor moment arm and restore hip biomechanics. His surgical pearls included the following:

- Medialization of the acetabulum to increase the abductor's moment arm.
- Control femoral anatomic anteversion to avoid impingement, micro separation, and instability.
- Greater trochanter advancement. This increases the abductor mechanical strength and joint reaction forces.

Although the current methods of soft tissue balancing in modern hip arthroplasty differ from Charnley's methods, the basic principles remain the same.[4,5]

The versatility of modern hip implants is effective to restore the hip biomechanics and result in a well balanced and stable hip arthroplasty. Knowledge of hip biomechanics, hip anatomy, and features of total hip implants are necessary to understand the surgical principles of hip replacement. Restoring the hip biomechanics with proper soft tissue balancing, limb length equality, and optimal implant positioning are the key surgical principles of total hip replacement.

Basic Biomechanical Concepts

The hip is the pivot upon which the human body is balanced in gait. The hip joint functions as a fulcrum, resulting in a state of equilibrium between body weight and the opposing hip abductors.[6] The length between the hip abductors and the femoral head is about half the distance of the lever arm between the femoral head and the body center of gravity. This possesses a biomechanical disadvantage of the hip abductors, which need to create a force at least twice the body weight to maintain the pelvis level when in a one-legged stance (Figure 18-1).

The estimated load or the joint reaction force on the femoral head and acetabulum in the stance phase of gait

Parvizi J, Klatt BA.
Essentials in Total Hip Arthroplasty (pp 147-152).

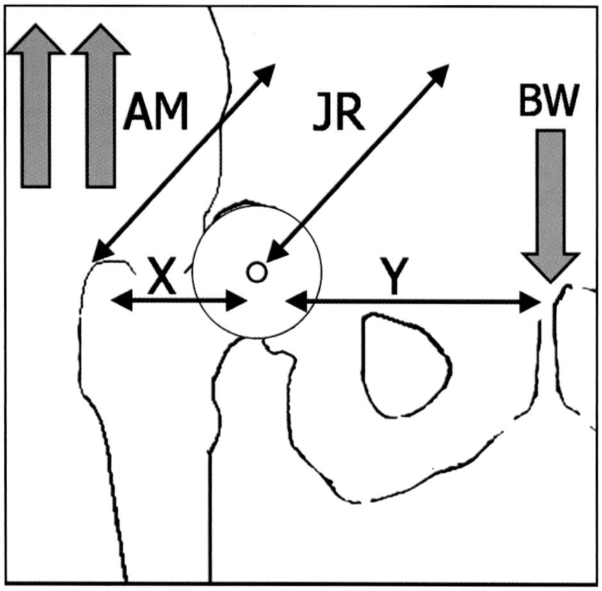

Figure 18-1. Hip biomechanics. X: The abductor's lever arm is the distance from the hip center to line of action of the abductors. Y: Distance between the hip center and the body weight. BW: Body weight. AM: Abductor's action force. JR: Resultant joint reaction force. The increase in the XY ratio (increase abductor lever arm) results in less joint reaction force of the hip. This is accomplished by medializing the acetabulum and increasing neck length or lateral offset. In THA, a decrease in JR leads to less wear.

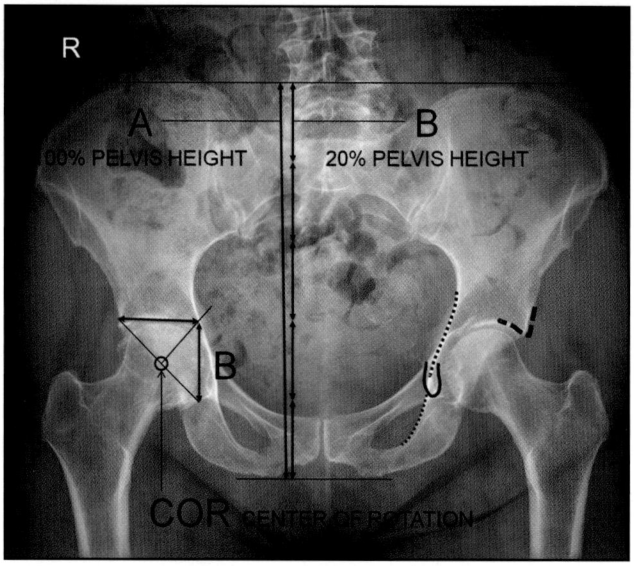

Figure 18-2. The distance from the ischial tuberosities to the iliac crest defines the pelvis height. Line A represents the pelvis height. Line B is 20% of the pelvis height. The true anatomic center of rotation can be located by drawing a right-angled triangle lateral to the tear drop. The triangle vertical and horizontal legs measure 20% of the pelvis height (line B). The midpoint of the hypotenuse of this right-angled triangle is the center of rotation of the hip. The tear drop, the ilioischial line, and the acetabular superolateral border are anatomical landmarks used also to determine the center of rotation.

is equal to the sum of the forces created by the abductors and the body weight, at least 3 times the body weight. The load during straight leg raise is estimated to be about the same. Excess body weight and physical activity significantly increase the forces around the hip joint.

The mechanical ability of the abductors is affected by the neck-shaft angle, neck length, and the hip center of rotation. Restoration of the normal center of rotation, the femoral lateral offset and leg lengths are an important goal to achieve in THA. The features of current implant designs available for THA allow a versatile use and recreation of hip biomechanics.[4]

Acetabular Component

The acetabular component should aim to restore the center of rotation of the hip.[7-9] A high, lateral, or posterior hip center is associated with increased joint reaction forces. An overmedialized acetabular component decreases the joint forces at the expense of bone loss, impingement, and hip instability if the hip center of rotation is not maintained. In clinical practice, the proper placement of the acetabular component may vary depending on the requirements of the reconstruction.

The apex of the acetabular component should be positioned just lateral to the teardrop. Ideally, the acetabular component should be covered at its superolateral margin by host bone with avoidance of overhang. The tear drop, the ilioischial line, and the acetabular superolateral border are helpful anatomical landmarks to determine the center of rotation. A more precise method to determine the true anatomic center of rotation is to draw a right-angled triangle starting 5 mm lateral to the tear drop. The triangle vertical leg should measure 20% of the pelvis height. At 90 degrees, the triangle horizontal leg is also 20% of the pelvis height. The midpoint of the hypotenuse of this right-angled triangle is the approximate center of rotation of the hip (Figure 18-2).

The orientation of the cup should be approximately 45 ± 10 degrees of inclination and 20 ± 10 degrees of anteversion. There are multiple methods used for assessment of adequate cup position, including radiographic, anatomical (bony and soft tissue landmarks), and computer-assisted surgery.[7,8,10,11] Cup position in terms of inclination and anteversion is an important factor for stability and hip range of motion. Acetabular malposition may lead to

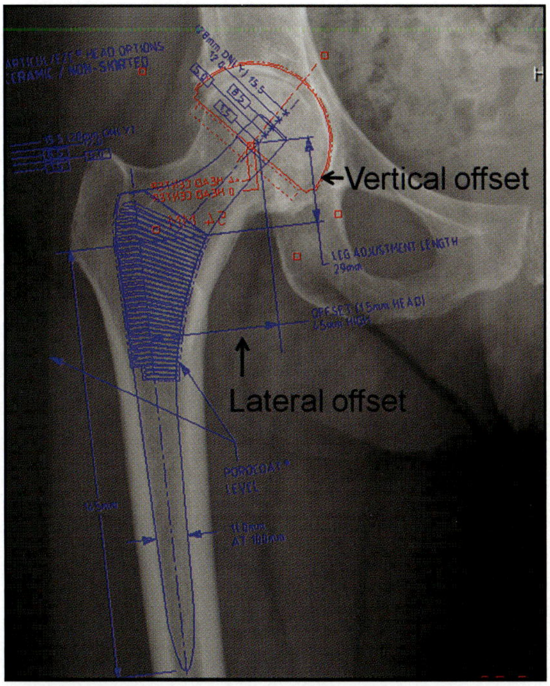

Figure 18-3. Digital preoperative templating allows planning for adequate level of femoral neck cut, restoration of lateral offset, and approximation of leg lengths equality.

instability, limb-length discrepancy, altered hip biomechanics, increased wear, and bony and component impingement.

A number of design features of modular acetabular implants can affect stability and range of motion. Relevant factors include acetabular liner geometry, depth, and the use of extended walls and constraints. The use of elevated rim liners in cementless acetabular fixation is relatively common and has led to controversy regarding their efficacy and indications. The proper use of elevated rim lines improves the rate of dislocations for revision hip arthroplasty. The improper use increases impingement and instability. Lateralized liners increase the lateral offset of the hip, improving soft tissue tensioning at the expense of increased joint reaction forces and acetabular stress.

Special Clinical Scenarios

1. Coxa profunda or acetabular protrusio. The acetabular component needs to be lateralized in these. During surgery, reaming does not extend to the full depth of the protruded wall. The use of the patient femoral head as autograft or morselized allograft and larger cups will help to place the acetabular component in a closer anatomic position lateral to the teardrop.
2. Acetabular dysplasia. The first step is to identify the true acetabulum. Localizing the ligamentum teres and following it to the proximal origin will help to localize the fovea, the transverse acetabular ligament, and the hip true center of rotation. Controlled medialization of the cup is recommended and will improve lateral coverage. In cases of high grade dislocation or in cases with large anterior and superior lateral defects, structural bone graft augmentation and reconstruction with cage or screws may be indicated. The use of high hip center with a smaller acetabular component is another option.

Femoral Component

The main objective on the femoral side is to equalize leg lengths, restore lateral offset, and avoid impingement and instability. Surgical planning should include templating of the femoral stem size, level of neck cut, lateral offset restoration, and leg length equalization. It is helpful to template both the affected and unaffected sides.[4]

The femoral component should be placed neutral within the medullary canal. A neutral stem will transmit the loading forces evenly within the femoral shaft and reduce stress. A varus or flexed femoral stem should be avoided, especially if cemented fixation is used. The version of the stem may be adjusted in cemented or modular neck implants to accommodate for a desired combined cup-stem anteversion goal.

The vertical height, lateral offset, and femoral version are important characteristics of the femoral component[4] (Figure 18-3).

Vertical Height

Vertical height or offset is determined primarily by the length of the prosthetic neck and the size of modular head used. In addition, the depth the implant is inserted into the femoral canal alters vertical height. The femoral neck-stem angle will affect both vertical and lateral offset. Reducing this angle increases lateral offset and abductors moment arm and decreases the vertical offset and length.

Lateral Offset

The definition of lateral offset is the distance from the center of the femoral head to a line through the axis of the distal part of the stem. Increased lateral offset can be achieved by doing the following:

1. Increasing the neck length. Increases leg length and lateral offset.
2. Reducing the neck-stem angle (127 degrees). Decreases leg lengths, increases lateral offset.
3. Medializing the neck of the femoral stem (dual offset implants). Increases lateral offset and does not change leg lengths. Femoral stems are manufactured with standard and high offset versions.

Femoral Version

Femoral version refers to the orientation of the neck in reference to the coronal plane. The normal femur is anteverted 10 to 15 degrees. Restoration of femoral neck version is important in achieving stability of the prosthetic joint. Cemented and uncemented stems with modular necks allow changing of the anteversion of the femoral implant if needed. Cementless stems are nearly fixed to the femoral anatomic version. Ranawat's concept of combined anteversion of the stem and cup should be approximately 35 to 45 degrees in females and 25 to 35 degrees in males.

The advances in modern bearing surfaces allowed the use of larger head sizes. The use of a large femoral head and trapezoidal femoral neck design increases the impingement-free range of motion. Larger head sizes provide greater range of motion through favorable head-neck ratios (≥2.0). This mechanical advantage decreases component impingement, increases range of motion to impingement, and increases the jump distance when component impingement occurs. In a well-positioned cup, larger heads improve hip stability.

Soft Tissue Balancing

Soft tissue balancing and adequate implant positioning are the key surgical principles of THA. The restoration of the femoral lateral offset and abductors tension are the main goals during soft tissue balancing.[12]

Increasing the lateral offset enhances the abductor's attachment moment arm. This biomechanical advantage decreases the magnitude of abductor force necessary for normal gait, and thereby decreases the joint reaction forces and polyethylene wear. The lack of offset restoration results in abductor muscle weakness, limping, and polyethylene wear. Lateral offset also plays an important role in hip stability by soft tissue (abductors) tension and by clearance of femoropelvic impingement.[11] A decreased lateral offset reduces the soft-tissue tension of the hip, leaving it prone to dislocation. Furthermore, the lack of lateral offset reduces the clearance between the femur and the pelvis, which may lead to dislocation through bony impingement.

Soft tissue balancing starts with systematic preoperative planning. Template the acetabulum near the anatomic hip center of rotation. Then, the goal of the femoral component template is to restore femoral lateral offset while maintaining equal limb lengths. This can be anticipated by measuring limb lengths discrepancy, femoral lateral offset, size of femoral component, and level of femoral neck cut as part of your routine surgical plan.[4]

Intraoperatively, limb lengths should be measured prior to dislocation of the hip. Once the acetabular component is implanted and has successfully restored the hip center of rotation, soft tissue balancing is primarily a function of the femoral stem design and position. The arthroplasty surgeon should know his or her options to increase the lateral femoral offset. Preoperative planning allows for templating of higher offset stem designs (medialized neck or reduced neck angle). This can be achieved with a medialized neck or reduced neck angle stems. Intraoperatively, the modular designs allow versatile use of neck size with the femoral head, which will increase length and offset. The use of lateralized liners will also increase the lateral offset and soft tissue tensioning.

Acetabular component position and impingement are assessed during intraoperative trialing. Once the femoral component is implanted, the hip is assessed for soft tissue tensioning, impingement within extreme hip range of motion, stability, and leg lengths. Soft tissue tensioning can be measured with custom external guides (prior to dislocation and after implant placement) or intraoperatively with tests such as the "Shuck test" (distract the femur in an inferior-distal direction to assess soft tissue tension).

Leg lengths can be assessed by palpating the medial malleoli in the decubitus supine position or by leg-to-leg comparison in decubitus lateralis position. The "dropkick test" is another technique to evaluate lengthening (the hip is held in extension while the knee is flexed to 90 degrees. If the extremity is lengthening, the extensor mechanism becomes taut and the knee tends to swing into extension).

Excessive lateral offset and overcorrection may predispose to lateral hip pain due to trochanteric irritation from a tight or stretched iliotibial band. In theory, high offset femoral stems will have higher stresses within the femoral neck and within the cement mantle on cemented stems.

Dynamic Impingement

Impingement with THA can be defined as the mechanical abutment between the prosthetic neck with the cup or liner (neck-on-cup implant impingement), or between the femoral trochanters with the pelvis (bone-on-bone impingement).[11] Dynamic impingement is a cause of hip instability, accelerated wear, aseptic loosening, and pain. Impingement associated with alternative hard-on-hard bearing surfaces may present with specific adverse outcomes. Ceramic-on-ceramic impingement is associated with an increased risk of ceramic fracture and squeaking. Metal-on-metal impingement may result in metallosis.

In the majority of cases, dynamic impingement is surgeon dependent. There are implant design factors and surgical technique factors; both of these elements should be controlled by the operating surgeon. Patients with a high dynamic pelvic tilt or with very flexible hips may reach dynamic impingement despite optimal hip arthroplasty balance and position.

Implant design factors include the femoral head-neck ratio and some features of the acetabular component. Surgical technique factors on the acetabular side are mostly related to the cup position (depth, anteversion, inclination). The femoral reconstruction variables include the level of the neck cut, the stem position, the lateral offset, and leg lengths (Table 18-1).

Table 18-1

Methods to Minimize Dynamic Impingement With Total Hip Arthroplasty

Implant design factors:

- Improved head-neck ratio
- Use large head available for acetabular size
- Avoid skirts on femoral heads
    - Use trapezoidal neck designs
    - Acetabular features
    - Avoid chamfer geometry of acetabular liners

Correct use of elevated rim liners (apex posterior inferior):

- Left hip 4 to 5 o' clock position
- Right hip 7 to 8 o' clock position

Surgical technique factors:

- Ranawat's combined stem and cup anteversion of 40 degrees in females and 20 degrees in males
- Acetabular inclination of 45 ± 10 degrees
- Acetabular anteversion of 20 ± 10 degrees (less for anterior approaches)
- Avoid excessive medialization of the cup
    - For medialized cups use a higher neck cut, longer femoral head, or high offset stem
- Minimize impingement by restoring leg length and lateral offset.
    - The lesser trochanter should not touch the ischium with limb in extension
    - The greater trochanter should not touch the ilium in external rotation and abduction
    - The greater trochanter should not touch the ilium in flexion, adduction and internal rotation
- Dysplastic hips use of stems with modular necks
- Remove acetabular osteophytes

References

1. Berry DJ, Harmsen WS, Cabanela ME, Morrey BF. Twenty-five-year survivorship of two thousand consecutive primary Charnley total hip replacements: factors affecting survivorship of acetabular and femoral components. *J Bone Joint Surg Am.* 2002;84-A(2):171-177.
2. Learmonth ID, Young C, Rorabeck C. The operation of the century: total hip replacement. *Lancet.* 2007;370(9597):1508-1519.
3. Morshed S, Bozic KJ, Ries MD, Malchau H, Colford JM Jr. Comparison of cemented and uncemented fixation in total hip replacement: a meta-analysis. *Acta Orthop.* 2007;78(3):315-326.
4. Bourne RB, Rorabeck CH. Soft tissue balancing: the hip. *J Arthroplasty.* 2002;17(4 suppl 1):17-22.
5. Charnley J. Arthroplasty of the hip. A new operation. *Lancet.* 1961;1(7187):1129-1132.
6. Radin EL. Biomechanics of the human hip. *Clin Orthop Relat Res.* 1980;(152):28-34.
7. D'Lima DD, Chen PC, Colwell CW Jr. Optimizing acetabular component position to minimize impingement and reduce contact stress. *J Bone Joint Surg Am.* 2001;83-A(suppl 2 pt 2):87-91.
8. Moskal JT, Capps SG. Improving the accuracy of acetabular component orientation: avoiding malposition. *J Am Acad Orthop Surg.* 2010;18(5):286-296.
9. Patil S, Bergula A, Chen PC, Colwell CW Jr, D'Lima DD. Polyethylene wear and acetabular component orientation. *J Bone Joint Surg Am.* 2003;85-A(suppl 4):56-63.
10. Barrack RL. Dislocation after total hip arthroplasty: implant design and orientation. *J Am Acad Orthop Surg.* 2003;11(2):89-99.

11. Malik A, Maheshwari A, Dorr LD. Impingement with total hip replacement. *J Bone Joint Surg Am.* 2007;89(8):1832-1842.
12. Austin MS, Hozack WJ, Sharkey PF, Rothman RH. Stability and leg length equality in total hip arthroplasty. *J Arthroplasty.* 2003;18(3 suppl 1):88-90.

19

Avoiding Complications

James Cashman, MD; Michael E. Ciminiello, MD; and James J. Purtill, MD

Total hip arthroplasty (THA) is one of the most successful operations in medicine. THA provides the patient with pain relief and improvement in function. When performed correctly, it is an operation that can be done with extraordinary precision and reproducibility and has become one of the most common procedures performed in orthopedic surgery today.

High expectations for THA outcomes drive both orthopedic surgeons and patients. While the complication rate is low, intraoperative problems can be catastrophic. Preoperative planning and attention to surgical detail will minimize the risk to the patient.

During hip replacement surgery, a thorough understanding of the complex neurovascular anatomy of the pelvis and proximal femur is required to minimize the risk of injury to these vital structures. Neurovascular injury can occur at any point during the operation. However, special care must be taken during surgical exposure, retractor placement, acetabular reaming, and screw placement to avoid these complications.

In addition to neurovascular injury, periprosthetic fracture is a potentially significant complication that may be encountered during THA. Neurovascular injury and intraoperative periprosthetic fracture are rare during total hip replacement. The incidence of these complications is higher for revision total hip replacement compared to primary procedures. As people live longer and older generations of THA implants need to be revised, avoiding these complications is ever more important.

Infection, instability, and leg length discrepancy are complications that are discussed in other sections of the text. Chapters 27 and 28 provide extensive information on the prevention and treatment of infection. A discussion of instability is provided in Chapter 28. Planning for and evaluating leg length discrepancy is discussed in Chapter 4. Proper preoperative planning and intraoperative assessment for limb length are essential in avoiding this complication.

Vascular Injury

Vascular injury during total hip replacement is one of the most dreaded complications in orthopedic surgery. Although rare, the surgeon must maintain a high index of suspicion should excessive bleeding occur during surgery or unexplained hypotension either intraoperatively or postoperatively. A change in neurovascular examination postoperatively may be the first symptom of a vascular injury; therefore, frequent clinical examination is necessary to make the diagnosis and intervene in a timely fashion.

The particular surgical approach chosen for THA places some vascular structures at more risk due to their proximity to the surgical field. In general terms, the structures at risk during hip replacement are the femoral artery and vein, obturator artery and vein, external iliac artery and vein, and profunda femoris branches more distally in the thigh.

There is increased risk of vascular injury during revision surgery where the normal anatomic landmarks may be altered. The presence of heterotopic bone, scar tissue, bony

Parvizi J, Klatt BA.
Essentials in Total Hip Arthroplasty (pp 153-159).

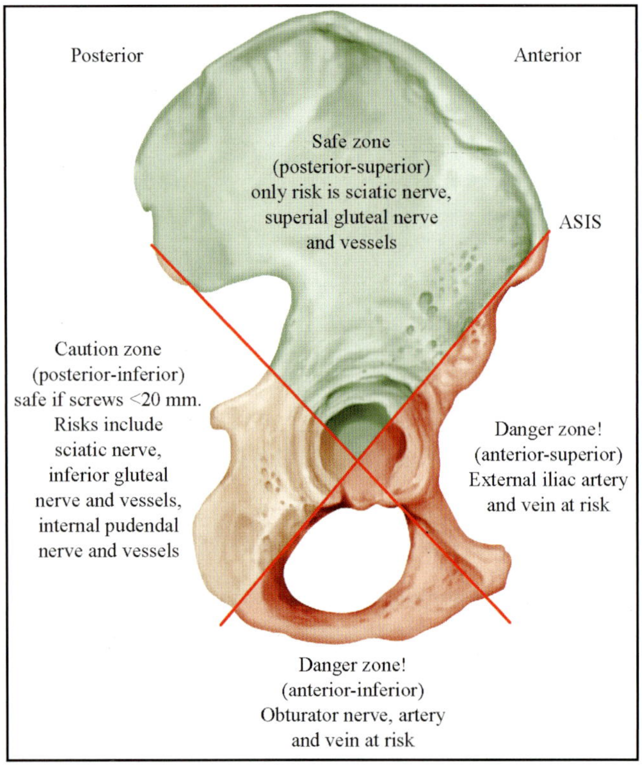

Figure 19-1. Recognition of the safe zones within the acetabulum allows for the safe placement of acetabular screws.

malunion secondary to previous trauma, congenital deformity, prior irradiation, and underlying peripheral vascular disease increase the risk of injury to local vascular structures.

Injury to a named vessel during THA is a rare complication with a reported prevalence between 0.2% and 0.3%.[1,2] Vascular injury has potentially severe implications. Shoenfield's review of 68 arthroplasties complicated by vascular injury reported a 7% and 15% mortality and amputation rate, respectively.[2,3]

Etiology of Vascular Injury

Patients with abnormal or altered anatomy are predisposed to sustaining an intraoperative vascular injury during THA. The presence of heterotopic ossification, excessive scar tissue, congenital deformity of the pelvis or femur, prior pelvic trauma, and radiation are some examples of this.

Vascular structures can be injured directly by retractors, acetabular reamers, scalpels, osteotomes, and adjacent osseous structures and indirectly as a result of stretch, torque, and compression.[2]

Excessive reaming of the medial wall has been reported to result in direct injury to the common iliac vein.[4] Errant placement of anterior acetabulum retractors may endanger the common femoral artery and vein. Retractors in the area of the medial femoral neck may result in injury to the medial and lateral circumflex femoral vessels.[1,2] Gentle, subperiosteal placement of these retractors and avoiding migration from a safe position is necessary to protect the neurovascular structures during hip replacement surgery. This is often difficult when the anatomy is altered by previous surgery, trauma, scar, heterotopic ossification, or previous irradiation.

Advances in implant design and an improved understanding of biologic fixation have lead to a marked increase in the use of cementless acetabular components. Screws can be used to augment cementless acetabular component fixation to the pelvis. Anatomical studies by both Keating et al[5] and Wasielewski et al[6] demonstrated the close proximity of the external iliac vessels, the obturator nerve and vessels, and superior and inferior vesicular venous plexus to the medial aspect of the acetabulum. A 4-quadrant system (Figure 19-1) for the safe placement of acetabular screws was also described by Wasielewski et al, and their recommendation was to avoid screw placement in the anterior-superior and anterior-inferior quadrants.[6] According to Lewallen,[2] the mechanical strength of screws placed through an acetabular shell into anterior-superior and anterior-inferior quadrants is poor and therefore there is no reason to risk neurovascular injury during primary total hip replacement. In revision cases where there may be posterior acetabular bone loss, screws into the anterior quadrants may be necessary. When this situation arises, Lewallen describes a technique where after careful dissection of the soft tissue off the anterior column, screws and drill bits may be passed under direct visualization and palpation.[2]

In addition to immediate, intraoperative damage to vascular structures with screws and retractors, there are reports of intrapelvic migration of components, bone cement, and screws secondary to trauma and component loosening with resultant laceration of the external iliac artery and ureter.[7,8]

Many patients undergoing total hip replacement have multiple comorbidities, including diabetes and peripheral vascular disease. Compression or kinking of atherosclerotic vessels has been implicated in vascular injury during total hip replacement. Arterial and venous thrombosis as well as embolism are well described in the literature.[9-11]

PRESENTATION, DIAGNOSIS, AND MANAGEMENT

The presentation of vascular injury is variable and depends on multiple factors. The type of injury in large part will determine when and how it presents clinically. Signs of injury may be obvious during surgery, more subtle in the several hours and days immediately after surgery, or delayed for months to years.[2,12]

Frank Hemorrhage

Massive, uncontrollable bleeding during surgery, usually immediately after instrumentation or placement of a retractor, is the cardinal sign that a major vessel within the operative field has been compromised. In addition to bleeding, an expanding, pulsating mass in the groin or thigh indicates vascular injury. This may become evident in the operating room (OR) or at any point in the patient's postoperative course.

Early recognition and prompt action is of paramount importance in the case of acute hemorrhage secondary to vascular injury. As with any bleeding, local control with pressure should be attempted first. If the injured vessel is within the pelvis or otherwise difficult to compress, direct pressure alone may be unsuccessful in controlling bleeding. Attempts at surgical ligation of visible vessels should be performed next. Prompt intraoperative consultation and intervention by a vascular surgeon is critical in saving the patient's life and limb. The question of whether to complete the THA in face of a vascular injury is a difficult one to answer and should be made in conjunction with the vascular surgeon.

When there is intraoperative vascular injury, the best course of action may be to close the hip and prepare the patient for a life-saving vascular surgical intervention. An on-table arteriogram, endovascular stenting or exploration, ligation, repair, and bypass of the injured vessel can then be performed acutely. Whichever intervention is necessary, time is not to be wasted.

Occult Hemorrhage

Unexplained hypotension in the OR may indicate vascular injury even in the absence of obvious hemorrhage. Although other causes are usually the culprit in this situation, the possibility should always be present in the surgeon's mind. There is a large space for blood to collect in the retroperitoneum and pelvis and lack of visible bleeding does not exclude the possibility that vascular injury has occurred.

Routine postoperative management of primary or revision THA includes monitoring of vital signs and neurovascular status. Hypotension, tachycardia, and low urine output with decreasing hemoglobin are signs of hemorrhagic shock. A change of neurovascular status such as pulse discrepancy or nerve palsy in the presence of hemorrhagic shock is concerning for vascular injury. Abdominal pain and swelling may be present with retroperitoneal bleeding. An urgent computed tomography (CT) of abdomen and pelvis with contrast should be obtained to evaluate for the presence of expanding retroperitoneal hematoma. Vascular surgical consultation and arteriogram should be obtained. Stenting, bypass, coiling, or chemoembolization of the involved vessels should be performed urgently.

Thrombosis and Embolism

Ischemic signs and symptoms may be the first indicator of vascular injury following total hip replacement. Vigilant neurovascular monitoring is imperative to make the diagnosis early. Early intervention in the setting of acute thromboses or embolism is necessary for normal limb function and survival.

Prior to entering the OR, the patient's neurovascular examination should be well documented and available in the medical record. Decreased temperature, pallor, a change in pulse, and a change in neurologic status of the limb are signs that raise concern for neurovascular injury. In the presence of an alteration in neurovascular status of the operated limb, a vascular surgery consult should be obtained along with arteriogram in preparation for early intervention.

Prevention

Careful preoperative planning and knowledge of each patient's risk factors for vascular complications may minimize risk of vascular injury during hip replacement. Preoperative evaluation by a vascular surgeon should be considered in cases where there is suspected or known peripheral vascular disease. In addition, a vascular or general surgeon may be needed when normal anatomic relationships are altered, such as acetabular protrusion, intrapelvic cement, or intrapelvic acetabular components. Lewallen, for example, suggests that intrapelvic mobilization of vessels may be performed prior to approaching the hip under the same anesthetic.[2]

Intraoperatively, a systematic, careful surgical approach and plan should be followed. Dissection should proceed with caution in situations where anatomic relationships are not normal. In revision situations, careful dissection of scar tissue and heterotopic bone minimizes but does not eliminate the risk of iatrogenic vascular compromise.

Precise, gentle retractor placement and attention to what all assistants are doing is essential. When retractors slip from their position, only the experienced operating surgeon should replace them.

Adherences to the principles of safe acetabular screw positioning and placement as well as acetabular reaming are vital to the safety of the operation. Avoidance of tearing and pulling fixed soft tissue, components, and other structures will help minimize the risk of injury to vascular structures.

In summary, it is far better to anticipate and plan for problems preoperatively, have contingency plans in place should they occur, and make every effort to avoid them in the OR.

Peripheral Nerve Injury

The sciatic, femoral, superior gluteal, and obturator nerves are 4 structures that may be damaged during THA. In general terms, these structures may be injured during dissection with retractor placement, from traction, or from ischemia. The particular surgical exposure has not been shown to influence rates of nerve palsy. Regardless of surgical approach, however, the femoral nerve is in close proximity to the anterior acetabular retractor while the sciatic nerve can be compromised by posterior acetabular retractors or during posterior surgical exposures. The superior gluteal nerve traverses the interval between the gluteus medius and minimus. It is at risk during the anterolateral exposure, especially if the gluteus medius split is posterior to the midpoint of the muscle or extended proximally more than 5 cm.

Iatrogenic peripheral nerve injury during THA is a relatively rare yet potentially debilitating complication. Nerve injury has been reported in 1% to 2% of all cases.[13] Clinically detectable sciatic nerve injury occurs in less than 1% of THAs.[14-16] Schmalzried and colleagues studied the results of over 3000 consecutive total hip replacements and identified postoperative lower extremity neuropathy in 1.7% overall and 1.3% of the primary arthroplasties.[17]

In addition, special situations may increase the risk of nerve injury. Nerve injury was found in 5.2% of patients undergoing primary THA for congenital dislocation or dysplasia of the hip and 3.2% after revisions for all diagnoses.[17]

Schmalzried et al reported that 90% of clinically evident neuropathy affected the sciatic nerve. In another study analyzing 440 THAs, Simmons and colleagues found transient femoral neuropathy in 2.7% of cases, all of which were associated with a Hardinge approach.[18]

Etiology of Peripheral Nerve Injury and Risk Factors

Much like vascular injury, peripheral nerves can be compromised at any point during the operation but are especially vulnerable when normal anatomic landmarks are absent secondary to previous surgery, heterotopic ossificiation, excessive scar tissue, prior irradiation, and pelvic/proximal femoral deformity.[18] Nerves can be injured directly during dissection and retraction or indirectly secondary to compression, excessive traction, lengthening, and ischemia.[2]

Entrapment of the sciatic nerve during application of cerclage wires has been reported.[19] The sciatic, femoral, and obturator nerves have all been reported to be at least in close proximity to, if not entirely encased in, extruded acetabular bone cement.[20-22] Improved biologic fixation has lead to a decrease in the use of cemented acetabular components; however, supplemental screw fixation outside of the "safe zones" described by Wasielewski et al is not recommended.[6]

Hematoma formation leading to sciatic and femoral nerve palsy associated with anticoagulation usually presents 1 or 2 days following surgery. There may be sudden, exquisite pain followed by nerve palsy. The diagnosis can be made clinically and confirmed with magnetic resonance imaging (MRI). Fleming et al reported that 4 out of 5 patients treated with decompression of the hematoma improved or completely recovered and the one treated expectantly did not.[23]

Presentation, Diagnosis, and Management

In nearly all instances, nerve palsy is evident immediately postoperatively, if not within the first 36 hours. New onset nerve palsy can be the first sign of vascular insult to the limb and therefore this must be ruled out. Clear and accurate documentation should accompany serial clinical, electromyographic, and nerve conduction examinations. Consultation with a neurologist and physiatrist should be considered early in the postoperative period.

The treatment of postoperative nerve palsy is dependent upon etiology. In 2 studies, a definable cause to the nerve palsy was present in less than 50% of cases.[17] If there is a hematoma thought to be causing the nerve palsy, urgent evacuation of hematoma has been shown to improve outcome.[24] When hardware, cables, cement, and wires are considered to be the cause of the nerve palsy, these offending agents should be removed.[2] When the affected limb has been lengthened significantly (2 to 4 cm), remove all constrictive bandages and flex the knee. This will alleviate tension on the sciatic nerve and the peroneal branch of the sciatic nerve.

Prevention

Careful surgical dissection, accurate retractor placement, and gentle retraction will minimize risk of nerve damage during hip replacement. Additionally, limiting the planned lengthening of the limb to less than 6% of the total length of the nerve or a total of 4 cm has been recommended to avoid nerve palsy.[2] Flexing the knee and extending the hip during surgical dissection via the posterior approach will decrease tension on the sciatic nerve. Avoiding screw placement into anterior-superior and anterior-inferior acetabular quadrants is recommended.[6] During relocation maneuvers, entrapment of soft tissue, which may include neurovascular structures, should be avoided.

Prognosis

Considerable variability exists in the extent of neurological recovery following nerve palsy after total hip replacement. This may be related to the etiology and severity of the initial injury.[2] The prognosis for femoral nerve palsy is better than that for sciatic nerve palsy.[25] Likewise, the prognosis for isolated peroneal nerve palsy is better than that for complete sciatic nerve palsy.[26] Schmalzried et al showed that good prognostic signs include retention of motor function with isolated sensory loss or motor recovery during the initial days after surgery.[17]

Intraoperative Periprosthetic Fracture

Periprosthetic femur fractures can present a broad spectrum of problems for both the patient and surgeon. Periprosthetic fractures can occur intraoperatively; in conjunction with trauma; or atraumatically in association with osteolyis, significant stress risers, and implant loosening.[27] Often it is a combination of these factors that leads to fracture. This discussion will focus on the management of intraoperative periprosthetic fractures during primary or revision THA.

Masri et al have described the mostly widely used classification system for periprosthetic femur fractures, which is known as the Vancouver classification.[28] The Vancouver classification of periprosthetic femur fractures consists of 3 types: Type A refers to a trochanteric fracture, either greater trochanter (AT) or lesser trochanter (AL); Type B refers to fracture around or just below the stem tip and is further subdivided into those in which the stem is well fixed (B_1), the stem is loose (B_2), and where the bone quality of the proximal femur is poor (B_3); Type C fractures are those that occur well below the tip of the stem. This classification is useful because it guides treatment with hardware and revision components.

Intraoperative femur fracture rates are highly dependent upon the type of implant being used. The estimated fracture rate when cemented primary femoral components are used ranges between 0.1% and 3.2%, and from 3% to 12% for revisions. The rate of femur fractures when uncemented femoral components are used in both primary and revision procedures ranges from 3% to 46%.[28-30]

Contributing Factors to Periprosthetic Fracture

Factors influencing femoral periprosthetic fracture can be divided into patient related, surgeon controlled, and implant related.[8] Patient related variables include osteoporosis, small size, deformity, osteolysis/loosening, prior surgical defects, trauma, and excessive loads. The exposure, method of implant and cement removal, bone preparation, implant sizing, and insertion are all surgeon-controlled factors. Finally, implant related variables include the number of sizes, proximal wedge effect, stem length, stem bow, instrumentation, fixation, and stem stiffness.[31]

Presentation, Diagnosis, and Management

A high index of suspicion and careful intraoperative inspection are fundamental to immediate diagnosis and treatment of most intraoperative periprosthetic femur fractures, both in primary and revision settings. Fractures of the femur may occur during dislocation, reaming/broaching, and during removal or impaction of the prosthesis. A sudden change in resistance, pitch, or position of the component while it is being inserted may indicate that an intraoperative fracture has occurred.

Cortical perforations may occur during femoral component removal, femoral preparation, or femoral component implantation. Perforations may be detected with surgical instruments such as curettes. Further evaluation may be accomplished with the use of fluoroscopy or intraoperative x-rays. Cortical perforation may necessitate the use of a longer femoral implant or bone graft struts. The femoral component should bypass a cortical defect by at least 2 cortical diameters. Cortical perforation weakens the femoral bone substantially and, left untreated, may lead to periprosthetic fracture.

The urge to not treat minor cracks in the cortex of the proximal femur should be resisted; when they occur, the fractures should be fully exposed to ensure there has not been propagation. The femoral component is removed. A cerclage cable is passed around the proximal femur above the lesser trochanter. The wire is tightened and the femoral component is impacted. A final tightening of the wire is followed by crimping of the wire-holding sleeve. If the femoral component is stable, the patient may be allowed protected weight bearing. If the femoral component is unstable, a long, cylindrical cementless stem or a cemented stem may be necessary. These fractures, when diagnosed and treated at the time of surgery, usually do not add significant morbidity to the operation or limit the patient's weight-bearing ability. However, if these fractures are left untreated, the force of weight bearing may cause a small cortical crack to propagate. This in turn may cause the prosthesis to loosen or may lead to a more substantial and displaced fracture. This may ultimately require revision surgery or a more extensive open reduction and internal fixation.

As with nondisplaced, minor, and proximal cracks, more substantial or displaced fractures should be fully exposed and the implant stability assessed. It may be necessary to use fluoroscopy or intraoperative x-ray to assess the extent of the fracture.

Unstable implants should be revised and alternative fixation techniques considered. The Vancouver classification guides surgical treatment. Type A fractures can be fixed rigidly with cables, plates, and screws and the implant left in place provided it is stable. Type B_1 fractures can be treated with either open reduction, internal fixation with a cable plate system with or without supplemental strut allografts, or revised with a long-stem prosthesis. Type B_2 fractures necessitate revision of the femoral component. Type B_3 fractures are best treated with proximal femoral replacement or proximal femoral composite allograft. Finally, Type C fractures are best treated with open reduction and internal fixation.

When these fractures are diagnosed postoperatively, in most cases the patient should return to the OR for appropriate treatment. The timing of surgical intervention is dependent on the availability of equipment, such as revision implants, and the overall condition of the patient. When return to the OR is delayed, the patient should not be allowed to weight bear through the affected limb.

Summary

Neurovascular injury and intraoperative periprosthetic fracture are rare during total hip replacement. The incidence of these complications is higher for revision procedures when compared to primary total hip replacement. As people live longer, older generations of THA implants need to be revised and avoiding these complications is ever more important.

Careful preoperative planning and meticulous surgical technique are imperative to avoiding these potentially catastrophic complications. Prompt recognition and early decisive action may be the difference between life and death.

References

1. Nachbur B, Meyer RP, Verkkala K, Zurcher R. The mechanisms of severe arterial injury in surgery of the hip joint. *Clin Orthop Relat Res.* 1979;(141):122-133.
2. Lewallen DG. Neurovascular injury associated with hip arthroplasty. *Instr Course Lect.* 1998;47:275-283.
3. Shoenfeld NA, Stuchin SA, Pearl R, Haveson S. The management of vascular injuries associated with total hip arthroplasty. *J Vasc Surg.* 1990;11(4):549-555.
4. Mallory TH, Jaffe SL, Eberle RW. False aneurysm of the common femoral artery after total hip arthroplasty. A case report. *Clin Orthop Relat Res.* 1997;(338):105-108.
5. Keating EM, Ritter MA, Faris PM. Structures at risk from medially placed acetabular screws. *J Bone Joint Surg Am.* 1990;72(4):509-511.
6. Wasielewski RC, Cooperstein LA, Kruger MP, Rubash HE. Acetabular anatomy and the transacetabular fixation of screws in total hip arthroplasty. *J Bone Joint Surg Am.* 1990;72(4):501-508.
7. Brentlinger A, Hunter JR. Perforation of the external iliac artery and ureter presenting as acute hemorrhagic cystitis after total hip replacement. Report of a case. *J Bone Joint Surg Am.* 1987;69(4):620-622.
8. Peterson CA, Lewallen DG. Periprosthetic fracture of the acetabulum after total hip arthroplasty. *J Bone Joint Surg Am.* 1996;78(8):1206-1213.
9. Aust JC, Bredenberg CE, Murray DG. Mechanisms of arterial injuries associated with total hip replacement. *Arch Surg.* 1981;116(3):345-349.
10. Parfenchuck TA, Young TR. Intraoperative arterial occlusion in total joint arthroplasty. *J Arthroplasty.* 1994;9(2):217-220.
11. Stubbs DH, Dorner DB, Johnston RC. Thrombosis of the iliofemoral artery during revision of a total hip replacement. A case report. *J Bone Joint Surg Am.* 1986;68(3):454-455.
12. Dorr LD, Conaty JP, Kohl R, Harvey JP Jr. False aneurysm of the femoral artery following total hip surgery. *J Bone Joint Surg* Am. 1974;56(5):1059-1062.
13. Farrell CM, Springer BD, Haidukewych GJ, Morrey BF. Motor nerve palsy following primary total hip arthroplasty. *J Bone Joint Surg Am.* 2005;87(12):2619-2625.
14. Brown GD, Swanson EA, Nercessian OA. Neurologic injuries after total hip arthroplasty. *Am J Orthop.* 2008;37(4):191-197.
15. Hurd JL, Potter HG, Dua V, Ranawat CS. Sciatic nerve palsy after primary total hip arthroplasty: a new perspective. *J Arthroplasty.* 2006;21(6):796-802.

16. Jolles BM, Bogoch ER. Posterior versus lateral surgical approach for total hip arthroplasty in adults with osteoarthritis. *Cochrane Database Syst Rev.* 2006;3:CD003828.
17. Schmalzried TP, Amstutz HC, Dorey FJ. Nerve palsy associated with total hip replacement. Risk factors and prognosis. *J Bone Joint Surg Am.* 1991;73(7):1074-1080.
18. Simmons C Jr, Izant TH, Rothman RH, Booth RE Jr, Balderston RA. Femoral neuropathy following total hip arthroplasty. Anatomic study, case reports, and literature review. *J Arthroplasty.* 1991;6(suppl):S57-66.
19. Mallory TH. Sciatic nerve entrapment secondary to trochanteric wiring following total hip arthroplasty. A case report. *Clin Orthop Relat Res.* 1983;(180):198-200.
20. Mahadevan D, Challand C, Keenan J. Cement extrusion during hip arthroplasty causing pain and obturator nerve impingement. *J Arthroplasty.* 2009;24(1):158, e1-3.
21. Birch R, Wilkinson MC, Vijayan KP, Gschmeissner S. Cement burn of the sciatic nerve. *J Bone Joint Surg Br.* 1992;74(5):731-733.
22. O'Brien S, Bennett D, Blair PH, Beverland DE. Femoral nerve compression after migration of bone cement to the groin after hip arthroplasty. *J Arthroplasty.* 2011;26(8):1571, e11-3.
23. Fleming RE Jr, Michelsen CB, Stinchfield FE. Sciatic paralysis. A complication of bleeding following hip surgery. *J Bone Joint Surg Am.* 1979;61(1):37-39.
24. Butt AJ, McCarthy T, Kelly IP, Glynn T, McCoy G. Sciatic nerve palsy secondary to postoperative haematoma in primary total hip replacement. *J Bone Joint Surg Br.* 2005;87(11):1465-1467.
25. Ahlgren SA, Elmqvist D, Ljung P. Nerve lesions after total hip replacement. *Acta Orthop Scand.* 1984;55(2):152-155.
26. Edwards BN, Tullos HS, Noble PC. Contributory factors and etiology of sciatic nerve palsy in total hip arthroplasty. *Clin Orthop Relat Res.* 1987;(218):136-141.
27. Mukundan C, Rayan F, Kheir E, Macdonald D. Management of late periprosthetic femur fractures: a retrospective cohort of 72 patients. *Int Orthop.* 2010;34(4):485-489.
28. Brady OH, Garbuz DS, Masri BA, Duncan CP. The reliability and validity of the Vancouver classification of femoral fractures after hip replacement. *J Arthroplasty.* 2000;15(1):59-62.
29. Morrey BF, Kavanagh BF. Complications with revision of the femoral component of total hip arthroplasty. Comparison between cemented and uncemented techniques. *J Arthroplasty.* 1992;7(1):71-79.
30. Masri BA, Meek RM, Duncan CP. Periprosthetic fractures evaluation and treatment. *Clin Orthop Relat Res.* 2004;(420):80-95.
31. Hu K, Zhang X, Zhu J, Wang C, Ji W, Bai X. Periprosthetic fractures may be more likely in cementless femoral stems with sharp edges. *Ir J Med Sci.* 2010;179(3):417-421.

20

Postoperative Management
Analgesia and Anticoagulation

Eric Schwenk, MD; Kishor Gandhi, MD, MPH; and Eugene R. Viscusi, MD

Although significant advances have been made in postoperative analgesia after total hip arthroplasty (THA), adequate pain control is still a challenge for many patients.[1] Over 50% of surgical patients name postoperative pain as a major concern.[2] In addition to creating patient dissatisfaction, postoperative pain can impair patient rehabilitation, a crucial component of regaining muscle strength and functional status back to normal. This, in turn, can delay discharge from the hospital. Effectively managing postoperative pain after THA improves both the physical and mental recovery of the patient.

Several options exist for postoperative analgesia in the THA patient. A multimodal approach (ie, one in which combinations of drugs and techniques with different mechanisms of action are utilized) can be very effective (Figure 20-1). This type of approach can limit the dependence on one particular class of drug and its associated side effects. The available modalities include neuraxial analgesia (injection of local anesthetics, opioids, or other agents into the spinal or epidural space), peripheral nerve blockade, and nonopioid (nonsteroidal anti-inflammatory drugs and antineuropathic drugs) as well as opioid drugs. Each of these techniques has its associated advantages and disadvantages, including side effects for which patients must be monitored. This chapter describes the various analgesia techniques for the THA patient in the postoperative period, emphasizing a multimodal approach, and includes some important points to consider when treating patients who are anticoagulated.

Neuraxial Analgesia

Spinal Analgesia

The use of local anesthetics (such as ropivacaine, bupivacaine, and tetracaine) in the intrathecal space is a well-established method of anesthesia for the surgical procedure in THA. Spinal anesthesia commonly used for total joint arthroplasty (TJA) involves the insertion of a spinal needle (Quincke, Sprotte, or Spinocan) into the intrathecal space of a seated or laterally positioned patient (Figure 20-2). Onset of anesthesia is rapid with this method and height of the spinal blockade depends on the baricity and volume of the local anesthetic and the patient's height and weight. In the case of unilateral hip arthroplasty, the combined spinal-epidural (CSE) technique is typically only needed in cases greater than 3 hours in length. If surgery requires extended duration beyond the time of the spinal anesthetic, the epidural may be activated to achieve extended duration. For shorter cases, spinal anesthesia is often sufficient for surgical anesthesia.

During the performance of spinal anesthesia, additives may be included in the intrathecal mix, such as opioids. The most commonly used opioids are morphine and fentanyl. Morphine has a higher degree of patient satisfaction when compared to fentanyl largely due to its prolonged analgesic effect. In one study, intrathecal morphine reduced the need

Parvizi J, Klatt BA.
Essentials in Total Hip Arthroplasty (pp 161-170).

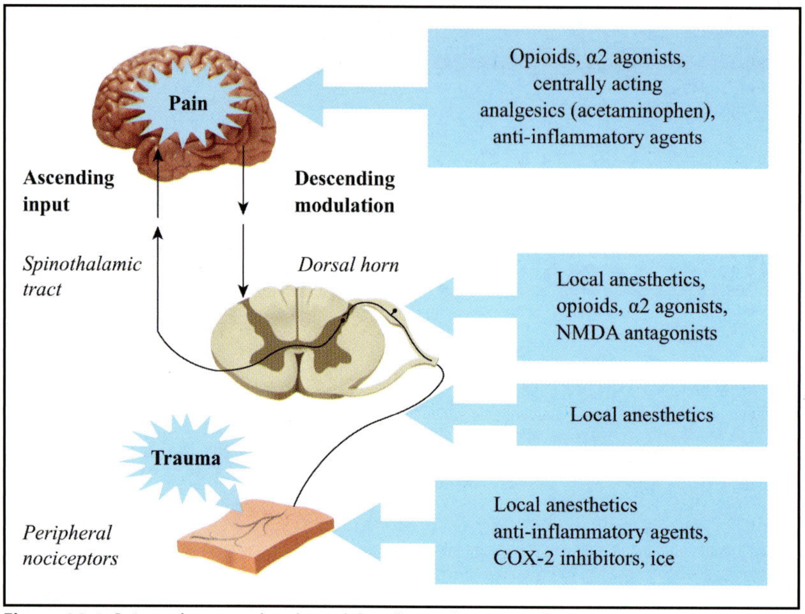

Figure 20-1. Pain pathways and multimodal analgesic therapy. (Adapted from Gottschalk A, Smith DS. New concepts in acute pain therapy: preemptive analgesia. *Am Fam Physician.* 2001;63(10):1979-1984.)

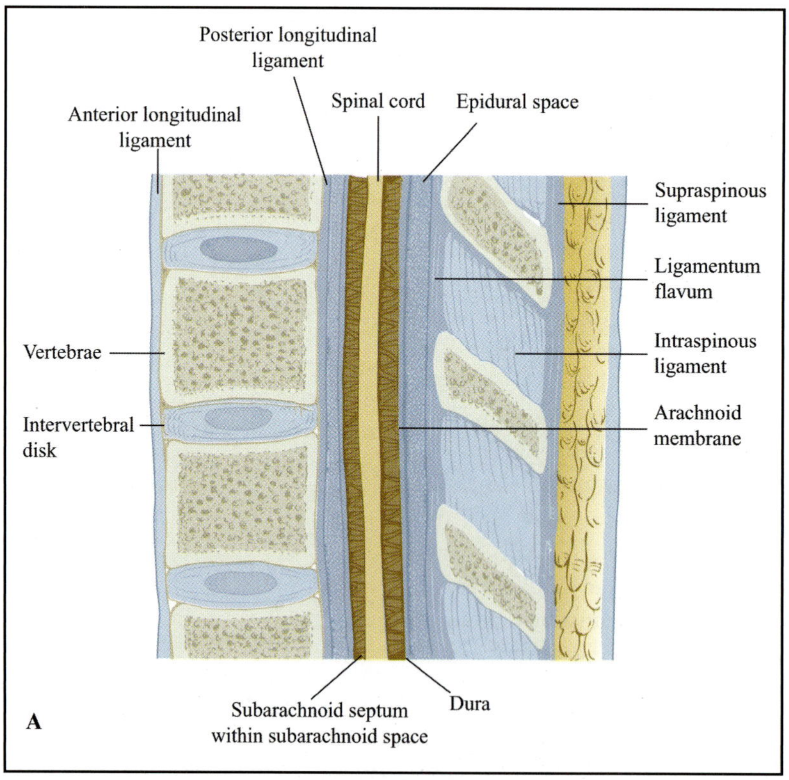

Figure 20-2. Layers encountered when entering the epidural and subarachnoid spaces.

for supplemental intravenous morphine after THA.[3] This was in contrast to total knee arthroplasty (TKA) patients, in whom even the largest intrathecal morphine dose did not provide adequate postoperative analgesia. As a result, postoperative pain after unilateral THA may effectively be managed with a single injection of opioid into the intrathecal space. Intrathecal morphine typically provides 12 to 18 hours of analgesia. Bilateral THA may require a CSE technique for adequate postoperative analgesia.

The most common side effects of intrathecal morphine as well as other opioids include pruritus, nausea, vomiting, urinary retention, sedation, and respiratory depression. Respiratory depression, the most serious of the side effects, is dose-dependent and typically manifests itself clinically as a decreased frequency of breathing, often accompanied by a compensatory increase in tidal volume. Clinicians must closely monitor patients for a decreased frequency of breathing, desaturations seen with pulse oximetry, or depressed level of consciousness. A lower dose of 100 μg of morphine added to the spinal anesthetic may be appropriate for some older patients in whom there is a higher concern for respiratory depression. However, caution must be used when intrathecal morphine is used for patients with obstructive sleep apnea or those prone to respiratory depression. Typical intrathecal morphine doses for THA of 200 μg generally provide effective analgesia and the side effect profile is generally well tolerated.

Clonidine, an $\alpha 2$ agonist, has been studied as an adjunct to local anesthetics used intrathecally. It potentiates the analgesia of local anesthetics in the intrathecal space and, when combined with morphine in an intrathecal regimen, results in significant improvements in postoperative pain and decreases intravenous morphine requirements during the first postoperative day.[4] Patients must be monitored for hypotension and bradycardia that result from intrathecal clonidine.

Epidural Analgesia

Epidural analgesia involves the insertion of a special needle (Hustead, Tuohy, or Crawford) into the epidural space, followed by injection of local anesthetic and/or opioid, or insertion of a catheter (see Figure 20-2). Commonly, a CSE technique is employed in which a one-time dose of local anesthetic is injected into the intrathecal space through a spinal needle that is inserted through the lumen of an epidural needle. This intrathecal injection provides surgical anesthesia for the procedure itself. The epidural catheter is inserted following the spinal procedure. The epidural catheter may then be used to provide continuous analgesia following THA. However, epidural catheters are not used nearly as frequently for postoperative analgesia after THA as they are after TKA. Patients undergoing THA typically report pain scores that are lower and of shorter duration compared to similar patients undergoing TKA.[5] As a result, epidural catheters are typically not needed after uncomplicated unilateral THA. However, various adjuvant agents, including epinephrine, ketamine, and opioids, can be injected into the epidural space as a one-time dose before the procedure to provide postoperative analgesia.

While continuous epidural analgesia may not be used routinely for uncomplicated THA, this technique should be considered when potent, nonopioid analgesia utilizing local anesthetics is desirable. Obstructive sleep apnea is an increasing concern among THA patients. Opioids in the postoperative period may increase the risk of respiratory depression. For these patients, epidural analgesia with local anesthetics may be warranted. An increasing number of THA patients are chronically taking opioids for control of osteoarthritis pain. Opioid-tolerant patients are at risk for uncontrolled postoperative pain and may be difficult to control with opioids alone. The use of local anesthetic techniques such as continuous epidural analgesia may be beneficial for these patients.

Epinephrine can be added to intensify the effect of local anesthetics or opioids by causing vasoconstriction of the vessels in the epidural space and therefore decreasing drug clearance from the epidural space.[6] The addition of epinephrine (5 μg/cc) allows for the usage of a larger maximum dose of local anesthetic agent. Ketamine, an N-methyl-D-aspartate (NMDA) receptor antagonist acting in the spinal cord, blocks peripheral afferent noxious stimulation and also may prevent central sensitization of nociceptors. One study showed that when given with a local anesthetic and an opioid, epidural ketamine reduces postoperative analgesic requirements after major surgery.[7]

Finally, opioids (typically morphine, hydromorphone, or fentanyl) can be injected into the epidural space as a one-time injection or via a continuous epidural catheter. They can be used with or without a local anesthetic. Compared with parenteral opioid use after surgery, continuous infusion of epidural opioid provides superior postoperative pain relief with a similar side effect profile.[8] However, continuous catheters come with their own set of problems, including failed or dislodged catheters, unilateral blocks, and incompatibility in patients who are anticoagulated. There is also the risk of epidural hematoma formation in anticoagulated patients, which has been associated with traumatic placement of the epidural needle or catheter, although it has also been reported to occur spontaneously.[9]

Another analgesic option for clinicians is extended-release epidural morphine (EREM). EREM (DepoDur [EKR Therapeutics, Inc, Bedminster, NJ]) utilizes a multivesicular, liposomal spherical particle (DepoFoam [Pacira Pharmaceuticals, Inc, Parsippany, NJ]) with internal aqueous chambers containing morphine, resulting in a gradual release and 48 hours of analgesia after a single epidural injection. Patients given EREM may have decreased supplemental opioid requirements in the postoperative period as well as superior analgesia for 48 hours.[10] Problems related to the epidural catheter itself or a patient-controlled analgesia (PCA) pump may be eliminated with EREM. In addition, EREM is compatible with anticoagulation therapy because it does not require an indwelling epidural catheter.

Similar to other opioids, the side effects of EREM include nausea and vomiting, pruritus, urinary retention, constipation, and respiratory depression. Of those patients experiencing respiratory depression after receiving EREM at recommended doses, almost all occurs in the first 24 hours of the postoperative period. The incidence of respiratory depression may be higher with EREM than standard PCA so patients should be monitored closely, particularly during the first 24 hours, and the lowest effective dose should be used.[11] In particular, caution should be exercised in the elderly and patients with obstructive sleep apnea.

Peripheral Nerve Blocks

Lumbar Plexus Block

The lumbar plexus block is a viable option for postoperative pain management in THA patients. The lumbar plexus arises from the second, third, and fourth lumbar spinal nerves and gives rise to the femoral, lateral femoral cutaneous, and obturator nerves. The femoral nerve innervates the quadriceps muscles, the skin of the anteromedial thigh, and the medial aspect of the leg below the knee and foot. The obturator nerve sends motor branches to the adductors of the hip and a highly variable cutaneous branch to the medial thigh or knee. The lateral femoral cutaneous nerve supplies the lateral thigh. Blockade of the lumbar plexus provides analgesia comparable to that of a continuous femoral nerve block but possibly with better ambulation.[12] Lumbar plexus blocks carry the risk of hematoma in the muscle sheath, retroperitoneal space, and kidney, as well as infection and inadvertent intrathecal or epidural injection.[13] Serious caution should be exercised in anticoagulated patients. Lumbar plexus blocks can be performed as single injections or as continuous blocks via a catheter.

Multimodal Nonopioid Agents

Nonsteroidal Anti-Inflammatory Drugs and Cyclooxygenase-2 Inhibitors

Research has shown that the use of nonopioid drugs in the preoperative period may reduce the possible effects of opioid-induced hyperalgesia in the postoperative period.[14] Opioid-induced hyperalgesia is a complex phenomenon that can follow rapid increases in opioids during or after surgery and can paradoxically result in lowering of a patient's pain threshold and lead to greater opioid requirements. Limiting opioids while maximizing the use of nonopioid drugs can minimize opioid-induced hyperalgesia.

Nonsteroidal anti-inflammatory drugs (NSAIDS) and cyclooxygenase-2 (COX-2) inhibitors given in the preoperative period can also create an "opioid-sparing effect" in the postoperative period. As a result, opioid-related side effects may decrease and patient satisfaction may increase as a result of better analgesia. NSAIDs and COX-2 inhibitors act in the peripheral nervous system by inhibiting prostaglandin synthesis and stimulation of nociceptors, while opioids exert their effects in the central nervous system (CNS). NSAIDs or COX-2 inhibitors can be used preoperatively to reduce the incidence of central and peripheral sensitization syndromes after surgery.[15] If not prevented, these syndromes can lead to increased opioid consumption and worse pain control postoperatively.

Preoperative use of NSAIDs such as ketorolac and ibuprofen can decrease postoperative pain intensity assessments and postoperative opioid consumption.[16] However, some surgeons are concerned about NSAID use prior to surgery due to the decrease in platelet aggregation, potentially increased bleeding time, and poor bone healing associated with drugs in this class. COX-2 inhibitors may reduce some of these problems.

There is now vast experience with the use of both selective and nonselective NSAIDs for THA analgesia. These agents are generally very safe and effective adjuncts in a multimodal analgesic platform and are widely accepted by the orthopedic community. Concerns about impaired healing and recovery with COX-2 inhibition have not been consistently demonstrated in clinical studies.[17] A meta-analysis

Table 20-1

NONOPIOID ANALGESICS AND SUGGESTED DOSING FOR TOTAL HIP ARTHROPLASTY PATIENTS

DRUG	DOSE	ROUTE OF ADMINISTRATION	TIME BEFORE SURGERY	TIME AFTER SURGERY
Acetaminophen	1 g	PO/IV	15 min	1 g every 4 to 6 hours (max 4 g in 24 hours)
NSAIDs				
Ketorolac	15 to 30 mg	PO/IV	1 to 2 hours	15 to 30 mg q6hrs
Ibuprofen	600 to 800 mg	PO/IV	1 to 2 hours	600 to 800 mg q6hrs
COX-2 inhibitors				
Celecoxib	200 to 400 mg	PO	1 hour	200 mg x 1 (2 hours after surgery)
Anti-neuropathics				
Gabapentin	600 to 1200 mg	PO	1 to 2 hours	100 to 200 mg BID
Pregabalin	75 to 150 mg	PO	1 hour	75 to 150 mg q12hrs

from 2005 recommended NSAIDs or COX-2 inhibitors for THA because they reduce pain and supplemental analgesic consumption.[16]

Gabapentin and Pregabalin

Gabapentin (Neurontin [Pfizer, New York, NY]) and pregabalin (Lyrica [Pfizer]), originally studied in patients with seizures and neuropathic pain syndromes, are beginning to play a role in postoperative pain. Some studies have shown that preoperative administration of gabapentin leads to decreased postoperative pain and opioid consumption, particularly in the first 24 hours after surgery.[18,19] Another study found that TKA patients, who typically experience more postoperative pain than THA patients, have improved analgesia and decreased anxiety after receiving 1200 mg of gabapentin preoperatively.[20] Although the effects of gabapentin at 6 months after surgery are not established,[21] it does seem to be a useful adjunct in the acute postoperative period.[22]

Pregabalin has been studied as well as a perioperative analgesic. Evidence suggests that pregabalin may reduce the incidence of chronic neuropathic pain after TJA as well as opioid consumption at 30 days postoperatively.[23] Another advantage of adding these and other nonopioid agents to a multimodal analgesia regimen is the ability to continue usage after discharge from the hospital (Table 20-1).

Ketamine

Ketamine is a phencyclidine derivative and an NMDA receptor antagonist and can reduce postoperative morphine consumption as well as nausea and vomiting.[24] A recent randomized, controlled trial found that intravenous ketamine has a morphine-sparing effect after THA, facilitating rehabilitation at 1 month postoperatively and possibly decreasing pain at 6 months. Although ketamine has the potential for psycho-cognitive side effects, the incidence did not differ significantly between the ketamine and placebo groups in that study.[25] Postoperative ketamine infusions may be particularly effective in opioid-tolerant patients who undergo surgery.[26] This mode of analgesia has been shown to significantly decrease postoperative opioid requirements in patients who are opioid tolerant.

Table 20-2

ORAL OPIOIDS AND SUGGESTED DOSING FOR TOTAL HIP ARTHROPLASTY PATIENTS IN THE POSTOPERATIVE PERIOD

DRUG	DOSAGE (MG)	FREQUENCY (HOURS)	DURATION (HOURS)
Codeine	50	q4 to 6	3.5
Hydromorphone	4	q3 to 4	3 to 4
Oxycodone	10	q4 to 6	4 to 6
Oxymorphone	5 to 10	q4 to 6	5 to 6
Hydrocodone/acetaminophen	10/500	q4 to 6	4 to 6

Adapted from Sinatra RS. Oral and parenteral opioid analgesics for acute pain management. In: Sinatra RS, de Leon-Casasola OA, Ginsberg B, Viscusi ER, eds. *Acute Pain Management.* New York: Cambridge University Press; 2009:188-203.

OPIOID ANALGESIA

Intravenous Patient-Controlled Analgesia

Intravenous PCA is the most widely used method of postoperative analgesia offered to patients after surgery.[27] It involves infusion pumps programmed to deliver patient-activated, fixed, and small doses of opioids with a lockout period as well as a maximum hourly dose. The most commonly utilized opioids include morphine, hydromorphone, and fentanyl. PCA provides a good option for patients who are willing to actively participate in their care and patient satisfaction is generally high with PCA. Opioid-related side effects, such as nausea and vomiting, pruritus, urinary retention, and respiratory depression, occur commonly with PCA. In addition, the elderly are especially vulnerable to confusion and delirium during PCA use.

As the prototype opioid agonist, morphine deserves some special consideration. It is a commonly used opioid in PCA therapy and is the opioid to which all others are compared. Intravenous morphine requires 15 to 30 minutes to take peak effect, which is slower than the highly lipid-soluble fentanyl and its derivatives. An additional important point to consider is the metabolism of morphine. Morphine-3-glucuronide and morphine-6-glucuronide, morphine's 2 major metabolites, are excreted principally by the kidneys. In patients with renal failure, elimination may be impaired and even small amounts of morphine can lead to respiratory depression. Therefore, extreme caution should be exercised before administering morphine to patients with renal failure.

Multimodal analgesic approaches typically involve one or more nonopioid drugs in combination with opioids. These other drugs often can help reduce opioid consumption and its associated side effects, as well as provide better pain control in the postoperative period.

Oral Opioids

Oral opioids are generally an important component of postoperative analgesia for the THA patient. Opioids commonly used in the postoperative period and during the transition to home include hydromorphone, oxycodone, oxymorphone, and hydrocodone (Table 20-2). Meperidine used to be commonly given for postoperative analgesia but has fallen out of favor partially due to the fact that one of its metabolites, normeperidine, causes CNS excitation and can cause seizures, particularly in renal failure patients.[28] Another limitation of meperidine involves its depression of myocardial contractility, a unique feature among opioid agonists. Finally, meperidine is associated with a high incidence of nausea and vomiting.

Hydromorphone is 5 times as potent as morphine with a slightly shorter duration of action. It is effective for moderate to severe pain and must be taken orally every 4 hours to maintain analgesia. Oxycodone is available as a sustained-release oral medication for treatment of moderate to severe pain. There has been abuse potential due to the ability of users to crush tablets and inject or snort the drug.[29] Recent formulation changes may make abuse by crushing more

Table 20-3

Postoperative Analgesia Options After Total Hip Arthroplasty and Their Compatibility With Anticoagulation

Technique	Compatible With Anticoagulation?
Neuraxial analgesia	No
Lumbar plexus block	Caution advised
Nonopioid analgesics	Yes
PCA	Yes
Oral opioids	Yes
Extended-release epidural morphine	Yes

difficult. For appropriate patients, it is a good analgesia option in the weeks following THA. Oxymorphone is a metabolite of oxycodone that is 10 times more potent than morphine and may cause significant nausea and vomiting. Physical dependence is a significant concern.[28] However, it is available as an immediate-release form that provides rapid analgesia, which can be useful for breakthrough pain. It is also available in an extended-release formulation. Hydrocodone is only available paired with either acetaminophen or aspirin. Its peak plasma concentration occurs after 80 minutes. As with several other oral opioids, abuse potential is high.

Anticoagulation in the Total Hip Arthroplasty Patient

Because of the increased risk of deep vein thrombosis (DVT) and pulmonary embolism (PE) in patients who undergo orthopedic procedures, THA patients are usually given anticoagulants during the perioperative period. For postoperative management of anticoagulation, the surgeon needs to choose a regimen based on guidance provided by the American Association of Orthopaedic Surgeons (AAOS) guidelines and the American College of Chest Physicians (ACCP) guidelines. The recommendations continue to evolve with a new focus on symptomatic events as an endpoint. Preventing symptomatic DVT and PE is to be balanced with preventing bleeding complications. Recent updates to the recommendations should be followed in the current literature. At time of press for this text, the most current guidelines serve as the recommended readings. With the most recent ACCP guidelines, there is finally a large amount of agreement with the AAOS guidelines.[30,31]

The choice of anticoagulation can influence the choice of postoperative analgesia technique (Table 20-3 and Table 20-4). In general, anticoagulated patients may safely take intravenous or oral opioids as well as multimodal agents, such as gabapentin, pregabalin, celecoxib, and acetaminophen. For patients receiving spinal or epidural analgesia, following American Society of Regional Anesthesia and Pain Medicine (ASRA) guidelines on anticoagulation is recommended.[32] Warfarin should be discontinued at least 3 days prior to the procedure and the international normalized ratio (INR) monitored prior to the performance of any neuraxial technique (spinal or epidural). Because of the risk of spinal and epidural hematoma formation, coagulation studies should return to normal prior to neuraxial needle placement. For similar reasons, patients taking clopidogrel (Plavix [Bristol-Myers Squibb, New York, NY]) should discontinue the medication 7 days before the procedure. Patients receiving unfractionated heparin for prophylaxis of DVTs in the hospital should receive their last dose 8 hours before receiving regional anesthesia. In addition, it is recommended that neuraxial techniques not be performed for a minimum of 10 to 12 hours after a prophylactic dose of low molecular weight heparin (LMWH) and 24 hours after a treatment dose (eg, 1 mg/kg of enoxaparin). At our institution, clinicians generally wait 24 hours after the last LMWH dose before performing neuraxial techniques. Aspirin alone is generally not a contraindication to spinal or epidural placement. Following these precautions may help reduce the risk of epidural hematoma formation. If the use of neuraxial techniques requires adjustment of

Table 20-4

Anticoagulation Monitors and Discontinuation Guidelines Before Neuraxial Analgesia

Agent	Coagulation Monitor PT	aPTT	Time to Effect	Discontinuation Before Regional Anesthesia
Intravenous heparin	↑	↑↑↑	Minutes	6 to 8 hours
Subcutaneous heparin	↑	↑↑↑	40 to 50 minutes	6 to 8 hours
LMWH	—	—	3 to 5 hours	24 hours
Warfarin	↑↑↑	↑	3 to 5 days	4 to 6 days
Dabigatran	↑↑↑	↑↑↑	0.5 to 2 hours	2.5 to 5 half-lives
Rivaroxaban	↑↑↑	↑↑↑	2 to 4 hours	2.5 to 5 half-lives
Antiplatelet Agents				
Aspirin	—	—	Hours	Not needed*
Clopidogrel	—	—	Hours	7 days
NSAIDs	—	—	Hours	Not needed*

*According to the 2010 ASRA guidelines, NSAIDs, including aspirin, do not create a level of risk that will interfere with neuraxial blockade. However, they recommend that neuraxial blockade not be performed in patients taking NSAIDs who will be given other medications that affect clotting mechanism in the early postoperative period.[26]

PTT is currently the recommended assay to test for the presence of dabigatran. There is no reliable test to detect the presence of rivaroxaban, although the PT may be increased.

antithrombotic therapy, it is advisable to carefully evaluate the associated cardiac risks and seek guidance from the patient's cardiologist or primary care provider.

Although current ASRA guidelines do not yet address the newer oral agents, a discussion of perioperative anticoagulants would not be complete without mention of dabigatran and rivaroxaban, which are becoming increasingly popular. Dabigatran (Pradaxa, Boehringer Ingelheim, UK) is an oral direct thrombin inhibitor primarily used in patients with a history of heparin-induced thrombocytopenia or with atrial fibrillation. It is used both for DVT and PE prophylaxis and in patients with atrial fibrillation for thrombus prophylaxis, as well as for secondary prevention of cardiac events in patients with acute coronary syndrome.[33] Peak plasma levels are reached in 30 to 120 minutes, which coincides with the maximum effect on clotting. The optimal timing of performance of neuraxial techniques in a patient receiving dabigatran is not clear but because its half-life is 14 to 17 hours, the safest approach would be to avoid neuraxial techniques until further data are available. If an atraumatic spinal anesthetic has been performed for THA, dabigatran may be given 4 hours after surgery for prophylaxis; epidural catheter placement is not recommended if postoperative dabigatran use is planned.[33]

Rivaroxaban (Xarelto, Janssen Pharmaceuticals, Leverkusen, Germany) is an oral factor Xa inhibitor approved for prevention of thromboembolism associated with THA. Peak levels are reached in 2 to 4 hours, which correspond to maximum anticoagulation effects; half-life is 5 to 9 hours. Performance of neuraxial techniques is not recommended in patients already taking it until further data are available. If an atraumatic spinal anesthetic is performed, rivaroxaban may be given 6 to 8 hours after the dose[33]; epidural catheters may be placed preoperatively in the setting of postoperative rivaroxaban administration but the catheter must be removed 24 hours after the previous dose and the next dose after removal may be safe after 4 hours.[34]

In addition to these suggestions, many physicians recommend caution when removing epidural catheters and will generally not remove a catheter from a patient whose INR is above 1.5. The 2010 ASRA guidelines recommend removing epidural catheters when the INR is less than 1.5,[31] as removal of the catheter may represent nearly as great a risk for hematoma as catheter insertion.[6] However, clinicians should always evaluate the risk/benefit ratio when applying guidelines in clinical practice. A recent large retrospective study reported the successful removal of epidural catheters in over 4000 patients whose mean INR was 1.9.[35] The risk, therefore, of taking measures to stop or reverse anticoagulation (ie, DVT, PE) so that the INR decreases to less than 1.5 for catheter removal may be greater than the risk of removing the catheter with an INR between 1.5 and 2.

Removal of epidural catheters in patients receiving LMWH is another potential source of confusion and potential problems. The ASRA guidelines state that epidural catheters may be safely maintained in patients receiving postoperative LMWH but that catheters should be removed a minimum of 10 to 12 hours after the last dose and at least 2 hours should elapse after catheter removal for the next dose.[31] We practice a cautious approach at our institution and remove our catheters 24 hours after the last LMWH dose.

Epidural hematomas can progress to cord compression, a serious risk of neuraxial analgesia. Symptoms of cord compression include severe back pain and, more commonly, lower extremity numbness or weakness, progressing to bowel or bladder dysfunction. Any delay in properly diagnosing symptoms of epidural hematoma can lead to irreversible spinal cord injury.

Lumbar plexus nerve blocks may be performed in THA patients who are anticoagulated. However, clinicians must be aware of the risk of muscle sheath, retroperitoneal, or renal hematoma.[13] If one chooses to perform this block for postoperative pain relief, he or she must carefully consider the benefits and risks.

Summary

Management of postoperative pain can lead to better outcomes after THA. Often, the best approach is a multimodal plan that utilizes combinations of drugs and various anesthetic techniques. This approach can limit the dependence on one particular class of drugs and its associated side effects. Particular attention should be given to anticoagulated patients when neuraxial and peripheral nerve blocks are utilized.

References

1. Apfelbaum JL, Chen C, Mehta SS, Gan TJ. Postoperative pain experience: results from a national survey suggest postoperative pain continues to be undermanaged. *Anesth Analg.* 2003;97:534-540.
2. Joshi GP, Ogunnaike BO. Consquences of inadequate postoperative pain relief and chronic persistent postoperative pain. *Anesth Clin N Am.* 2005;23:21-36.
3. Rathmell JP, Pino CA, Taylor R, Patrin T, Viani BA. Intrathecal morphine for postoperative analgesia: a randomized, controlled, dose-ranging study after hip and knee arthroplasty. *Anesth Analg.* 2003;97:1452-7.
4. Sites BD, Beach M, Biggs R, Rohan C, Wiley C, Rassias A, Gregory J, Fanciullo G. Intrathecal clonidine added to a bupivacaine-morphine spinal anesthetic improves postoperative analgesia for total knee arthroplasty. *Anesth Analg.* 2003;96:1083-1088.
5. Salmon P, Hall GH, Peerbhoy D, Shenkin A, Parker C. Recovery from hip and knee arthroplasty: patients' perspective on pain, function, quality of life, and well-being up to 6 months postoperatively. *Arch Phys Med Rehabil.* 2001;82:360-366.
6. Bernards CM. Epidural and spinal anesthesia. In: Barash PG, Cullen BF, Stoelting RK, Cahalan MK, Stock MC, eds. *Clinical Anesthesia.* 6th ed. Philadelphia, PA: Lippincott Williams & Wilkins; 2009:927-954.
7. Chia YY, Liu K, Liu YC, Chang HC, Wong CS. Adding Ketamine in a Multimodal Patient-Controlled Epidural Regimen Reduces Postoperative Pain and Analgesic Consumption. *Anesth Analg.* 1998;86:1245-1249.
8. Singelyn FJ, Deyaert M, Joris D, Pendeville E, Gouverneur JM. Effects of intravenous patient-controlled analgesia with morphine, continuous epidural analgesia, and continuous three-in-one block on postoperative pain and knee rehabilitation after total knee arthroplasty. *Anesth Analg.* 1998;87:88-92.
9. Lo CC, Chen JY, Lo YK, Lai PH, Lin YT. Spontaneous spinal epidural hematoma: a case report and review of the literatures. *Acta Neurol Taiwan.* 2012;21:31-34.
10. Viscusi ER, Martin G, Hartrick CT, Singla N, Manvelian G. Forty-eight hours of postoperative pain relief after total hip arthroplasty with a novel, extended-release epidural morphine formulation. *Anesthesiology.* 2005;102:1014-1022.
11. Sumida S, Lesley MR, Hanna MN, Kumar K, Wu CL. Meta-analysis of the effect of extended-release epidural morphine versus intravenous patient-controlled analgesia on respiratory depression. *J Opioid Manag.* 2009;5:301-305.
12. Ilfeld BM, Mariano ER, Madison SJ, et al. Continuous femoral versus posterior lumbar plexus nerve blocks for analgesia after hip arthroplasty: a randomized, controlled study. *Anesth Analg.* 2011;113:897-903.

13. Tsui BCH, Rosenquist RW. Peripheral nerve blockade. In: Barash PG, Cullen BF, Stoelting RK, Cahalan MK, Stock MC, eds. *Clinical Anesthesia.* 6th ed. Philadelphia, PA: Lippincott Williams & Wilkins; 2009:955-1002.
14. Mercadante S, Ferrera P, Villari P, Arcuri E. Hyperalgesia: an emerging iatrogenic syndrome. *J Pain Symptom Manag.* 2003;26:769-775.
15. Samad TA, Moore KA, Sapirstein A, et al. Interleukin-1β-mediated induction of Cox-2 in the CNS contributes to inflammatory pain hypersensitivity. *Nature.* 2001;410:471-475.
16. Fischer HB, Simanski CJP. A procedure-specific systematic review and consensus recommendations for analgesia after total hip replacement. *Anaesthesia.* 2005;60:1189–1202.
17. Abdul-Hadi O, Parvizi J, Austin MS, Viscusi E, Einhorn T. Nonsteroidal anti-inflammatory drugs in orthopaedics. *J Bone Joint Surg Am.* 2009;91:2020-2027.
18. Turan A, White PF, Karamanlioglu B, et al. Gabapentin: an alternative to the cyclooxygenase-2 inhibitors for perioperative pain management. *Anesth Analg.* 2006;102:175-181.
19. Seib RK, Paul JE. Preoperative gabapentin for postoperative analgesia: a meta-analysis. *Can J Anesth.* 2006;53:461-469.
20. Menigaux C, Adam F, Guignard B, Sessler DI, Chauvin M. Preoperative gabapentin decreases anxiety and improves early functional recovery from knee surgery. *Anesth Analg.* 2005;100:1394-1399.
21. Clarke H, Pereira S, Kennedy D, et al. Adding Gabapentin to a multimodal regimen does not reduce acute pain, opioid consumption or chronic pain after total hip arthroplasty. *Acta Anaesthesiol Scand.* 2009;53:1073-1083.
22. Hurley RW, Cohen SP, Williams KA, Rowlingson AJ, Wu CL. The analgesic effects of perioperative gabapentin on postoperative pain: a meta-analysis. *Reg Anesth Pain Med.* 2006;31:237-247.
23. Buvanendran A, Kroin JS, Della Valle CJ, Kari M, Moric M, Tuman KJ. Perioperative oral pregabalin reduces chronic pain after total knee arthroplasty: a prospective, randomized, controlled trial. *Anesth Analg.* 2010;110:199-207.
24. Bell RF, Dahl JB, Moore RA, Kalso EA. Perioperative ketamine for acute postoperative pain (review). *Acta Anaesthesiol Scand.* 2005;49:1405-1428.
25. Remerand F, Le Tendre C, Baud A, et al. The early and delayed analgesic effects of ketamine after total hip arthroplasty: a prospective, randomized, controlled double-blind study. *Anesth Analg.* 2009;109:1963–1971.
26. Urban MK, Ya Deau JT, Wukovits B, Lipnitsky JY. Ketamine as an adjunct to postoperative pain mangement in opioid tolerant patients after spinal fusions: a prospective randomized trial. *HSS J.* 2008;4:62-65.
27. Grass JA. Patient-controlled analgesia. *Anesth Analg.* 2005;101:S44-S61.
28. Stoelting RK, Hillier SC. *Pharmacology and Physiology in Anesthetic Practice.* 4th ed. Philadelphia, PA: Lippincott Williams & Wilkins; 2006:103-104.
29. Stoelting RK, Hillier SC. *Pharmacology and Physiology in Anesthetic Practice.* 4th ed. Philadelphia, PA: Lippincott Williams & Wilkins; 2006:116.
30. Falck-Ytter Y, Francis CW, Johanson NA, et al. Prevention of VTE in orthopedic surgery patients: antithrombotic therapy and prevention of thrombosis. 9th ed. American College of Chest Physicians evidenced-based clinical practice guidelines. *Chest.* 2012;141;e278S-e325S.
31. Parvizi J, Azzam K, Rothman RH. Deep venous thrombosis prophylaxis for total joint arthroplasty: american academy of orthopaedic surgeons guidelines. *J Arthroplasty.* 2008;23(7 suppl):2-5.
32. Horlocker TT, Wedel DJ, Rowlingson JC, et al. regional anesthesia in the patient receiving antithrombotic or thrombolytic therapy. American society of regional anesthesia and pain medicine evidence-based guidelines. 3rd ed. *Reg Anesth Pain Med.* 2010;35:64-101.
33. Llau JV, Ferrandis R. New anticoagulants and regional anesthesia. *Curr Opin Anesthesiol.* 2009;22:661-666.
34. Rosencher N, Bonnet MP, Sessler DI. Selected new antithrombotic agents and neuraxial anaesthesia for major orthopaedic surgery: management strategies. *Anaesthesia.* 2007;62:1154-1160.
35. Liu SS, Buvanendran A, Viscusi ER, et al. Uncomplicated removal of epidural catheters in 4,365 patients with international normalized ratio greater than 1.4 during initiation of warfarin therapy. *Reg Anesth Pain Med.* 2011;36:231-235.

21

Controversies in Total Hip Arthroplasty

Thomas K. John, MD; Benjamin Bender, MD; and Javad Parvizi, MD, FRCS

In the United States, almost 400,000 total hip replacements are performed annually, and in Europe the estimation is that more than 600,000 hip replacement procedures are performed. These numbers are expected to rise in the upcoming years due to aging population, expanding indications, heightened patient expectations, and rapid growth of revision procedures.[1,2]

Many controversies surround hip arthroplasty; in this chapter we will review several controversies. Ever since the earliest attempts in total hip arthroplasty (THA) by Gluck in Germany in 1891 using ivory to replace the femoral head to the advances pioneered by Charnley nearly a century later with metals and bone cement, controversies have brewed within the field whether it be about the surgical technique, materials used, instrumentation, or perioperative care. While literature exists that looks at each of the above categories in detail, few indulge the debate within each topic.

Hip Precautions

Current dogma in routine postoperative care in primary THA teaches the implementation of hip precautions. Dislocation following primary THA remains a major challenge and leads to lengthy hospital stay, rehabilitation, and incidence of reoperation.[3,4] Etiology is commonly attributed to component malpositioning, soft tissue-related factors, and surgical approach.[5] Average incidence of dislocation after a primary THA is approximately 3% with several contributing factors: history of prior surgery, posterior surgical approach, malpositioning of one or both components, femoral impingement on the pelvis, impingement of the neck of the femoral component on the margin of the socket, inadequate soft tissue tension, weak adductor muscles, avulsion or nonunion of the greater trochanter, and noncompliance or extremes of positioning during the postoperative period.[6]

With most dislocations occurring within the first 3 months, proponents of routine postoperative restrictions argue that dislocations are often precipitated by extreme positioning of the hip during a period when the patient is still regaining optimal muscle control and strength. As such, personnel involved in the postoperative care of the total hip patient are routinely advised to ensure avoidance of extreme positions via the use of an abduction pillow, a pillow between the legs during sleep, use of a high chair, elevated toilet seat, avoiding driving as well as being a passenger, and the need to sleep in a supine position for up to 6 weeks.[4] These imposing restrictions, while often viewed as necessary, are received by the patient population as largely discouraging for postoperative mobilization.

Very few studies have been done in this area. The largest randomized, prospective study by Peak et al[5] looked at 303 THAs done through an anterolateral approach with the patient groups split into restricted and unrestricted groups. It was found that the patients in the unrestricted group were much more satisfied, performed more daily activities, incurred savings of $655 per patient, and had a dislocation rate of 0.33% within the entire group. As such, the surgeon is faced with new data that fail to show a clear benefit of implementing restrictive precautions at the cost of faster time to rehabilitation.

Parvizi J, Klatt BA.
Essentials in Total Hip Arthroplasty (pp 171-180).

Hip Resurfacing

Hip resurfacing, the alternative to THA, brings with it a new set of controversies. Developed as an attractive alternative that would spare femoral bone stock, a small amount of diseased bone is removed from the femoral head where a metal cap is placed anatomically congruent to the indigenous head along with a metallic acetabular component. The closely related, limited femoral head resurfacing employs a similar technique while sparing the acetabulum. Although this concept faced an initial decline in popularity in the last few decades mainly due to poor design, inappropriate materials, and poor instrumentation,[7] the constantly evolving field of metal implants has allowed for the resurgence of its use. A recent study of 1140 patients who underwent hybrid metal-on-metal hip resurfacing revealed a 95.2% survival rate at 5 years before conversion to THA.[8]

Opponents argue that in order to be a "viable" alternative to the standard THA, it must offer a distinct improvement or advantage over the existing gold standard of treatment, even for select indications. Complications in hip resurfacing result from implant malpositioning mainly from surgeon inexperience, technical difficulty, complex instrumentation, and risk of femoral neck fracture. Furthermore, it is argued that compared to the standard total hip, it cannot restore hip biomechanics and limb length.[9]

This raises the vital question: For whom should hip resurfacing be done and for whom should hip resurfacing not be done? Currently accepted indications include patients with primary osteoarthritis, osteonecrosis, developmental dysplasia of the hip, rheumatoid arthritis, post-traumatic arthritis, patients with high rates of dislocation, and patients with retained hardware. Absolute contraindications include patients with inadequate femoral head, neck, or acetabular bone stock. Relative contraindications have included patients with body mass index (BMI) greater than 35, tall patients, females, and those with femoral head cysts greater than 1 cm.

The dearth of long-term studies have led to some surgeons recommending the limitation of its use to patients less than 60 years of age with good bone stock,[10] with some narrowing the group to young active males, who are traditionally at risk for failure of THA.[11] Schmalzried et al[12] looked at 147 consecutive hips that underwent metal-on-metal resurfacing, concluding a stringent selection criteria predicted a favorable postoperative outcome, some of which included patients with earlier stage disease with disease limited to the articular cartilage. Using the arthritic hip grading system that took into account preoperative Harris hip score, occurrence of mild to moderate postoperative pain, preoperative range of motion (ROM), postoperative ROM, pre-and postoperative hip center of rotation, pre-and postoperative horizontal femoral offset, limb-length discrepancy, and acetabular radiolucencies, those with a higher hip grade or lesser arthritic changes did better.

This brings up another point to consider: the role of dual energy x-ray absorptiometry (DEXA) scan. It has been argued that the DEXA scan can assess the adequacy of the femoral head bone stock preoperatively and in subsequent postoperative follow-up of the patient in addition to detecting any evidence of stress shielding around the femoral component.[13,14] To date, no prospective, large-scale study has been conducted evaluating the role of DEXA scans. However, it has been shown to play a key role when using resurfacing to treat osteonecrosis of the femoral head due to concerns of placing an implant onto nonviable bone.[15]

The potential of systemic metal ion elevation is also an ongoing source of concern.[16,17] It is unclear what the consequences of elevated ion levels are. Ziaee et al[18] showed that cobalt and chromium ions are able to cross the placenta in pregnant women, and while the study suggested that the placenta plays a modulatory effect in total ion transfer, the mean cord blood level of cobalt, for example, was significantly higher than in the control group.

In recent years it has been determined that vertical positioning of the acetabular component leads to edge loading and extensive metal ion release with systemic and in particular local toxicity. Periarticular muscle destruction, particularly abductor mechanism, is seen to occur in patients with failed metal-on-metal resurfacing of THA.

Cement Usage

Using the Charnley fixation system, acrylic cement became the standard for femoral component fixation and while the latest trend has seen a draw away from using cemented stems, it is still widely used. Features universal to the femoral component include the need for a high strength superalloy, wide medial and lateral borders to load the proximal cement mantle in compression, and minimization of sharp edges, among others. Typical failures are seen at the prosthetic-cement junction mainly due to the debonding process and subsequent fracture of the cement. Developers have tried to ameliorate this by modifying the surface with texturing, precoating the stem with polymethylmethacrylate (PMMA), etc. The problem with a roughened stem is that when debonding and loosening occurs, a textured surface generates more debris than a polished surface.

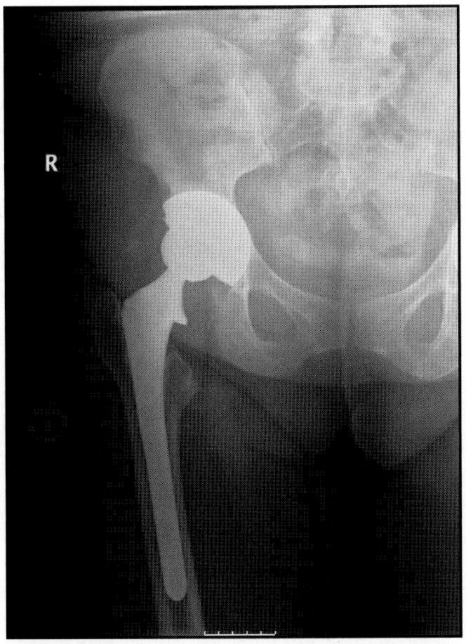

Figure 21-1. Stress shielding of the proximal femur caused by extensively coated femoral stem with diaphyseal engagement.

Cementless stems with porous surfaces were a product stemming from the problems seen with cemented stems—mainly loosening—and bone loss from fragmented cement. This led to the development of porous metal surfaces to allow for bony ingrowth as long as immediate stability and intimate bony contact were ensured. Made from titanium or cobalt chrome, the cementless stems are either anatomic or straight in terms of its stem shape. The anatomic shape affords a posterior bow that requires overreaming of the canal, and if the stem is not placed correctly down the canal, it can impinge on the anterior cortex, causing postoperative thigh pain. In addition, extensively coated femoral stems have been known to cause undesirable proximal bone wasting from stress shielding, particularly at the proximal level (Figure 21-1). Extensive bone ingrowth, while providing a stable construct, also poses a major obstacle when trying to extract the component, often causing unnecessary damage to the surrounding bone stock at explantation. Cemented components, despite modifications in design, have not substantially improved long-term survival, allowing for an increasing trend toward the use of cementless components.

Which is better? The revision burden for cemented prostheses from 1979 to 2000 was 7.4% while for uncemented implants, the rate was 17.9%.[19] With first-generation cementing techniques, radiographic 10-year follow-up revealed up to 30% to 40% femoral loosening rates, which were substantially reduced with third-generation techniques, with loosening rates reported at 10%.[20] Opponents to cemented prostheses identify debonding, aseptic femoral loosening, and sheer difficulty of revision arthroplasty. With cementless prosthesis, critics agree that 10- to 15-year follow-up studies show very low rates of aseptic loosening around 0% to 11%, and problems with polyethylene wear and osteolysis remain at the forefront of the debate. Furthermore, manufacturing cost of cementless components far outweigh its cemented counterpart.

Nonetheless, the vast majority of studies report no significant differences in long-term mortality rates between cemented and cementless THAs.[21-23] Uncemented prostheses have been connected to a significant amount of thigh pain, poorer function, and greater dependence on walking aids.[24]

Surgical Approaches

Essentially, all approaches require careful planning and positioning of the patient that allows for optimal visualization and access to the operative site. Several options exist for the surgical approach to the reconstruction of the hip along with advantages and disadvantages of each. The current debate suggests that a more anterior or direct lateral approach may decrease the overall risk for dislocation in the postoperative patient, whereas a posterior approach affords better early functional outcome because it does not violate the abductor mechanism.

In recent years, the direct anterior approach has gained popularity mostly because of its potential to not violate the abductor mechanism and afford lower instability than the posterior approach. Randomized studies evaluating the role of direct anterior approach, performed either through a Watson-Jones interval or Smith-Petersen approach, is currently underway with some presentations in meetings that suggest better early functional outcome for the direct anterior approach.

The classic posterior approach, also known as the Southern-Moore approach, extends from the posterior-superior iliac spine to the posterior border of the trochanter then down 13 cm along the femoral shaft, splitting the gluteus maximus, innervated by the inferior gluteal nerve. A subtle variant, the posterolateral approach, also known as the Langenback-Kocher approach, lies from the posterior-superior iliac spine to the trochanter tip, hip held at 45 degrees—ideal for THA, visualization of the acetabulum, and pelvic fractures. The biggest benefit of the posterior approach and its variant is the preservation of the abductor muscles, which in turn translates to better postoperative functional outcomes. The main problem with the posterior approach, however, remains its rather high rate of dislocation following primary THA.[3,25] Among various factors include approach, component positioning, as well as the soft tissue status. Soft tissue repair following the posterior approach in a study of 56 revision THAs has shown a reduction in dislocation rate from 10% in the group without repair to 1.9% in the group with repair.[26] Alternatives such as a modified posterior approach described by Williams et al[27] that preserved the piriformis, labrum, and capsule has been shown to decrease the dislocation rate compared to conventional techniques.[28]

One needs to keep in mind the variations of each approach such as the 2-incision anterior, anterolateral, direct lateral, as well as the transtrochanteric approaches, each with its own benefits and pitfalls. Whether one chooses between the posterior or anterior approach forces the surgeon to choose between risking abductor dysfunction versus a potential dislocation.

Minimally Invasive Surgery

The concept of minimally invasive surgery (MIS) was introduced to orthopedics in the 1970s by Watanabe in association with arthroscopy. MIS is defined as a surgical technique performed through a short skin incision to minimize injury to muscles and/or bones. MIS does not necessarily stand for a short scar, but refers to minimum damage to soft tissues, particularly muscles and their insertions. Every injury to a muscle or its attachment is associated with decreased muscle strength and impaired proprioception. Muscle protection translates into accelerated rehabilitation, which in turn enables the patient to be discharged from the surgical ward and start rehabilitation potentially faster. In a standard surgical approach, size of the incision is dictated by the requirements during the surgery; with the minimally invasive techniques, the size of the surgical approach is much more of a fixed parameter. Currently accepted MIS approaches include the miniposterior, anterolateral, the 2-incision, and the direct anterior approach. Marred by complications even at the hands of the most experienced surgeon, problems are often attributed to poor component positioning, wound complications, heterotopic bone formation, surgeon inexperience, low case volume, and inexperience with the procedure itself.[29,30] Often times these approaches are scaled down versions of traditional approaches. The miniposterior approach involves an incision near the tip of the trochanter, splitting the fascia over the gluteus maximus, and breaching the medius into the joint. This approach often sacrifices the piriformis tendon and part of the short external rotators.[31] In a study, comparison to the standard posterior approach showed significantly shorter time and lower risk of nerve palsy, and aseptic loosening was observed.[32] Other studies,[33,34] however, have shown no improvement in early postoperative outcomes, surgical times, estimated blood loss, length of stay, or disposition at discharge with the miniposterior approach. In some series, higher incidence of complication has been observed with MIS approach as it compromises visualization and may lead to component malpositioning (Figure 21-2).

The minianterolateral approach is a modification to the Hardinge and Watson-Jones approaches to the hip with an oblique incision over the greater trochanter about 2 cm above the tip proceeding caudally, splitting the tensor fascia lata (TFL) and the gluteus medius. Studies have shown no or slightly longer operating time, less blood loss, less length of stay, and less need for placement in rehabilitation.[31,35,36]

The 2-incision approach utilizes a small direct anterior approach for visualization of the acetabulum and a miniposterior approach for access to the femur and must be done with aid of fluoroscopy. The fluoroscope is used to locate the anterior incision over the femoral neck 2 to 3 finger breadths below the anterior-superior iliac spine. The incision is made parallel to the TFL and the sartorius. For the posterior incision, the piriformis fossa is palpated and a small stab wound is made and extended in line with the femoral neck for approximately 1.25 inches. Without fluoroscopy, the anterior incision is made along the medial border of the TFL and centered at the lower margin of the greater trochanter. One of the main problems as reported by Berger et al[37] is the incidence of femoral shaft fractures from inserting a tapered, wedge-shaped stem without direct visualization.

The direct anterior approach may represent the truest minimally invasive approach with a true internervous plane. A modification of the Smith-Petersen approach, the incision is made between the TFL, innervated by the superior gluteal nerve, and the sartorius, innervated by the femoral nerve. A longitudinal incision is made at the anterior edge of the greater trochanter to access the hip joint. Potential problems that have been reported include dislocation, femoral fracture, hematoma, infection, and injury to the lateral cutaneous femoral nerve.[38,39] The latter can be avoided using a more lateral approach, closer to the trochanter. Nakata et al[40] reported significantly improved single-leg stance, faster 50 m walking time, and improvement in the use of walking aids in comparison to the group with the miniposterior approach.

Which of these is most practical in terms of minimally invasive approach to the hip? The results are far-reaching in implying it is largely dependent on surgeon comfort, experience, patient selection, and technique. Each comes

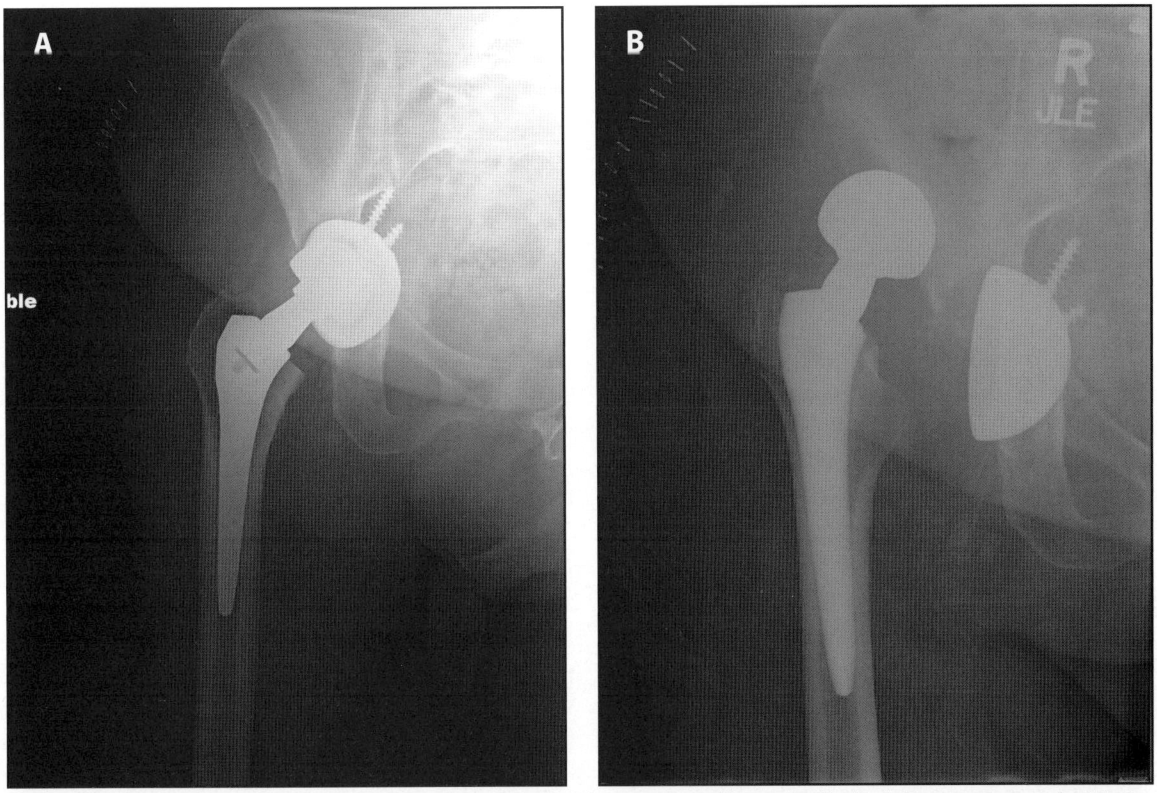

Figure 21-2. THA performed using minimally invasive approach. (A) Pelvic reaming with poor visualization led to component malpositioning with pelvic discontinuity. (B) Acetabular component migrated and hip dislocated on postoperative day 2. Early revision with cage construct was required.

with its own complications and benefits, and surgeons widely agree the true benefit at this stage remains largely cosmetic. No matter which approach is done, it is most important that visualization enables the surgeon to position the hip implants appropriately.

Deep Vein Thrombosis

Venous thromboembolism (VTE) has long been a problem facing the practice of THA. Hemostasis in the human body is a physiological balance between coagulation and fibrinolysis, traced back to the intrinsic and extrinsic pathways of the coagulation cascade, ending with the formation of fibrin, the main player in the formation of clots.

Virchow described the 3 conditions that predisposed a patient to VTE: venous stasis, endothelial injury, and hypercoagulability.[41] Endothelial injury is commonly seen with hip surgery with kinking of the femoral vein during positioning and manipulation of the lower extremity. This in turn leads to local trauma, excessive venodilation, disruption of the endothelium—which ultimately turns on the coagulation cascade—and platelet activators that lead to clot. It is thought that thermal injury that occurs with the use of bone cement can also lead to clot formation. Venous stasis impedes blood flow, bringing platelets in contact with the endothelium, preventing dilution of activated clotting factors, retarding inflow of clotting factor inhibitors, and allowing clotting factors to aggregate. This is seen in THA during immobilization intra- and postoperatively, tourniquet use, postoperative swelling, and positioning. Hypercoagulability is seen with primary causes such as protein C or S deficiencies. With blood loss, a reduction of antithrombin III is seen along with the inhibition of the endogenous fibrinolytic system. In THA, increase in fibrinopeptide A, prothrombin F1.2, and thrombin-antithrombin complexes are seen during femoral reaming, which ultimately result in the formation of clot.

Prophylaxis has always been a source of debate with no real consensus reached within the specialty of orthopedic surgery, let alone for THA. It can include either mechanical or chemical methods. However, few recent medical studies currently exist that aim to form a consensus in VTE prophylaxis.[42,43] Mechanical methods include graduated compression stockings, foot pumps, and intermittent pneumatic compression devices. Chemical methods include aspirin, warfarin, heparin, low molecular weight heparin (LMWH), and fondaparinux, among others. Among these, the most commonly used are warfarin and LMWH. Earlier studies by Coventry[44] et al reported a reduced prevalence from 3.4% fatal PE to 0.05% in patients given warfarin compared to controls in 2012 postoperative THA patients, while Amstutz et al[45] reported an incidence of 0.5% symptomatic/nonfatal PE on 3000 THA patients after 3 weeks of postoperative warfarin use.

Similar efficacy has been reported with LMWH as well. Clagett et al[46] evaluated 3016 total hip patients treated with LMWH perioperatively and noted a 15% prevalence of deep vein thrombosis (DVT). Hull et al[47] reported a DVT prevalence between 10% to 13% in total joints patients when treated with LMWH, and 24% with warfarin. However, they noted almost twice the incidence of bleeding complications, 2.8% with LMWH compared to 1.5% with warfarin, and wound hematoma complications of 5.8% with LMWH and 2.5% with warfarin. Colwell et al[48] found similar rates of DVT incidence with LMWH and warfarin, but once again found nearly doubled rates of bleeding complications with LMWH, when compared to warfarin. Proponents of LMWH use point out the marked ease of use with no need for monitoring proved reduction of DVT, and low to no incidence of herapin-induced thrombocytopenia seen with heparin. Warfarin, on the other hand, requires monitoring of the international normalized ratio and pertinent dose adjustments. Furthermore, the initial delay in reaching therapeutic levels also complicates its use. Ultimately, current practice in routine postoperative prophylaxis for THA remains surgeon preference.

Two bodies have evaluated the literature and provided guidelines for prevention of VTE following total joint arthroplasty. The American College of Chest Physicians (ACCP) mostly endorse chemical prophylaxis while the guidelines proposed by the American Academy of Orthopaedic Surgeons (AAOS) accept aspirin and mechanical prophylaxis for prevention of VTE following total joint arthroplasty. The most recent version of the AACP guidelines endorses aspirin and mechanical prophylaxis as acceptable modalities for prevention of VTE.[49]

Computer Navigation

Successful hip reconstruction to restore normal hip biomechanics requires accurate placement of implants. Of all the factors associated with dislocation rates following THA, component malposition is probably the most manageable.[50] Computer-aided navigation for THA came into play during the late 1990s when computed tomography (CT) became advanced in its accuracy and ability to produce reconstruction images of quality. Navigation systems initially involved massive robots that were often intrusive to the surgical domain. This was followed by passive systems that kept track of the patient locations, the surgical tools, and employed preoperative CT images, fluoroscopy, or image-free techniques.

The position of the acetabular cup and the femoral stem is the most important, with the safe zone for the cup alignment being defined as 40 to 50 degrees of abduction and 15 to 25 degrees of anteversion. Conventional techniques rely on the surgeon's experience and the assumption that the trunk and pelvis remain in a known orientation, which does not always remain constant.

Navigation systems rely on a pelvic coordinate system that uses the bony landmarks to determine the acetabular cup orientation.

Proponents of navigation in THA cite the dramatic improvement in the precision of cup placement.[51-54] As such, results from computer-aided navigation have shown a dramatic reduction of outliers and excellent axial alignment for THA patients. In addition, significant improvements in soft tissue management and avoidance of large incisions have led to a decrease in subsequent revision surgeries. However, opponents argue the difficulty in the learning curve, with initial measurements and assessments frequently being inaccurate. Furthermore, for the sake of smaller incisions and potentially accurate measurements, operative time is also lengthened, raising other concerns as higher rates of intraoperative development of venous thromboembolism.

Bearing Surfaces

With more THAs performed now than ever, improving longevity of these implants while maintaining a reasonable cost has become more of a concern. Within the past 2 decades, more THAs have been performed using metal-on-metal or ceramic-on-ceramic bearing surfaces. With the recent withdrawal of a metal-on-metal resurfacing (ASR [DePuy, Raynham, MA]), popularity of metal-on-metal has waned rapidly, leaving ceramic-on-ceramic as the only hard bearing surface for use. Highly cross-linked polyethylene (XLPE) remains the most popular alternative of bearing surface, so much so that it has largely replaced conventional polyethylene. Although wear performance of alternative bearing surfaces are encouraging, some concerns with these bearing surfaces remain. Cross-linking of polyethylene leads to a reduction in mechanical properties of this material that may predispose XLPE to fatigue fractures. Thus,

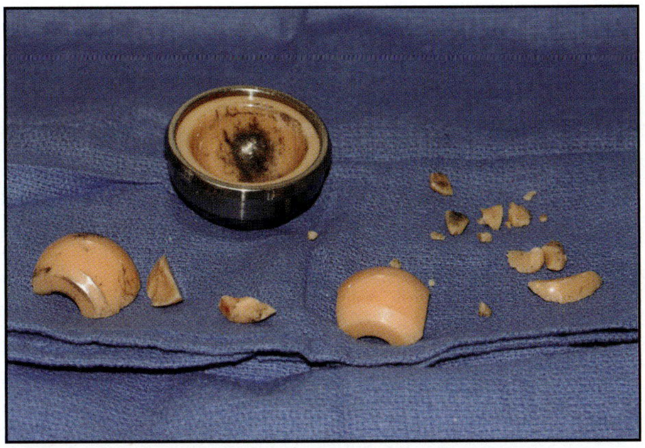

Figure 21-3. Fracture of ceramic-on-ceramic bearing surface.

appropriate positioning of the acetabular component to avoid edge loading appears to be very important when XLPE is used.

Ceramic-on-ceramic bearing surfaces such as alumina and zirconia are ideal bearing surfaces due to the material properties of hardness and high resistance to roughening when used as a bearing surface. Ceramic-on-ceramic, despite its extremely low in vivo wear rate, carries 2 disadvantages. One issue is that its low toughness can result in fracture of the bearing surface when used in THA (Figure 21-3). Recent improvements that have focused on increasing chemical purity and on reducing grain size have substantially reduced the incidence of ceramic fractures. The other issue with a ceramic-on-ceramic bearing surface relates to squeaking that is thought to occur after 1% to 7% of THA performed using ceramic-on-ceramic bearing surface.[55] The exact etiology of squeaking is not known but it is thought to relate to edge loading of the component and patch wear (stripe wear),[56] and/or impingement between femoral neck and the acetabular rim, leading to generation of metal particles and their transfer to the bearing surface. Although squeaking can occur after any type of ceramic-on-ceramic bearing surface, the highest incidence of squeaking has been reported with the use of Trident (Stryker, Mahwah, NJ) acetabular component and Accolade (Stryker) femoral stem. One of the causes of squeaking and clicking may be component malpositioning, although this is not the primary reason.[57]

Metal-on-metal bearing surfaces were introduced as an alternative to the metal-on-polyethylene surfaces, and the metal-on-metal coupling has succeeded in generating substantially lower wear debris. Although various different types of metals can be used, the degree of success relies primarily on the size (larger femoral heads) and surface finish, largely based on the level of fluid film lubrication it achieves.

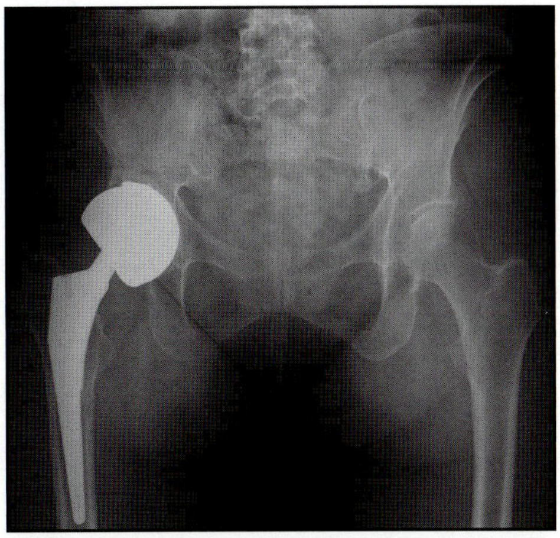

Figure 21-4. Patient with large head metal-on-metal THA. The vertical positioning of the acetabular component lead to elevation of systemic metal ions and local destruction of the abductor muscles.

Passuti et al[58] reported only 5 cases of unusual osteolysis and 10 cases of impingement after a 7-year follow-up of 2614 THAs with metal-on-metal bearing surfaces. Nonetheless, one of the major problems that persists is the effect of metal allergy since the metallic components used in alloys are biologically active. Metal-on-metal bearings are similar to hip resurfacing in that vertical positioning of the acetabular component leads to edge loading and extensive metal ion release with systemic and in particular local toxicity (Figure 21-4). Periarticular muscle destruction, particularly abductor mechanism, has occurred in patients with failed metal-on-metal THA.

Metal Allergy

While conventional THA has done exceedingly well in patients, increased scrutiny has been given to those patients who have been getting them earlier in life, which translates to longer exposure to the prosthesis. One of the major prevalent concerns is the breakdown of the metals used in implants. Metal alloys undergo corrosive wear and produce soluble ions while metal and polyethylene components break down, producing a collection of particles in regional lymph nodes and the spleen, in one instance displaying sinus histiocytosis containing cobalt chrome and titanium particles.[59] It is theorized that the wear debris from the bone-implant surface induces a phagocytic response and ultimately cytokine release. Metal ion release in serum has also been cited as a rising issue. Clarke et al[17] reported an increased level of metal ion release in patients who underwent resurfacing compared to those receiving a 28-mm metal prosthetic head, while larger studies by Antoniou et al[60] and Daniel et al[61] reported no significant difference in the amount of metal ion in whole blood at 1-year follow-up between resurfacing or prosthetic implants.

Metal-on-metal bearing surface and its relation to carcinogenesis have long been reported as a potential concern, although the incidence of malignant tumor at implant sites are low as reported in a cohort of 10,785 THAs that found no increase in leukemia or lymphoma.[62] The International Agency for Research on Cancer went so far as to conclude there was inadequate evidence to cite a link between orthopedic implants and carcinogenicity. However, Visuri et al[63] have recently reported on an increase in the prevalence of melanoma and prostate cancer in patients who have undergone THA.

A type IV hypersensitivity with lymphocyte infiltrations in periprosthetic tissue as a reaction to metal-on-metal articulation has been identified as aseptic lymphocyte dominated vasculitis associated lesion (ALVAL). Hypersensitivity to metal-on-metal bearing surfaces has also been reported when large amounts of metallic debris contribute to metal sensitization. The wear debris contributes to the accumulation of T lymphocytes and an absence of B lymphocytes. This may also play a part in reports of dermal hypersensitivity seen in up to 10% of all patients with some having positive titanium ointment skin tests in the context of a failed total hip implant.[64,65]

While there are numerous current reports on the presence of ions in serum tests and explore the possible link to cancer, there is no current evidence that significantly substantiates any of these claims that would preclude one from employing any of the currently used implants. Further data accumulation is imperative in this area of THA as well as most other sources of controversy to settle any sound debate.

In recent years, the issue of systemic and local toxicity of metal ions released from metal-on-metal bearing surface or even corroded trunnion of femoral stem has been explored further. It is known that metal ions released from bearing surface or corroded surface result in adverse local reaction and destruction of muscle and bone. The use of metal-on-metal bearing surface has declined sharply with the recognition of this problem. What remains a puzzle is how to detect patients who may be at risk of metal hypersensitivity. It is known that patch testing of the skin does not have much of a role in identifying patients with metal hypersensitivity. There are a number of patients with cutaneous sensitivity who have well-functioning metal prostheses. On the other hand, patients with metal-on-metal failure or metal hypersensitivity may not manifest cutaneous reaction to the culprit metal, mostly nickel. In recent years and because of concern with metal hypersensitivity, most surgeons will utilize titanium implants and ceramic-on-ceramic or ceramic-on-polyethylene bearing surfaces in patients with reported metal hypersensitivity. One of the diagnostic tests used to evaluate patients with suspected metal hypersensitivity is the lymphocyte transformation test (LTT), which involves culturing of the lymphocytes from the patient with suspected metal hypersensitivity and exposure of the lymphocyte to various allergens, such as nickel and cobalt. A test is positive when proliferation of the lymphocyte in the presence of allergen is considerably elevated. Although still used by some institutions, the LTT is believed to be a very crude test and suffers accuracy for diagnosis of metal hypersensitivity. There is currently a dire need for a better understanding of the metal hypersensitivity phenomenon and design of tests that can help detect and diagnose this problem when it occurs.

References

1. Mendenhall S. 2006 hip and knee implant review. *Orthop Net News.* 2006;17:1-16.
2. Eingartner C. Current trends in total hip arthroplasty. *Ortop Traumatol Rehabil.* 2007;9(1):8.
3. Woo RY, Morrey BF. Dislocations after total hip arthroplasty. *J Bone Joint Surg Am.* 1982;64(9):1295-1306.
4. Talbot NJ, Brown JH, Treble NJ. Early dislocation after total hip arthroplasty: are postoperative restrictions necessary? *J Arthroplasty.* 2002;17(8):1006-1008.
5. Peak EL, Parvizi J, Ciminiello M, et al. The role of patient restrictions in reducing the prevalence of early dislocation following total hip arthroplasty. A randomized, prospective study. *J Bone Joint Surg Am.* 2005;87(2):247-253.
6. Harkess JWCJ, John R. *Arthroplasty of the Hip.* 11th ed. Philadelphia, PA: Mosby; 2008.
7. Rechl H, Pilge H, Rudert M. [Development of hip resurfacing]. *Orthopade.* 2008;37(7):626-633.
8. Hoberg M, Le Duff MJ, Amstutz HC. [Metal-on-metal hybrid hip resurfacing: development and current state]. *Orthopade.* 2008;37(7):679-684.
9. Slover JD, Rubash HE. Hip resurfacing arthroplasty: time to consider it again? No. *Instr Course Lect.* 2008;57:267-271.
10. Mont MA, Ragland PS, Etienne G, Seyler TM, Schmalzried TP. Hip resurfacing arthroplasty. *J Am Acad Orthop Surg.* 2006;14(8):454-463.
11. Schmalzried TP. The optimal metal-metal arthroplasty is still a total hip arthroplasty: in opposition. *J Arthroplasty.* 2006;21(4 suppl 1):77-79.
12. Schmalzried TP, Silva M, de la Rosa MA, Choi ES, Fowble VA. Optimizing patient selection and outcomes with total hip resurfacing. *Clin Orthop Relat Res.* 2005;441:200-204.

13. Harty JA, Devitt B, Harty LC, Molloy M, McGuinness A. Dual energy x-ray absorptiometry analysis of peri-prosthetic stress shielding in the Birmingham resurfacing hip replacement. *Arch Orthop Trauma Surg.* 2005;125(10):693-695.

14. Murray JR, Cooke NJ, Rawlings D, Holland JP, McCaskie AW. A reliable DEXA measurement technique for metal-on-metal hip resurfacing. *Acta Orthop.* 2005;76(2):177-181.

15. Thorey F, Reck F, Windhagen H, von Lewinski G. Influence of bone density on total hip resurfacing arthroplasty in patients with osteonecrosis of the femoral head: a radiological analysis. *Technol Health Care.* 2008;16(3):151-158.

16. Shetty VD, Villar RN. Development and problems of metal-on-metal hip arthroplasty. *Proc Inst Mech Eng [H].* 2006;220(2):371-377.

17. Clarke MT, Lee PT, Arora A, Villar RN. Levels of metal ions after small- and large-diameter metal-on-metal hip arthroplasty. *J Bone Joint Surg Br.* 2003;85(6):913-917.

18. Ziaee H, Daniel J, Datta AK, Blunt S, McMinn DJ. Transplacental transfer of cobalt and chromium in patients with metal-on-metal hip arthroplasty: a controlled study. *J Bone Joint Surg Br.* 2007;89(3):301-305.

19. Malchau H, Herberts P, Eisler T, Garellick G, Söderman P. The Swedish Total Hip Replacement Register. *J Bone Joint Surg Am.* 2002;84-A(suppl 2):2-20.

20. Buckwalter AE, Callaghan JJ, Liu SS, et al. Results of Charnley total hip arthroplasty with use of improved femoral cementing techniques. a concise follow-up, at a minimum of twenty-five years, of a previous report. *J Bone Joint Surg Am.* 2006;88(7):1481-1485.

21. Khan RJ, MacDowell A, Crossman P, et al. Cemented or uncemented hemiarthroplasty for displaced intracapsular femoral neck fractures. *Int Orthop.* 2002;26(4):229-232.

22. Khan RJ, MacDowell A, Crossman P, Keene GS. Cemented or uncemented hemiarthroplasty for displaced intracapsular fractures of the hip--a systematic review. *Injury.* 2002;33(1):13-17.

23. Sonne-Holm S, Walter S, Jensen JS. Moore hemi-arthroplasty with and without bone cement in femoral neck fractures. A clinical controlled trial. *Acta Orthop Scand.* 1982;53(6):953-956.

24. Emery RJ, Broughton NS, Desai K, Bulstrode CJ, Thomas TL. Bipolar hemiarthroplasty for subcapital fracture of the femoral neck. A prospective randomised trial of cemented Thompson and uncemented Moore stems. *J Bone Joint Surg Br.* 1991;73(2):322-324.

25. Mahomed NN, Barrett JA, Katz JN, et al. Rates and outcomes of primary and revision total hip replacement in the United States medicare population. *J Bone Joint Surg Am.* 2003;85-A(1):27-32.

26. Suh KT, Roh HL, Moon KP, Shin JK, Lee JS. Posterior Approach With Posterior Soft Tissue Repair in Revision Total Hip Arthroplasty. *J Arthroplasty.* 2008;23(8):1197-1203.

27. Williams CR, Kernohan JG, Sherry PG. A more stable posterior approach for hemiarthroplasty of the hip. *Injury.* 1997;28(4):279-281.

28. Martinez AA, Herrera A, Cuenca J, Panisello JJ, Tabuenca A. Comparison of two different posterior approachs for hemiarthroplasty of the hip. *Arch Orthop Trauma Surg.* 2002;122(1):51-52.

29. Fehring TK, Mason JB. Catastrophic complications of minimally invasive hip surgery. A series of three cases. *J Bone Joint Surg Am.* 2005;87(4):711-714.

30. Feinblatt JS, Berend KR, Lombardi AV, Jr. Severe symptomatic heterotopic ossification and dislocation: a complication after two-incision minimally invasive total hip arthroplasty. *J Arthroplasty.* 2005;20(6):802-806.

31. Vail TP, Callaghan JJ. Minimal incision total hip arthroplasty. *J Am Acad Orthop Surg.* 2007;15(12):707-715.

32. Wright JM, Crockett HC, Delgado S, Lyman S, Madsen M, Sculco TP. Mini-incision for total hip arthroplasty: a prospective, controlled investigation with 5-year follow-up evaluation. *J Arthroplasty.* 2004;19(5):538-545.

33. Ogonda L, Wilson R, Archbold P, et al. A minimal-incision technique in total hip arthroplasty does not improve early postoperative outcomes. A prospective, randomized, controlled trial. *J Bone Joint Surg Am.* 2005;87(4):701-710.

34. Woolson ST, Mow CS, Syquia JF, Lannin JV, Schurman DJ. Comparison of primary total hip replacements performed with a standard incision or a mini-incision. *J Bone Joint Surg Am.* 2004;86-A(7):1353-1358.

35. Howell JR, Masri BA, Duncan CP. Minimally invasive versus standard incision anterolateral hip replacement: a comparative study. *Orthop Clin North Am.* 2004;35(2):153-162.

36. Berger RA. Mini-incision total hip replacement using an anterolateral approach: technique and results. *Orthop Clin North Am.* 2004;35(2):143-151.

37. Berger RA. Total hip arthroplasty using the minimally invasive two-incision approach. *Clin Orthop Relat Res.* 2003(417):232-241.

38. Kennon RE, Keggi JM, Wetmore RS, Zatorski LE, Huo MH, Keggi KJ. Total hip arthroplasty through a minimally invasive anterior surgical approach. *J Bone Joint Surg Am.* 2003;85-A(suppl 4):39-48.

39. Kennon R, Keggi J, Zatorski LE, Keggi KJ. Anterior approach for total hip arthroplasty: beyond the minimally invasive technique. *J Bone Joint Surg Am.* 2004;86-A(suppl 2):91-97.

40. Nakata K, Nishikawa M, Yamamoto K, Hirota S, Yoshikawa H. A clinical comparative study of the direct anterior with mini-posterior approach two consecutive series. *J Arthroplasty.* 2009;24(5):698-704.

41. Brotman DJ, Deitcher SR, Lip GY, Matzdorff AC. Virchow's triad revisited. *South Med J.* 2004;97(2):213-214.

42. Geerts WH, Bergqvist D, Pineo GF, et al. Prevention of venous thromboembolism: American College of Chest Physicians evidence-based clinical practice guidelines (8th Edition). *Chest.* 2008;133(6 suppl):381S-453S.

43. Prevention and treatment of venous thromboembolism. International Consensus Statement (guidelines according to scientific evidence). *Int Angiol.* 2006;25(2):101-161.

44. Coventry MB, Beckenbaugh RD, Nolan DR, Ilstrup DM. 2,012 total hip arthroplasties. A study of postoperative course and early complications. *J Bone Joint Surg Am.* 1974;56(2):273-284.

45. Amstutz HC, Friscia DA, Dorey F, Carney BT. Warfarin prophylaxis to prevent mortality from pulmonary embolism after total hip replacement. *J Bone Joint Surg Am.* 1989;71(3):321-326.

46. Clagett GP, Anderson FA Jr, Geerts W, et al. Prevention of venous thromboembolism. *Chest.* 1998;114(5 suppl):531S-560S.

47. Hull RD, Pineo GF, Francis C, et al. Low-molecular-weight heparin prophylaxis using dalteparin extended out-of-hospital vs in-hospital warfarin/out-of-hospital placebo in hip arthroplasty patients: a double-blind, randomized comparison. North American Fragmin Trial Investigators. *Arch Intern Med.* 2000;160(14):2208-2215.

48. Colwell CW Jr, Collis DK, Paulson R, et al. Comparison of enoxaparin and warfarin for the prevention of venous thromboembolic disease after total hip arthroplasty. Evaluation during hospitalization and three months after discharge. *J Bone Joint Surg Am.* 1999;81(7):932-940.

49. American College of Chest Physicians Evidence-Based Clinical Practice Guidelines. Prevention of VTE in orthopaedic surgery patients. Antithrombotic therapy and prevention of thrombosis, 9th ed. *Chest.* 2012;141(2 suppl):e278s-e325s.

50. Lin F, Lim D, Wixson RL, Milos S, Hendrix RW, Makhsous M. Validation of a computer navigation system and a CT method for determination of the orientation of implanted acetabular cup in total hip arthroplasty: a cadaver study. *Clin Biomech (Bristol, Avon).* 2008;23(8):1004-1011.

51. Gandhi R, Marchie A, Farrokhyar F, Mahomed N. Computer navigation in total hip replacement: a meta-analysis. *Int Orthop.* 2009;33(3):593-597.

52. Ulrich SD, Bonutti PM, Seyler TM, Marker DR, Jones LC, Mont MA. Outcomes-based evaluations supporting computer-assisted surgery and minimally invasive surgery for total hip arthroplasty. *Expert Rev Med Devices.* 2007;4(6):873-883.

53. Ecker TM, Tannast M, Murphy SB. Computed tomography-based surgical navigation for hip arthroplasty. *Clin Orthop Relat Res.* 2007;465:100-105.

54. Haaker RG, Tiedjen K, Ottersbach A, Rubenthaler F, Stockheim M, Stiehl JB. Comparison of conventional versus computer-navigated acetabular component insertion. *J Arthroplasty.* 2007;22(2):151-159.

55. Restrepo C, Parvizi J, Kurtz SM, Sharkey PF, Hozack WJ, Rothman RH. The noisy ceramic hip: is component malpositioning the cause? *J Arthroplasty.* 2008;23(5):643-649.

56. Yoo JJ, Kim YM, Yoon KS, et al. Contemporary alumina-on-alumina total hip arthroplasty performed in patients younger than forty years: a 5-year minimum follow-up study. *J Biomed Mater Res B Appl Biomater.* 2006;78(1):70-75.

57. Walter WL, O'Toole GC, Walter WK, Ellis A, Zicat BA. Squeaking in ceramic-on-ceramic hips: the importance of acetabular component orientation. *J Arthroplasty.* 2007;22(4):496-503.

58. Passuti N, Terver S. [Metal on metal bearing surfaces in total hip arthroplasty: a survey of material incidents]. *Rev Chir Orthop Reparatrice Appar Mot.* 2007;93(3):288-312.

59. Albores-Saavedra J, Vuitch F, Delgado R, Wiley E, Hagler H. Sinus histiocytosis of pelvic lymph nodes after hip replacement. A histiocytic proliferation induced by cobalt-chromium and titanium. *Am J Surg Pathol.* 1994;18(1):83-90.

60. Antoniou J, Zukor DJ, Mwale F, Minarik W, Petit A, Huk OL. Metal ion levels in the blood of patients after hip resurfacing: a comparison between twenty-eight and thirty-six-millimeter-head metal-on-metal prostheses. *J Bone Joint Surg Am.* 2008;90(suppl 3):142-148.

61. Daniel J, Ziaee H, Salama A, Pradhan C, McMinn DJ. The effect of the diameter of metal-on-metal bearings on systemic exposure to cobalt and chromium. *J Bone Joint Surg Br.* 2006;88(4):443-448.

62. Mathiesen EB, Ahlbom A, Bermann G, Lindgren JU. Total hip replacement and cancer. A cohort study. *J Bone Joint Surg Br.* 1995;77(3):345-350.

63. Visuri TI, Pukkala E, Pulkkinen P, Paavolainen P. Cancer incidence and causes of death among total hip replacement patients: a review based on Nordic cohorts with a special emphasis on metal-on-metal bearings. *Proc Inst Mech Eng [H].* 2006;220(2):399-407.

64. Lalor PA, Gray AB, Wright S, Railton GT, Freeman MA, Revell PA. Contact sensitivity to titanium in a hip prosthesis? *Contact Dermatitis.* 1990;23(3):193-194.

65. Lalor PA, Revell PA, Gray AB, Wright S, Railton GT, Freeman MA. Sensitivity to titanium. A cause of implant failure? *J Bone Joint Surg Br.* 1991;73(1):25-28.

22

Outcomes of Primary and Complex Primary Hips

Sanaz Hariri, MD and Henrik Malchau, MD, PhD

A recent article in *Lancet* declared total hip replacement "the operation of the century,"[1] and it is widely recognized that joint pain and functional status significantly improve after total hip arthroplasty (THA). In fact, most patients with THAs report significant pain relief within 1 week after surgery. Furthermore, postoperatively, THA patients have improved scores in other health-related quality of life dimensions such as social function, mental health, and vitality.[2-4] It is important to identify those factors that may predispose certain patients to less favorable outcomes with the hopes that modifiable risk factors can be altered. The variables surrounding THAs are too numerous to include in one chapter, but what follows is a review of selected patient, implant, surgeon, and systems issues that can affect the outcomes of THA.

We will talk about factors affecting THA outcomes in general. However, it is incumbent on each surgeon to be updated on the latest data regarding his or her specific implants of choice. To stay up to date on factors that may affect their surgical outcomes, surgeons should both read the peer-reviewed literature and access annual reports from national registries, such as those in Australia, Norway, and Sweden, which are readily available online. Registries are valuable in that they generate statistically valid information even on less commonly occurring conditions and newer implants. Registries offer analysis for specific cohorts that could help inform decisions regarding the best procedure and implant for patients based on their diagnosis or demographics. Furthermore, registries allow centers to compare their outcomes to others. Departments with consistently higher proportions of complications should analyze themselves with a thorough review of their protocols, operative techniques, and implant choices.[5]

Patient-Related Factors

Obesity

Obesity certainly predisposes one to needing THA for osteoarthritis but it may also adversely affect THA results.[6,7] A biomechanical study found that the strain in the cement mantle increased linearly with increases in body weight between 45 and 91 kg. These increased strains can exceed the fatigue limit of cement, particularly when there is a pore in the cement or a sharp corner of the prosthesis, creating a stress riser.[8] Morbid obesity is strongly associated with postoperative prolonged wound drainage after THA. This is clinically significant because each day of wound drainage increases the risk of wound infection by 42%.[9] Highly obese THA patients indeed show a trend toward a higher infection rate and their odds ratio for risk of infection is 4.3, but this difference does not reach statistical significance.[10]

Obesity seems to affect the outcomes of women in particular. For example, the incidence rate ratio for infection comparing obese with nonobese women was 16.1, but obesity in men did not appear to increase their infection rate. Both obese men and women had a higher incidence of dislocation than their nonobese counterparts but the relative

Parvizi J, Klatt BA.
Essentials in Total Hip Arthroplasty (pp 181-189).

rate increase due to obesity was greater in women than in men (rate ratio 3.0 versus 1.8).[11]

Some studies conclude that obesity should not be a relative contraindication for THAs. At 6 and 18 months follow-up, it was shown that for every 1 point increase in body mass index (BMI), the Harris hip score (HHS) dropped on average 0.25 or 0.35 points, respectively. Although this effect was statistically significant, the clinical effect is quite small given that the mean HHS improvement at 18 months was 43. BMI was not a significant predictor for any of the Short Form 36 (SF-36) component scores.[12] At minimum 10-year follow-up, it has been shown that there is no significant difference in clinical and radiological outcomes, intraoperative and postoperative complications, survivorship, or rate of revision in obese versus nonobese patients.[13,14]

Age

The data on age as a predictor of outcome are also mixed. Advanced age has been found to be associated with increased in-hospital development of major medical complications and mortality.[15,16] Two Swedish studies found that age did not predict the preoperative Western Ontario and McMaster Universities Osteoarthritis Index (WOMAC) and SF-36 scores of THA patients, but younger patients gained more function postoperatively than older patients and reached a higher absolute mean SF-36 score, except for pain.[17,18] However, a Canadian study found that when adjusting for potential confounding effects, age was not a significant determinant of postoperative pain or function.[19,20]

The risk of revision may be affected by age. According to the Australian Hip Registry, neither age nor gender alone significantly affects the risk for revision in primary THAs. However, they found a difference in risk of revision between age groups within gender groups. Females 75 years or older had a significantly lower revision rate than females under the age of 55. The opposite was found in the male population. Men 75 years or older had a significantly higher revision rate than men under the age of 55.[21] The Swedish Hip Registry reported that women had a 30% smaller revision risk than men, but they had lower EuroQoL-5 Dimension (EQ-5D) scores and were less satisfied with their THA than men at 1-year follow-up.[5]

Comorbid Conditions, Functional Status, and Expectations

Patients with lower preoperative physical function do not achieve the same function and pain level postoperatively as those with higher preoperative function.[22] The inability to walk longer than 10 min preoperatively significantly decreases one's chance of being able to walk more than 60 min postoperatively. Having hip flexion range of less than 70 degrees significantly reduces the chance that one will have flexion range of greater than 90 degrees postoperatively. However, complete or almost complete alleviation of pain was achieved in over 80% of patients at 10 years postoperatively regardless of their preoperative functional status.[23] The number of comorbidities preoperatively did not predict a worse WOMAC function or SF-36 physical function score postoperatively.[18]

A patient's preoperative psychological status has been examined. While 44% of THA patients have over-threshold hospital anxiety and depression (HAD) and 55% of THA patients have over-threshold HAD subscale scores, depression and anxiety did not affect functional outcome postoperatively in one study.[24] However, the Swedish Hip Registry reported that patients with high anxiety have significantly more pain preoperatively and significantly worse pain relief, satisfaction, mobility, and EQ-5D gains postoperatively.[5,25]

Patient preoperative expectations may be self-fulfilling. Expectation of complete pain relief was an independent predictor of better physical function and pain improvement at 6 months postoperatively. Expectation of low risk of complications independently predicted greater postoperative satisfaction. Expectations did not correlate to preoperative functional health status.[26]

Implant-Related Factors

Cemented Versus Uncemented

The debate between cemented versus uncemented prostheses is ongoing. There are clearly geographic preferences, with the United States favoring uncemented whereas Europeans are more apt to cement their prostheses. Yet, according to the Swedish Hip Registry, the rate of uncemented THAs has increased over the last decade with the introduction of new articulations, highly cross-linked polyethylene, improved liner fixation, and good long-term results for certain uncemented stems. Cement is currently the most common fixation method for patients under the age of 50 in Sweden. Overall, in Sweden the proportion of all-uncemented THAs has increased from 7.3% in 2005 to 9.9% in 2006.[5]

In the 1980s and 1990s, there were concerns particularly regarding wear and osteolysis in uncemented THAs (Figure 22-1). In the early days of uncemented implants, Rothman and Cohn asked in 1990: "Should the contemporary hip surgeon abandon the proved dependability of

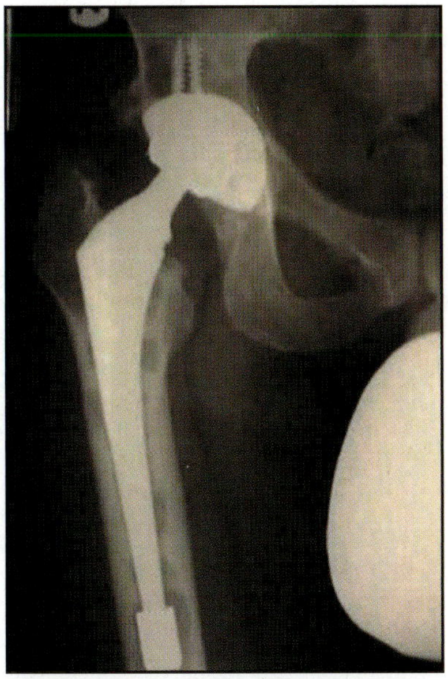

Figure 22-1. Wear has lead to extensive osteolysis around both the acetabular and femoral components of this uncemented THA.

cemented fixation for the theoretically appealing but as yet unproved technology of cementless fixation?" They conceded that cement provides immediate strong implant fixation resulting in early pain relief. However, they worried that cement demonstrates progressive loss of fixation with time whereas biologic fixation is theoretically permanent.[27]

A recent systematic review and meta-analysis of the published literature compared cemented and uncemented fixation in THA. Overall, there was no difference in failure (defined as revision) between the groups. Subgroup analysis, however, showed superior survival rates in cemented fixation in studies including patients of all ages as compared to those studies that only studied younger (≤55 years old) patients. Year of publication was associated with improved survival of uncemented implants relative to cemented implants (ie, uncemented fixation showed relative superiority with time).[28]

The Australian Hip Registry reported that the risk of revision is significantly higher for cementless compared to both hybrid and cemented THAs. There was no difference in revision risk between cemented and hybrid THAs. However, when stratified for age, patients younger than 55 years old showed no difference in revision risk between cementless, cemented, or hybrid fixation.[21] The Swedish Hip Registry found that cemented fixation yielded the smallest number of revisions at long-term follow-up. In fact, they reported a 27-year survival of 77.3% when examining 70,000 cemented THAs.[5]

Stem Design and Surface Finish

Uncemented Stems

There is debate as to whether hydroxyapatite (HA) coating of femoral stems offers any advantage to porous coating or grit blasting alone in cementless fixation. When comparing stems (porous-coated or roughened) with or without HA coating, there is no significant difference in clinical, radiographic, or survivorship outcomes.[29-33]

Cemented Stems

Since Charnley's original polished flatback femoral component, implant companies have introduced polymethylmethacrylate (PMMA) precoating and increased surface roughness in hopes of increasing the metal-cement bond and thus reducing aseptic loosening in cemented stems. One study compared PMMA precoat and satin finish stems using identical stem geometries, identical acetabular components, one surgeon, and the same operative technique for the 2 groups. At a minimum 2-year follow-up, the cemented stem precoat population had significantly more radiographic and debonding failures than the satin finish population. Based on this finding, the group discontinued use of that precoat stem and is following the precoat group carefully for radiographic evidence of debonding.[34]

A biomechanical study found that rough cemented stems have significantly less axial, anterior-posterior, and rotational migration than polished stems.[35] However, clinical studies have shown a higher rate of aseptic loosening, debonding, subsidence, metallic shedding, and massive femoral osteolysis and metallosis in rough, textured stems as compared to satin-finish stems.[36-38] At a minimum 10-year follow-up, one study reported that polished stems (roughness 0.1 μm Ra) did not require revision nor did they demonstrate radiographic evidence of loosening, but 5.4% of them demonstrated osteolysis distal to the trochanters. Two percent of matte stems (roughness 0.8 μm Ra) and 9.2% of the grit-blasted stems (roughness 2.1 μm Ra) were revised for aseptic loosening.[39]

The combination of roughened and precoated femoral components has a considerably higher and earlier rate of failure compared to smooth stems.[40] A retrospective study of a grit-blasted PMMA precoated femoral stem showed an alarming 12% aseptic loosening rate of the femoral component at an average of 31 months postoperatively, with all having been revised or pending revision. The mechanism of failure was theorized as such: the smooth finish and cylindric shape of the distal stem allowed cement-prosthesis debonding. Once the stem was loose, the roughened proximal portion of the stem generated a large amount of cement debris, leading to rapid failure.[41] However, a prospective randomized study of smooth-Ra 17 versus rough-Ra 170 stems at a minimum 5-year follow-up showed no significant difference in revision rate for aseptic loosening.[42]

A surgeon shared his 27-year experience with cemented femoral components. He began with the polished Charnley stem and reported a revision rate of 2.4% for aseptic loosening at about 20-year follow-up. He later began implanting a proximal precoat stem that had a 1.5% early loosening rate with significant bone lysis (minimum 2-year follow-up) that increased to a 3.2% revision rate (all also associated with significant bone loss) just 3 years later. In the end, the surgeon returned to a polished stem with a geometry almost identical to the Charnley stem.[43]

Collar and Taper

One can choose between collared and collarless implants when performing cemented THAs. Biomechanical studies have shown that calcar-collar contact reduced peak strains in the proximal cement.[8,44] In a randomized clinical trial, the collarless hips lost significantly more medial femoral neck cortical bone and had a higher incidence of radiolucent lines in femoral Gruen zone VI as compared to collarless hips. There was no difference in the incidence of stem subsidence or osteolysis. Clinical scores and incidence of pain did not differ between the 2 groups.[45] Another randomized study found similar HHSs without a difference in incidence or magnitude of pain at an average of 9.6 years follow-up. There was no significant difference in survival rates between the 2 groups.[46]

The taper of the stem also can affect cement strain. Early studies showed that cement strains were highest at the most proximal portions of the cement mantle and near the tip of the femoral component. These were also, predictably, common sites of cement debonding and cement mantle failure.[8,47] In a biomechanical cadaver study, a moderately tapered stem had peak strains located at the most proximal stem regions whereas a dramatically tapered stem had peak strains located at the middle of the stem. Minimizing cement strain at the crucial proximal and distal areas could theoretically reduce cement-prosthesis debonding.[48]

Surgical Technique and Postoperative Care

Surgical Volume

It was reported in 2001 that patients treated with primary THAs by surgeons who performed >50 primary THAs in Medicare patients per year had a lower dislocation rate than those whose surgeons performed 5 or less per year.[49] Patients who had their revision THAs done by high-volume surgeons (>12 revisions/year) were more satisfied than those who had low-volume surgeons.[50]

Surgical Approach

Historically, the posterior approach is thought to have a higher dislocation rate but a lower rate of postoperative limp. Gait analysis has shown that patients who had the anterolateral approach deviated from normal gait with respect to increased trunk inclination, reduced sagittal plan range of motion, and greater loading asymmetry, whereas several of the posterolateral patients had near-normal gait patterns.[51] In a clinical study, limp of any severity was seen in 29% of anterolateral approach patients compared to 17% of posterior approach patients.[19] When compared to the anterolateral group, at 2-month follow-up the posterior group had significantly less need for assistance in walking 10 feet and in walking one block. Over time, the differences diminished but the ability to walk one block without assistance remained significantly higher for the posterior group.[52]

An extensive literature review encompassing 14 studies with 13,203 primary THAs found the combined dislocation rate to be 1.27% for the transtrochanteric approach, 3.23% for the posterior approach (3.95% without posterior repair, 2.03% with posterior repair), 2.18% for the anterolateral approach, and 0.55% for the direct lateral approach.[53] A recent review of 21,047 primary THAs placed from 1969 to 1999 found a cumulative 10-year dislocation rate of 3.1% with an anterolateral approach, 3.4% with the transtrochanteric approach, and 6.9% with the posterolateral approach.[54]

A careful repair of the capsule and short external rotators during the posterior approach decreases the dislocation rate.[55] When the posterior capsule and short external rotators are repaired to the greater trochanter with nonabsorbable suture, 0.85% dislocation has been reported.[56] Studying the posterolateral approach, one group found a 4.8% early dislocation rate (within the first 6 months postoperatively) for those with a complete posterior capsulectomy versus a 0.7% early dislocation rate in those with a formal posterior capsular repair.[57] In a meta-analysis of studies using the posterior approach, there was a 4.46% dislocation rate in those without soft tissue repair as compared to 0.49% in those with a soft tissue repair, translating into an 8.21 times greater relative risk of dislocation when not performing a soft tissue repair.[58]

Using a hip simulator, it was demonstrated that femoral heads >32 mm in diameter (namely 38- and 44-mm heads) had greater range of motion (ROM), virtually no component-to-component impingement, and a significant increase in flexion before dislocation.[59] A larger femoral head diameter has been found to decrease the risk of postoperative dislocation, particularly in hips placed via the posterolateral approach. Overall, the relative risk of dislocation is 1.7 for 22-mm heads when compared to 32-mm heads, and 1.3 for 28 mm compared with 32-mm heads.[54] The cup abduction angle dictates the effect of increasing the femoral head size. When the shell is within its acceptable range of abduction, increasing femoral head size may improve joint stability while higher cup abduction angles minimize this effect on joint stability.[60]

Component Positioning

Component position affects the dislocation rate and direction. Hips are at the lowest risk for dislocation when radiological anteversion of the cup is 15 degrees and abduction is 45 degrees. In a study of primary THAs via an anterolateral approach, patients with anterior dislocations had significantly greater cup anteversion (17 degrees) and greater cup abduction (48 degrees) than those with posterior dislocations (anteversion 11 degrees, abduction 42 degrees).[61] Even if a stem or cup alone is in its proper position, dislocation may occur as predicted by the sum of the anteversions. The sum of cup and stem anteversion in anteriorly dislocated hips was significantly greater than that in nondislocated hips. The sum of cup and stem anteversion in posteriorly dislocated hips was significantly less than the sum in nondislocated hips.[62] In hips placed via a posterolateral approach, those that experienced a posterior dislocation had significantly lower cup anteversion than those that did not dislocate. Seventy-eight percent of the hips that dislocated posteriorly had cup anteversion less than 20 degrees.[63]

A relatively vertical cup positioning can have adverse effects specific to the bearing surface implanted. There is debate whether an increased cup abduction angle and anteversion predisposes ceramic-on-ceramic hips to "squeaking." Restrepo et al found no correlation between noisy components and cup position.[64] Walter et al found that, when compared to quiet hips, significantly fewer squeaking hips had acetabular shells that were placed in a range of 25 degrees +/- 10 degrees of anteversion and 45 degrees +/- 10 degrees of abduction.[65]

A steep cup may dramatically increase serum cobalt and chromium levels in certain metal-on-metal THA patients.[66] In a simulator study of metal-on-metal hips, THAs with a steep cup angle (55 degrees) had a 5-fold, significantly higher long-term steady-state wear than cups placed at 45 degrees of abduction.[67] Increased cup abduction angles lead to superior and lateral head penetration, increasing polyethylene (PE) wear rates.[68] In a study of ceramic-on-PE and metal-on-PE articulations, cup inclination was the single greatest factor affecting wear rates with cups greater than 45 degrees of abduction exhibiting higher PE wear rates.[69] In fact, one study demonstrated a 40% increase in mean linear PE wear in THAs with a cup abduction angle of ≥45 degrees.[70]

Postoperative Restrictions

It is controversial whether restrictions above the usual ROM positional precautions are useful. In THAs via an anterolateral approach, a group of patients were given restrictions above the usual hip ROM restrictions: abduction pillow placed in the operating room before bed transfer, pillows to maintain abduction while in bed, elevated toilet seats and chairs, no sleeping on their sides, and no driving or riding in automobiles. There were no dislocations in the group that did not have these restrictions (in fact, one patient in the restricted group dislocated). Furthermore, the unrestricted group returned to work sooner and had a higher level of satisfaction with the pace of their recovery than the restricted group (and had $650 per patient less additional expenditure).[71]

Postoperative weight-bearing restrictions are also of questionable value. The theoretical argument for immediate loading is that functional recovery may be hastened while reducing periprosthetic demineralization. However, there is concern that implant stability and ingrowth may be jeopardized. It has been found that when solid initial fixation is obtained intraoperatively and radiographically in uncemented femoral components, bone ingrowth fixation occurs reliably whether patients are made partial or full weight-bearing postoperatively.[72,73]

Systems Issues

Hospital case volume correlates with THA outcomes. For both primary and revision THAs, as hospital volume (THAs/year) increases, there is a significant trend toward lower inpatient mortality, less discharges to extended care facilities, and a lower incidence of prolonged length of stay. For primary THAs, low-volume hospitals (LVHs) were defined as 1 to 40 cases/year; very high-volume hospitals (VHVHs) were defined as >140 cases/year. For revision THAs, LVHs were defined as 1 to 10 cases/year; VHVHs were defined as >46 cases/year.[74,75] Another study similarly found that the risk of death for primary THAs is lower in hospitals performing >100 primary THAs/year as compared with those in hospitals in which 10 or fewer primary THAs were performed per year.[49] Patients who had primary THAs at high-volume centers (>100 THAs/year) were more satisfied with their primary THA than those at low-volume centers.[50]

Specialty orthopedic hospitals have recently emerged and are quite controversial. Supporters argue that their focused approach improves outcomes and reduces cost. Opponents argue that they attract the most profitable patients with the least comorbidities without fulfilling societal obligations, such as emergency services and charity care. Both may be correct. Specialty orthopedic hospitals have indeed been found to attract patients with less comorbidities and who live in more affluent areas than their counterparts in general hospitals. However, even when adjusting for patient characteristics and procedural volume, the odds of adverse outcomes occurring are significantly lower in specialty hospitals than in general hospitals. The authors hypothesize that perhaps individual orthopedic surgeon procedural volumes, the expertise and experience of ancillary staff, and/or organizational factors (eg, clinical pathways) explain these findings.[76]

THA cases with major resident participation resulted on average in a 20-minute longer case duration. However, the transfusion rate, hospital length of stay, complication rate, technical error rate, and minimum 1-year follow-up HHS were no different than those cases in which there was no major resident participation.[77]

Waiting for a THA does lead to poorer physical function preoperatively, but the effect of that wait on postoperative function is controversial.[78] In Sweden, it was found that there was no difference in postoperative SF-36 or WOMAC scores between patients who had to wait less than or more than 3 months for surgery.[17] However, a Canadian study found that waiting time for THAs is detrimental to outcomes as measured by the WOMAC questionnaire. The odds of achieving a better-than-expected functional outcome decreased by 8% with each additional month spent waiting for a THA. Waiting times longer than 6 months resulted in a 50% decrease in the odds of achieving a better-than-expected outcome when compared to those who waited <6 months. It is hypothesized that prolonged waits may result in muscle atrophy, tissue contractures, and deterioration in the patient's medical condition that may not be recoverable after surgery.[79]

Summary

Primary THAs are well known to have overall excellent results, but it is important to identify risk factors predisposing certain patients to poorer outcomes. While the data are somewhat mixed about the effects of patient-related factors on postoperative outcomes, advanced age, obesity, and comorbid medical conditions are not absolute contraindications for THAs and in some studies have been shown to not adversely affect outcomes. Higher patient expectations for recovery may be self-fulfilling as these patients have better postoperative function. In terms of implant selection, there seems to be no clear advantage to either cemented versus uncemented and collar versus collarless stems. Hydroxylapatite coating of press-fit stems offer no advantage. PMMA precoated, roughened cemented stems can lead to early debonding, aseptic failure, and massive osteolysis.

Repairing the posterior capsule and short external rotators has decreased the risk of dislocation associated with the posterolateral approach. The anterolateral approach is associated with more gait dysfunction postoperatively than the posterolateral approach. Component malpositioning, particularly of the cup, predisposes patients to dislocation and increases wear rates. Surgeons and hospitals with higher THA case volumes and orthopedic specialty hospitals have better patient outcomes than low-volume surgeons and hospitals and general hospitals. Waiting time for THAs may or may not affect postoperative functional outcomes.

Arthroplasty instrumentation has evolved to the point that today we have a number of well-designed implants that can reproducibly achieve bony ingrowth. With that said, cement techniques are still useful in certain populations as demonstrated by registry data. The next step in improving THA patient outcomes must be improved surgical technique, particularly focusing on cup position. Steep cup inclinations can compromise THA outcomes in a number of ways depending on the particular bearing surface combination. Navigation might someday be a useful tool in helping the surgeon reliably achieve cup abduction angles less than 55 degrees.

References

1. Learmonth ID, Young C, Rorabeck C. The operation of the century: total hip replacement. *Lancet.* 2007;370(9597):1508-1519.
2. Jones CA, Beaupre LA, Johnston DW, Suarez-Almazor ME. Total joint arthroplasties: current concepts of patient outcomes after surgery. *Rheum Dis Clin North Am.* 2007;33(1):71-86.
3. Ng CY, Ballantyne JA, Brenkel IJ. Quality of life and functional outcome after primary total hip replacement. A five-year follow-up. *J Bone Joint Surg Br.* 2007;89(7):868-873.
4. Ethgen O, Bruyere O, Richy F, Dardennes C, Reginster JY. Health-related quality of life in total hip and total knee arthroplasty. A qualitative and systematic review of the literature. *J Bone Joint Surg Am.* 2004;86-A(5):963-974.
5. Sahlgrenska University Hospital. Swedish hip arthroplasty register: annual report; 2006.
6. Bourne R, Mukhi S, Zhu N, Keresteci M, Marin M. Role of obesity on the risk for total hip or knee arthroplasty. *Clin Orthop Relat Res.* 2007;465:185-188.
7. Karlson EW, Mandl LA, Aweh GN, Sangha O, Liang MH, Grodstein F. Total hip replacement due to osteoarthritis: the importance of age, obesity, and other modifiable risk factors. *Am J Med.* 2003;114(2):93-98.
8. O'Connor DO, Burke DW, Jasty M, Sedlacek RC, Harris WH. In vitro measurement of strain in the bone cement surrounding the femoral component of total hip replacements during simulated gait and stair-climbing. *J Orthop Res.* 1996;14(5):769-777.
9. Patel VP, Walsh M, Sehgal B, Preston C, DeWal H, Di Cesare PE. Factors associated with prolonged wound drainage after primary total hip and knee arthroplasty. *J Bone Joint Surg Am.* 2007;89(1):33-38.
10. Namba RS, Paxton L, Fithian DC, Stone ML. Obesity and perioperative morbidity in total hip and total knee arthroplasty patients. *J Arthroplasty.* 2005;20(7 suppl 3):46-50.
11. Lubbeke A, Stern R, Garavaglia G, Zurcher L, Hoffmeyer P. Differences in outcomes of obese women and men undergoing primary total hip arthroplasty. *Arthritis Rheum.* 2007;57(2):327-334.
12. Moran M, Walmsley P, Gray A, Brenkel IJ. Does body mass index affect the early outcome of primary total hip arthroplasty? *J Arthroplasty.* 2005;20(7):866-869.
13. McLaughlin JR, Lee KR. The outcome of total hip replacement in obese and non-obese patients at 10- to 18-years. *J Bone Joint Surg Br.* 2006;88(10):1286-1292.
14. Haverkamp D, de Man FH, de Jong PT, van Stralen RA, Marti RK. Is the long-term outcome of cemented THA jeopardized by patients being overweight? *Clin Orthop Relat Res.* 2008;466(5):1162-1168.
15. Parvizi J, Mui A, Purtill JJ, Sharkey PF, Hozack WJ, Rothman RH. Total joint arthroplasty: when do fatal or near-fatal complications occur? *J Bone Joint Surg Am.* 2007;89(1):27-32.
16. Zhan C, Kaczmarek R, Loyo-Berrios N, Sangl J, Bright RA. Incidence and short-term outcomes of primary and revision hip replacement in the United States. *J Bone Joint Surg Am.* 2007;89(3):526-533.
17. Nilsdotter AK, Lohmander LS. Age and waiting time as predictors of outcome after total hip replacement for osteoarthritis. *Rheumatology (Oxford).* 2002;41(11):1261-1267.
18. Nilsdotter AK, Petersson IF, Roos EM, Lohmander LS. Predictors of patient relevant outcome after total hip replacement for osteoarthritis: a prospective study. *Ann Rheum Dis.* 2003;62(10):923-930.
19. Ritter MA, Harty LD, Keating ME, Faris PM, Meding JB. A clinical comparison of the anterolateral and posterolateral approaches to the hip. *Clin Orthop Relat Res.* 2001;(385):95-99.
20. Jones CA, Voaklander DC, Johnston DW, Suarez-Almazor ME. The effect of age on pain, function, and quality of life after total hip and knee arthroplasty. *Arch Intern Med.* 2001;161(3):454-460.
21. Australian Orthopaedic Association. National joint replacement registry: hip and knee arthroplasty, annual report; 2008.
22. Fortin PR, Clarke AE, Joseph L, et al. Outcomes of total hip and knee replacement: preoperative functional status predicts outcomes at six months after surgery. *Arthritis Rheum.* 1999;42(8):1722-1728.
23. Roder C, Staub LP, Eggli S, Dietrich D, Busato A, Muller U. Influence of preoperative functional status on outcome after total hip arthroplasty. *J Bone Joint Surg Am.* 2007;89(1):11-17.
24. Caracciolo B, Giaquinto S. Self-perceived distress and self-perceived functional recovery after recent total hip and knee arthroplasty. *Arch Gerontol Geriatr.* 2005;41(2):177-181.
25. Rolfson J, Dahlberg O, Nilsson J, Malchau H, Garellick G. Determining outcomes in total hip replacement surgery. *J Bone Joint Surg Br.* 2008;91(2):157-161.
26. Mahomed NN, Liang MH, Cook EF, et al. The importance of patient expectations in predicting functional outcomes after total joint arthroplasty. *J Rheumatol.* 2002;29(6):1273-1279.
27. Rothman RH, Cohn JC. Cemented versus cementless total hip arthroplasty. A critical review. *Clin Orthop Relat Res.* 1990;(254):153-169.
28. Morshed S, Bozic KJ, Ries MD, Malchau H, Colford JM Jr. Comparison of cemented and uncemented fixation in total hip replacement: a meta-analysis. *Acta Orthop.* 2007;78(3):315-326.
29. Yee AJ, Kreder HK, Bookman I, Davey JR. A randomized trial of hydroxyapatite coated prostheses in total hip arthroplasty. *Clin Orthop Relat Res.* 1999;(366):120-132.
30. Kim YH, Kim JS, Oh SH, Kim JM. Comparison of porous-coated titanium femoral stems with and without hydroxyapatite coating. *J Bone Joint Surg Am.* 2003;85-A(9):1682-1688.
31. Rorabeck CH. Tapered hydroxyapatite-coated press-fit stems: any added value? *J Arthroplasty.* 2006;21(4 suppl 1):85-88.
32. Lee JM, Lee CW. Comparison of hydroxyapatite-coated and non-hydroxyapatite-coated noncemented total hip arthroplasty in same patients. *J Arthroplasty.* 2007;22(7):1019-1023.

33. Paulsen A, Pedersen AB, Johnsen SP, Riis A, Lucht U, Overgaard S. Effect of hydroxyapatite coating on risk of revision after primary total hip arthroplasty in younger patients: findings from the Danish Hip Arthroplasty Registry. *Acta Orthop.* 2007;78(5):622-628.
34. Vaughn BK, Fuller E, Peterson R, Capps SG. Influence of surface finish in total hip arthroplasty. *J Arthroplasty.* 2003;18(7 suppl 1):110-115.
35. Ebramzadeh E, Sangiorgio SN, Longjohn DB, Buhari CF, Dorr LD. Initial stability of cemented femoral stems as a function of surface finish, collar, and stem size. *J Bone Joint Surg Am.* 2004;86-A(1):106-115.
36. Gonzalez Della Valle A, Rana A, Nestor B, Bostrom M, Westrich G, Salvati EA. Metallic shedding, surface finish changes, and extensive femoral osteolysis in the loose Spectron EF stem. *Clin Orthop Relat Res.* 2006;442:165-170.
37. Della Valle AG, Zoppi A, Peterson MG, Salvati EA. A rough surface finish adversely affects the survivorship of a cemented femoral stem. *Clin Orthop Relat Res.* 2005;(436):158-163.
38. Collis DK, Mohler CG. Comparison of clinical outcomes in total hip arthroplasty using rough and polished cemented stems with essentially the same geometry. *J Bone Joint Surg Am.* 2002;84-A(4):586-592.
39. Firestone DE, Callaghan JJ, Liu SS, Goetz DD, Sullivan PM, Vittetoe DA, et al. Total hip arthroplasty with a cemented, polished, collared femoral stem and a cementless acetabular component. A follow-up study at a minimum of ten years. *J Bone Joint Surg Am.* 2007;89(1):126-132.
40. Ong A, Wong KL, Lai M, Garino JP, Steinberg ME. Early failure of precoated femoral components in primary total hip arthroplasty. *J Bone Joint Surg Am.* 2002;84-A(5):786-792.
41. Sylvain GM, Kassab S, Coutts R, Santore R. Early failure of a roughened surface, precoated femoral component in total hip arthroplasty. *J Arthroplasty.* 2001;16(2):141-148.
42. Rasquinha VJ, Ranawat CS, Dua V, Ranawat AS, Rodriguez JA. A prospective, randomized, double-blind study of smooth versus rough stems using cement fixation: minimum 5-year follow-up. *J Arthroplasty.* 2004;19(7 suppl 2):2-9.
43. Collis DK, Mohler CG. Loosening rates and bone lysis with rough finished and polished stems. *Clin Orthop Relat Res.* 1998;(355):113-122.
44. Harrington MA Jr, O'Connor DO, Lozynsky AJ, Kovach I, Harris WH. Effects of femoral neck length, stem size, and body weight on strains in the proximal cement mantle. *J Bone Joint Surg Am.* 2002;84-A(4):573-579.
45. Meding JB, Ritter MA, Keating EM, Faris PM, Edmondson K. A comparison of collared and collarless femoral components in primary cemented total hip arthroplasty: a randomized clinical trial. *J Arthroplasty.* 1999;14(2):123-130.
46. Settecerri JJ, Kelley SS, Rand JA, Fitzgerald RH Jr. Collar versus collarless cemented HD-II femoral prostheses. *Clin Orthop Relat Res.* 2002;(398):146-152.
47. Jasty M, Maloney WJ, Bragdon CR, O'Connor DO, Haire T, Harris WH. The initiation of failure in cemented femoral components of hip arthroplasties. *J Bone Joint Surg Br.* 1991;73(4):551-558.
48. Peters CL, Bachus KN, Craig MA, Higginbotham TO. The effect of femoral prosthesis design on cement strain in cemented total hip arthroplasty. *J Arthroplasty.* 2001;16(2):216-224.
49. Katz JN, Losina E, Barrett J, et al. Association between hospital and surgeon procedure volume and outcomes of total hip replacement in the United States medicare population. *J Bone Joint Surg Am.* 2001;83-A(11):1622-1629.
50. Katz JN, Phillips CB, Baron JA, et al. Association of hospital and surgeon volume of total hip replacement with functional status and satisfaction three years following surgery. *Arthritis Rheum.* 2003;48(2):560-568.
51. Madsen MS, Ritter MA, Morris HH, et al. The effect of total hip arthroplasty surgical approach on gait. *J Orthop Res.* 2004;22(1):44-50.
52. Zimmerma S, Hawkes WG, Hudson JI, et al. Outcomes of surgical management of total HIP replacement in patients aged 65 years and older: cemented versus cementless femoral components and lateral or anterolateral versus posterior anatomical approach. *J Orthop Res.* 2002;20(2):182-191.
53. Masonis JL, Bourne RB. Surgical approach, abductor function, and total hip arthroplasty dislocation. *Clin Orthop Relat Res.* 2002;(405):46-53.
54. Berry DJ, von Knoch M, Schleck CD, Harmsen WS. Effect of femoral head diameter and operative approach on risk of dislocation after primary total hip arthroplasty. *J Bone Joint Surg Am.* 2005;87(11):2456-2463.
55. Khan RJ, Yao F, Li M, Nivbrant B, Wood D. Capsular-enhanced repair of the short external rotators after total hip arthroplasty. *J Arthroplasty.* 2007;22(6):840-843.
56. Weeden SH, Paprosky WG, Bowling JW. The early dislocation rate in primary total hip arthroplasty following the posterior approach with posterior soft-tissue repair. *J Arthroplasty.* 2003;18(6):709-713.
57. White RE Jr, Forness TJ, Allman JK, Junick DW. Effect of posterior capsular repair on early dislocation in primary total hip replacement. *Clin Orthop Relat Res.* 2001;(393):163-167.
58. Kwon MS, Kuskowski M, Mulhall KJ, Macaulay W, Brown TE, Saleh KJ. Does surgical approach affect total hip arthroplasty dislocation rates? *Clin Orthop Relat Res.* 2006;447:34-38.
59. Burroughs BR, Hallstrom B, Golladay GJ, Hoeffel D, Harris WH. Range of motion and stability in total hip arthroplasty with 28-, 32-, 38-, and 44-mm femoral head sizes. *J Arthroplasty.* 2005;20(1):11-19.
60. Crowninshield RD, Maloney WJ, Wentz DH, Humphrey SM, Blanchard CR. Biomechanics of large femoral heads: what they do and don't do. *Clin Orthop Relat Res.* 2004;(429):102-107.
61. Biedermann R, Tonin A, Krismer M, Rachbauer F, Eibl G, Stockl B. Reducing the risk of dislocation after total hip arthroplasty: the effect of orientation of the acetabular component. *J Bone Joint Surg Br.* 2005;87(6):762-769.
62. Komeno M, Hasegawa M, Sudo A, Uchida A. Computed tomographic evaluation of component position on dislocation after total hip arthroplasty. *Orthopedics.* 2006;29(12):1104-1108.
63. Nishii T, Sugano N, Miki H, Koyama T, Takao M, Yoshikawa H. Influence of component positions on dislocation: computed tomographic evaluations in a consecutive series of total hip arthroplasty. *J Arthroplasty.* 2004;19(2):162-166.

64. Restrepo C, Parvizi J, Kurtz SM, Sharkey PF, Hozack WJ, Rothman RH. The noisy ceramic hip: is component malpositioning the cause? *J Arthroplasty.* 2008;23(5):643-649.

65. Walter WL, O'toole GC, Walter WK, Ellis A, Zicat BA. Squeaking in ceramic-on-ceramic hips: the importance of acetabular component orientation. *J Arthroplasty.* 2007;22(4):496-503.

66. Brodner W, Grubl A, Jankovsky R, Meisinger V, Lehr S, Gottsauner-Wolf F. Cup inclination and serum concentration of cobalt and chromium after metal-on-metal total hip arthroplasty. J Arthroplasty. 2004;19(8 suppl 3):66-70.

67. Williams S, Leslie I, Isaac G, Jin Z, Ingham E, Fisher J. Tribology and wear of metal-on-metal hip prostheses: influence of cup angle and head position. *J Bone Joint Surg Am.* 2008;90(suppl 3):111-117.

68. Hirakawa K, Mitsugi N, Koshino T, Saito T, Hirasawa Y, Kubo T. Effect of acetabular cup position and orientation in cemented total hip arthroplasty. *Clin Orthop Relat Res.* 2001;(388):135-142.

69. Wan Z, Boutary M, Dorr LD. The influence of acetabular component position on wear in total hip arthroplasty. *J Arthroplasty.* 2008;23(1):51-56.

70. Patil S, Bergula A, Chen PC, Colwell CW Jr, D'Lima DD. Polyethylene wear and acetabular component orientation. *J Bone Joint Surg Am.* 2003;85-A(suppl 4):56-63.

71. Peak EL, Parvizi J, Ciminiello M, Purtill JJ, Sharkey PF, Hozack WJ, et al. The role of patient restrictions in reducing the prevalence of early dislocation following total hip arthroplasty. A randomized, prospective study. *J Bone Joint Surg Am.* 2005;87(2):247-253.

72. Woolson ST, Adler NS. The effect of partial or full weight bearing ambulation after cementless total hip arthroplasty. *J Arthroplasty.* 2002;17(7):820-825.

73. Boden H, Adolphson P. No adverse effects of early weight bearing after uncemented total hip arthroplasty: a randomized study of 20 patients. *Acta Orthop Scand.* 2004;75(1):21-29.

74. Doro C, Dimick J, Wainess R, Upchurch G, Urquhart A. Hospital volume and inpatient mortality outcomes of total hip arthroplasty in the United States. *J Arthroplasty.* 2006;21(6 suppl 2):10-16.

75. Mitsuyasu S, Hagihara A, Horiguchi H, Nobutomo K. Relationship between total arthroplasty case volume and patient outcome in an acute care payment system in Japan. *J Arthroplasty.* 2006;21(5):656-663.

76. Cram P, Vaughan-Sarrazin MS, Wolf B, Katz JN, Rosenthal GE. A comparison of total hip and knee replacement in specialty and general hospitals. *J Bone Joint Surg Am.* 2007;89(8):1675-1684.

77. Robinson RP. The impact of resident teaching on total hip arthroplasty. *Clin Orthop Relat Res.* 2007;465:196-201.

78. Fielden JM, Cumming JM, Horne JG, Devane PA, Slack A, Gallagher LM. Waiting for hip arthroplasty: economic costs and health outcomes. *J Arthroplasty.* 2005;20(8):990-997.

79. Garbuz DS, Xu M, Duncan CP, Masri BA, Sobolev B. Delays worsen quality of life outcome of primary total hip arthroplasty. *Clin Orthop Relat Res.* 2006;447:79-84.

Cement

Improved protocol in cement handling and introduction of the third-generation cementing technique have significantly reduced the porosity of the cement mantle and increased their structural strength. This should reduce the chances of cement mantle fracture and subsequent implant loosening. Initiation and propagation of the cracks in the cement mantle, one of the primary mechanisms of failure of cemented stems, are observed with 90% occurring in locations where the mantle was incomplete or less than 1-mm thick. Cement mantle with uniform 3-mm thickness reduces cement cracking and the subsequent loosening of the components.

Interfaces

The control of surface properties using different kinds of treatments or coatings with the intention of achieving a good bone ingrowth in cementless components may reduce the chance of loosening. Adequate protection of substrate from corrosion and no delamination in biochemical and biomechanical environments are 2 essential requirements of the coatings. Adding porous tantalum on the outer surface of the cups seems promising, but the results of the hydroxyapatite (HA) coated components are not good; cell-mediated HA resorption seems to be the main mechanism for loss of HA coating. Although screws may increase bone ingrowth in their vicinity, the frequently observed granulomas with the deepest penetration into the periprosthetic bone were along the screw-bone interface. Due to this, some surgeons think that screws and screw holes should be avoided in younger patients if possible.

Miscellaneous

Malignant Cells Infiltration

The inflammatory reaction to a metastatic tumor includes the presence and activation of macrophages, giant cells, and leukocytes and is associated with necrosis of bone. The activation of these inflammatory cells may be an important mechanism in the development of aseptic loosening. The diagnosis of malignant disease made by histological studies after revision for either presumed infection or aseptic loosening suggests the potential for secondary malignant disease to mimic both septic and aseptic loosening.[25] One should maintain a high index of suspicion and consider metastatic disease as a differential diagnosis in cases of aseptic loosening, particularly when there is rapid progression of symptoms, the history is atypical, or the patient has a history of malignant disease.

Genetic

Recently, Malik et al reported that aseptic loosening and deep infection of total hip replacement may be due to the genetic influence of candidate susceptibility genes, as progression of loosening and osteolysis varies between individuals with apparently identical total joint replacements.[26,27]

References

1. Berry DJ, Harmsen WS, Cabanela ME, Morrey BF. Twenty-five-year survivorship of two thousand consecutive primary Charnley total hip replacements: factors affecting survivorship of acetabular and femoral components. *J Bone Joint Surg Am.* 2002;84-A(2):171-177.
2. Callaghan JJ, Templeton JE, Liu SS, et al. Results of Charnley total hip arthroplasty at a minimum of thirty years. A concise follow-up of a previous report. *J Bone Joint Surg Am.* 2004;86-A(4):690-695.
3. Mahomed NN, Barrett JA, Katz JN, et al. Rates and outcomes of primary and revision total hip replacement in the United States medicare population. *J Bone Joint Surg Am.* 2003;85-A(1):27-32.
4. Clohisy JC, Calvert G, Tull F, McDonald D, Maloney WJ. Reasons for revision hip surgery: a retrospective review. *Clin Orthop Relat Res.* 2004;(429):188-192.
5. Ulrich SD, Seyler TM, Bennett D, et al. Total hip arthroplasties: what are the reasons for revision? *Int Orthop.* 2008;32(5):597-604.
6. Dobzyniak M, Fehring TK, Odum S. Early failure in total hip arthroplasty. *Clin Orthop Relat Res.* 2006;447:76-78.
7. Nelson CL, McLaren AC, McLaren SG, Johnson JW, Smeltzer MS. Is aseptic loosening truly aseptic? *Clin Orthop Relat Res.* 2005;(437):25-30.
8. Munger P, Roder C, ckermann-Liebrich U, Busato A. Patient-related risk factors leading to aseptic stem loosening in total hip arthroplasty: a case-control study of 5,035 patients. *Acta Orthop.* 2006;77(4):567-574.
9. Flugsrud GB, Nordsletten L, Espehaug B, Havelin LI, Meyer HE. The effect of middle-age body weight and physical activity on the risk of early revision hip arthroplasty: a cohort study of 1,535 individuals. *Acta Orthop.* 2007;78(1):99-107.
10. Malchau H, Herberts P, Ahnfelt L. Prognosis of total hip replacement in Sweden. Follow-up of 92,675 operations performed 1978-1990. *Acta Orthop Scand.* 1993;64(5):497-506.
11. McAuley JP, Szuszczewicz ES, Young A, Engh CA Sr. Total hip arthroplasty in patients 50 years and younger. *Clin Orthop Relat Res.* 2004;(418):119-125.
12. Kim YH, Oh SH, Kim JS, Koo KH. Contemporary total hip arthroplasty with and without cement in patients with osteonecrosis of the femoral head. *J Bone Joint Surg Am.* 2003;85-A(4):675-681.
13. Mont MA, Seyler TM, Plate JF, Delanois RE, Parvizi J. Uncemented total hip arthroplasty in young adults with osteonecrosis of the femoral head: a comparative study. *J Bone Joint Surg Am.* 2006;88(suppl 3):104-109.

14. McLaughlin JR, Lee KR. The outcome of total hip replacement in obese and non-obese patients at 10- to 18-years. *J Bone Joint Surg Br.* 2006;88(10):1286-1292.

15. Malik MH, Gray J, Kay PR. Early aseptic loosening of cemented total hip arthroplasty: the influence of non-steroidal anti-inflammatory drugs and smoking. *Int Orthop.* 2004;28(4):211-213.

16. Espehaug B, Havelin LI, Engesaeter LB, Langeland N, Vollset SE. Patient-related risk factors for early revision of total hip replacements. A population register-based case-control study of 674 revised hips. *Acta Orthop Scand.* 1997;68(3):207-215.

17. Katz JN, Losina E, Barrett J, et al. Association between hospital and surgeon procedure volume and outcomes of total hip replacement in the United States medicare population. *J Bone Joint Surg Am.* 2001;83-A(11):1622-1629.

18. Losina E, Barrett J, Mahomed NN, Baron JA, Katz JN. Early failures of total hip replacement: effect of surgeon volume. *Arthritis Rheum.* 2004;50(4):1338-1343.

19. Sharkey PF, Shastri S, Teloken MA, Parvizi J, Hozack WJ, Rothman RH. Relationship between surgical volume and early outcomes of total hip arthroplasty: do results continue to get better? *J Arthroplasty.* 2004;19(6):694-699.

20. Clohisy JC, Frazier E, Hirayama T, bu-Amer Y. RANKL is an essential cytokine mediator of polymethylmethacrylate particle-induced osteoclastogenesis. *J Orthop Res.* 2003;21(2):202-212.

21. Purdue PE, Koulouvaris P, Potter HG, Nestor BJ, Sculco TP. The cellular and molecular biology of periprosthetic osteolysis. *Clin Orthop Relat Res.* 2007;454:251-261.

22. Holt G, Murnaghan C, Reilly J, Meek RM. The biology of aseptic osteolysis. *Clin Orthop Relat Res.* 2007;460:240-252.

23. Hallab N, Merritt K, Jacobs JJ. Metal sensitivity in patients with orthopaedic implants. *J Bone Joint Surg Am.* 2001;83-A(3):428-436.

24. Bradford L, Baker D, Ries MD, Pruitt LA. Fatigue crack propagation resistance of highly crosslinked polyethylene. *Clin Orthop Relat Res.* 2004;(429):68-72.

25. O'Shea K, Kearns SR, Blaney A, Murray P, Smyth HA, McElwain JP. Periprosthetic malignancy as a mode of failure in total hip arthroplasty. *J Arthroplasty.* 2006;21(6):926-930.

26. Malik MH, Jury F, Bayat A, Ollier WE, Kay PR. Genetic susceptibility to total hip arthroplasty failure: a preliminary study on the influence of matrix metalloproteinase 1, interleukin 6 polymorphisms and vitamin D receptor. *Ann Rheum Dis.* 2007;66(8):1116-1120.

27. Malik MH, Bayat A, Jury F, Kay PR, Ollier WE. Genetic susceptibility to total hip arthroplasty failure--positive association with mannose-binding lectin. *J Arthroplasty.* 2007;22(2):265-270.

24

Osteonecrosis of the Hip

Lawrence P. Lai, MD, MS; Thorsten M. Seyler, MD; and Michael A. Mont, MD

Osteonecrosis, also referred to as avascular necrosis, atraumatic necrosis, ischemic necrosis, or aseptic necrosis, is a musculoskeletal condition in which death of bone occurs. It most often affects weight-bearing joints with poor access to blood flow. Consequently, the most common areas of occurrence are the hip followed by the knee, shoulder, and ankle. In 1925, Haenisch first described a case of osteonecrosis in an adult patient who suffered ischemic necrosis of the femoral head.[1] Since then, the knowledge regarding hip osteonecrosis has substantially improved. The disease prevalence is 10,000 to 20,000 new cases per year. Hip osteonecrosis can affect patients of any age. However, patients living in their third decade are especially prone to the disease.[2] If untreated, approximately 80% of affected hips will progress and eventually develop painful osteoarthritis and require surgical intervention.[2] This includes 59% to 66% of asymptomatic hips.[3,4] There is a wide spectrum of treatment options ranging from nonoperative pharmacotherapies to surgeries, which remove the necrotic bones, to replacing the joints. The optimal treatment, of course, depends on the stage of the disease and the age of the patient. However, most of the patients are eventually referred to orthopedic surgeons. In the United States, up to 10% of hip replacements performed involve osteonecrosis.[5]

This chapter provides a synopsis of hip osteonecrosis. The chapter will describe the etiology and pathophysiology of the disease, and then discuss the diagnosis and present a treatment algorithm. Treatment options, both nonoperative and operative, will be discussed.

Etiology and Associated Risk Factors

There are many risk factors for osteonecrosis of the hip but they commonly involve disruption of the blood flow to the hip. Hip injuries are the most common direct cause of hip osteonecrosis. Traumatic events such as femoral fractures and dislocations can lead to severed blood vessels and ischemia. Because of poor redundancy of blood flow to the femoral head, any damage to the major blood vessels, particularly the lateral epiphyseal arteries, the nutrient artery entering the femur, and the ligamentum teres artery, may cut the blood flow in a substantial area.

In addition to trauma, some systemic diseases that interrupt the blood flow or change the hemodynamics can also lead to hip osteonecrosis. These include Caisson disease, Gaucher's disease, coagulopathies, and some autoimmune diseases. Caisson disease, also known as decompression sickness, is a syndrome caused by sudden atmospheric pressure changes. The nitrogen in the bloodstream is released rapidly and forms gas bubbles that can damage blood vessels. Because the blood vessels to the hip are less capable of sustaining injury, blood flow in the hip area is likely to be interrupted.[6] Gaucher's disease is one of the lysosomal storage diseases caused by a deficiency in an enzyme, glucocerebrosidase, that normally breaks down the fat glucocerebroside. As a result, fat accumulates in the organs, including the bone marrow. Gaucher's disease can also affect

Parvizi J, Klatt BA.
Essentials in Total Hip Arthroplasty (pp 197-213).

Table 24-1

Risk Factors Associated With Osteonecrosis

Direct Risk Factors
• Trauma (fracture, dislocation, burns) • Caisson disease • Gaucher's disease • Coagulapathies (thrombophilia, hypofibrinolysis, Factor V Leiden, Protein C and S deficiencies, antithrombin III deficiency) • Autoimmune (systemic lupus erythematosus, rheumatoid arthritis, polymyalgia rheumatica) • Pregnancy • Iatrogenic (postradiation, chemotherapy) • Organ transplants • Hypersensitivity reactions • Leukemia • Sickle cell disease • HIV • SARS • Gastrointestinal disorders and liver dysfunction
Indirect Risk Factors
• Corticosteroid use • Alcohol consumption • Cigarette smoking

blood supply to the hip through infarction. The incidence of hip osteonecrosis in Gaucher's disease can reach 30% according to a Gaucher registry.[7] Coagulopathies such as thrombophilia, hypofibrinolysis, and sickle cell disease may lead to ischemia and subsequent osteonecrosis. Autoimmune diseases such as systemic lupus erythematosus, rheumatoid arthritis, and polymyalgia rheumatica are all possible risk factors for osteonecrosis. Although the exact relationship between whether these conditions cause the disease or result specifically from the treatment of the disease (corticosteroids or other agents) is not known.

The pathogenetic mechanisms of indirect causes have not been clearly defined. Corticosteroid use, alcohol consumption, and tobacco use are the most studied factors in osteonecrosis. In 1957, Pietrograndi first described the development of osteonecrosis following corticosteroid therapy.[8] Since then, studies have shown that a corticosteroid dose >2 g for approximately 2 to 3 months is likely to increase the risk of osteonecrosis.[9] The disease usually leads to symptoms 3 to 24 months after the initial use of corticosteroids.[10-12]

In regards to alcohol consumption, studies in Japan demonstrated a positive association between alcohol consumption and this disease.[13,14] Alcohol consumption of greater than 400 mL per week increased the risk for osteonecrosis by over 11 times compared to nondrinkers.[13] The exact mechanism is not yet understood. One possible pathway is that hyperlipidemia, resulting from liver damage due to excessive alcohol intake, may lead to fat emboli.

The same studies on alcohol consumption and osteonecrosis also examined smoking as a risk factor.[13,14] Smoking increases the risk of osteonecrosis with a minimum dose of 20 pack-years.[14] Smoking may cause vessel damage, which may lead to osteonecrosis.

Other reported risk factors for osteonecrosis are postradiation, human immunodeficiency virus, and severe acute respiratory syndrome (Table 24-1). Many studies have examined human immunodeficiency virus as a risk factor for osteonecrosis. However, the rate seems to be low with only 0.12% to 4.4% of patients with the disease developing osteonecrosis.[15-20] Severe acute respiratory syndrome was a recently discovered risk factor. Reports of corticosteroid usage to treat this syndrome and the increased incidence of osteonecrosis began to appear in 2004, less than 2 years after severe acute respiratory syndrome was first reported.[21] Understanding risk factors can help with the diagnosis and treatment of osteonecrosis.

Pathophysiology

The natural history of hip osteonecrosis depends on the affected area, which will affect symptoms. If the size is small, affecting less than 15% of the femoral head, and the patient is asymptomatic, the lesion may heal spontaneously.[3] However, if the lesion is larger than 15% of the femoral head, a repair process leading to collapse usually occurs. First, the repair begins in reaction to the lesion but necrotic tissue is partially absorbed. Reactive bone is laid down on dead trabeculae, which forms a sclerotic area with inflammation. Bone reabsorption and fibrosis then occur. Microfractures can develop in areas of dead bone. As the microfractures progress, subchondral fractures occur. This will lead to collapse of the femoral head and eventually painful osteoarthritis.

The description of the pathogenesis of osteonecrosis of the hip can either be extraosseous or intraosseous. An extraosseous process occurs when the blood flow to the hip

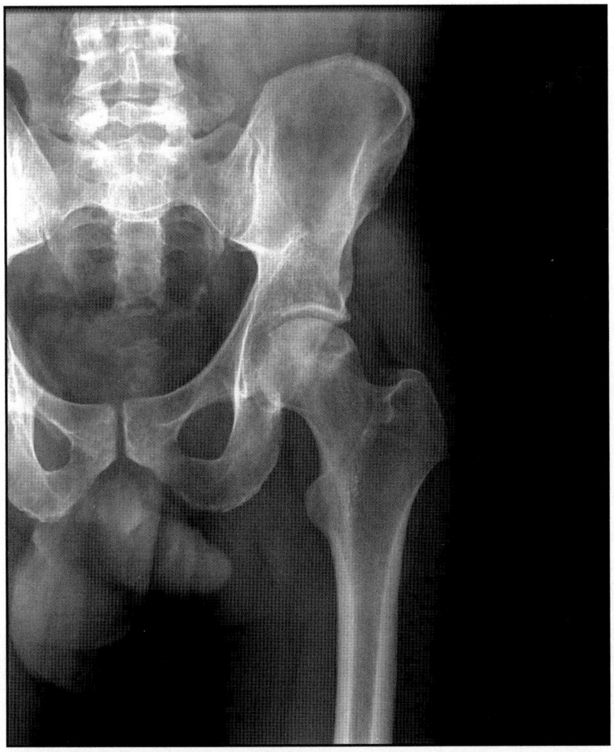

Figure 24-1. Roentgenogram of hip osteonecrosis.

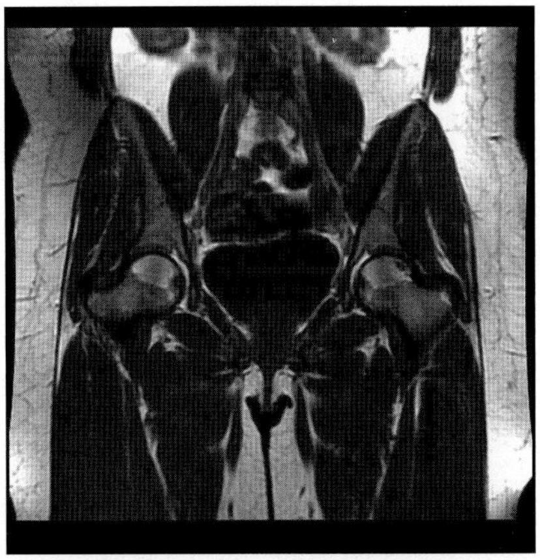

Figure 24-2. Magnetic resonance image of hip osteonecrosis.

is compromised. On the other hand, intraosseous processes involve the bone marrow (eg, a hyperlipidemic condition that results in bone death). Embolization of the vasculature and increased intraosseous pressure are possible mechanisms that decrease or even shut down blood flow.

McCarthy summarized the importance of blood flow to the bone.[22] When circulatory disorders occur, ischemia follows. As a result, changes occur that lead first to the death of hematopoetic and fatty marrow elements, which then occlude the vascular supply and eventually lead to bone death. Studies on bone blood flow are important to decrease or even prevent bone ischemia so steps can be taken at the vascular level to treat osteonecrosis.

Another way to try to understand the pathogenesis of osteonecrosis is to study its possible genetic basis. A study on patients who have COL2A1, a type II collagen gene, may have an increased risk for osteonecrosis.[23] Similarly, a gene on the same chromosome as COL2A1 was found to be associated with familial osteonecrosis.[24] Other genes that affect coagulation may increase the risk for osteonecrosis.[25] Genes affecting lipid transport and metabolism may be involved.[26] Genes controlling molecular production of increased catalase and decreased nitric oxide may be associated with a higher risk for osteonecrosis.[27,28] In contradistinction, a recently described drug resistance gene may lower the risk for the disease.[29] Understanding the genetic factors may eventually help screen for osteonecrosis and thus delay the progression of disease.

Diagnosis

The typical symptom of hip osteonecrosis is groin pain that is exacerbated with ambulation.[30] The pain is described as deep and throbbing and sometimes can even radiate to the knees. Onset can be acute and intermittent. On physical examination, limitation of internal rotation in both extension and flexion can be found. However, in asymptomatic cases, osteonecrosis may be evident only on radiographic examination. The main imaging modalities to aid in the diagnosis of hip osteonecrosis are standard radiographs and magnetic resonance imaging (MRI) (Figures 24-1 and 24-2). A Japanese study developed criteria to diagnose femoral head atraumatic osteonecrosis using radiographic tools.[31] Major criteria included femoral head collapse, demarcating sclerosis, a crescent sign (see Figure 24-1), and low-intensity bands on T1-weighted images. Minor criteria included femoral head collapse with joint space narrowing, mottled sclerosis, acetabular involvement, and homogenous or inhomogeneous low intensity without the T1-weighted band patterns. Other radiographic studies that have been used but with limited applications in the diagnosis of hip osteonecrosis include bone scans (Figure 24-3), positron emission tomography, and computed tomography (CT) scans (Figure 24-4).

Radiographs are also used to stage the progression of the disease. In 1974, Kerboul developed a method to measure the extent of necrosis of the femoral head on the anterior-posterior and lateral roentgenograms called the

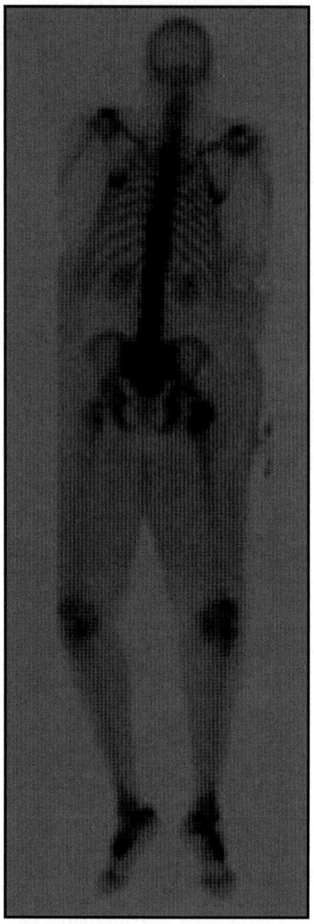

Figure 24-3. Bone scan of hip osteonecrosis.

Kerboul angle.[32] In this method, an arc of the affected necrotic area of the femoral head is determined on the anterior-posterior and lateral roentgenograms. Summing up these 2 angles gives a combined necrotic angle. Small lesions (<15% of the femoral head) corresponded to less than 150 degrees of the combined necrotic angle. Medium lesions (15% to 30% of the femoral head) corresponded to 150 to 250 degrees. Large lesions (>30% femoral head involvement) corresponded to >250 degrees. Kerboul angle >250 degrees has been used to diagnose or predict collapse of the femoral head.[33]

A nonimaging technique in the diagnosis of hip osteonecrosis includes arthroscopy. Arthroscopy was shown to be useful in staging of the disease when imaging techniques were not convincing.[34] A study showed that arthroscopy detected postcollapse of the femoral head that was not evident on roentgenograms or MRI.[35]

Classification Systems

Ficat and Arlet were the first to introduce a radiolographical classification system where 3 stages were described.[36] Later, a fourth stage was added and the revised classification system is the most commonly used classification today. In this system, stage I is defined as normal radiographic findings. Cysts and sclerosis begin to appear in stage II. Stage III is characterized by a crescentic line caused by a subchondral fracture also known as the crescent sign (see Figure 24-1). Stage IV is the end stage with femoral head flattening and acetabular osteophytes.

Steinberg incorporated data acquired from MRI and bone scans in disease classification.[37] In this new classification system, stage 0 is normal. Stage I represents normal radiographs but abnormal technetium bone scans or MRIs. Stage II shows progression to sclerosis while stage III is characterized by the crescent sign. Stage IV demonstrates femoral head collapse. Acetabular changes occur in stage V, and stage VI represents advanced osteoarthritic changes.

The Association Research Circulation Osseous group (ARCO) further developed a classification system based on the Steinberg classification system.[38,39] Stage 0 is normal. Stage 1 demonstrates normal radiographic and CT images but at least bone scan or MRI positive with subclassification of A, B, and C depending on involved area, length of crescent sign, and femoral head collapse. Stage 2 represents sclerosis and osteolysis with the same subclassifications as stage 1. Stage 3 shows the crescent sign with the same subclassifications as stage 1. Stage 4 demonstrates osteoarthritis and acetabular involvement.

The Japanese Orthopaedic Association also developed a classification system for hip osteonecrosis.[40,41] The distinctive feature of this classification is that the location of the lesion was assessed. Lesions less than one-third of the medial weight-bearing zone, lesions between one-third to two-thirds, and lesions greater than two-thirds are classified as types 1A, 1B, and 1C, respectively. Type 2 represents femoral head flattening. Type 3 involves cyst formation and is also subcategorized into 3A for a medial weight-bearing zone and 3B for a lateral zone.

Table 24-2 gives an overview of the main radiographic classification systems. Other classifications have been developed but not used widely.[10,42-47] Combining clinical and radiographical information, Figure 24-5 shows a possible algorithm when staging for osteonecrosis.

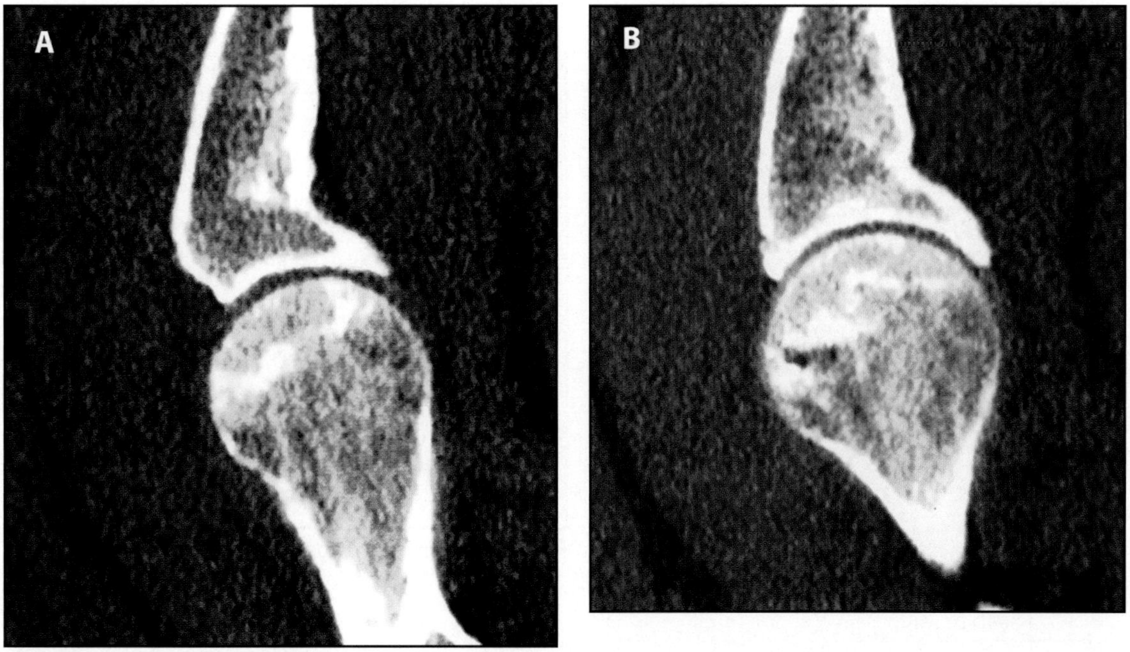

Figure 24-4. Computed tomography of osteonecrosis.

Treatment

Treatment options include nonoperative and operative depending on the causes and radiographic stage of the disease. Nonoperative treatments typically target risk factors. Operative treatments are often reserved for more advanced stages of the disease.

Nonoperative Treatment

Nonoperative treatment includes pharmacological agents such as lipid-lowering agents, anticoagulants, prostacyclin analogues, and bisphosphonates (Table 24-3).

Cholesterol-lowering agents, particularly the statins, act by reducing the enzyme of HMG-CoA reductase that is involved in cholesterol synthesis[48] and thus lowering blood lipid levels. An elevated blood lipid level has been shown to be a risk factor for osteonecrosis. Other cholesterol-lowering agents include bile acid sequestrants, niacin, gemfibrozil, probucol, and clofibrate. Their effectiveness in the treatment of hip osteonecrosis warrants further study.

Anticoagulants, such as heparin and lovenox, are useful in treating hip osteonecrosis associated or caused by coagulopathies as previously discussed. The main obstacles in using these drugs, however, are that monitoring of bleeding time and adjusting for therapeutic dosing is necessary.

Prostacyclin analogues, such as iloprost, inhibit the aggregation of platelets and reduce hypertension. Reducing blood pressure would ideally enhance blood flow to the ischemic bone areas, which may lead to revascularization. This modality needs further study.

The mechanism of bisphosphonates is to decrease osteoclastic activity in the bone formation process and thus to promote the osteoblastic process, which is thought to help bone healing in osteonecrosis. This modality has been promising in some short-term studies but needs further evaluation.

Other nonsurgical treatments include physical therapy with assisted weight-bearing, extracorporeal shock wave therapy, magnetic field therapy, and hyperbaric oxygen treatment.[49] Assisted weight-bearing strategies were thought to reduce stress on the weight-bearing portion of the femoral head to allow repair of the osteonecrotic lesions. However, a study has shown unsuccessful results in 80% of the cases.[50] Because of this, other nonoperative modalities are being examined such as extracorporeal shock wave therapy, pulsed electromagnetic field therapy, and hyperbaric oxygen treatment (Table 24-4).

In initial studies, extracorporeal shock wave therapy has been promising.[51,52] One possible mechanism is that the shock wave treatment may alter the analgesic effect by increasing pain threshold and thus allowing alteration of the vascularity of the affected areas of the femoral head.

Table 24-2

Radiographic Classification of Hip Osteonecrosis

Stage	Explanation
Ficat and Arlet[36]	
I	Normal
II	Cystic or sclerotic lesions
III	Crescent sign (subchondral fracture)
IV	Osteoarthritis
Steinberg[37]	
0	Normal
I	Normal x-ray with abnormal bone scan or MRI
II	Cystic or sclerotic lesions
III	Crescent sign
IV	Femoral head flattening
V	Acetabular involvement
VI	Advanced osteoarthritis
ARCO[37]	
0	Normal
1	X-ray and CT normal. At least one other imaging modality positive
2	Sclerosis, osteolysis, focal porosis
3	Crescent sign
4	Osteoarthritis
Japanese Orthopaedic Association[37]	
1	Demarcation line, subdivided into 1A, 1B, 1C in relation to weight-bearing area
2	Flattening of femoral head
3	Cystic lesions subdivided into 3A (medial) and 3B (lateral)
Marcus and Enneking[81]	
1	Normal
2	Area of peripheral infarct on x-ray
3	Crescent sign
4	Flattened femoral head
5	Cartilage wear with medial osteophyte formation
6	End-stage osteoarthritis

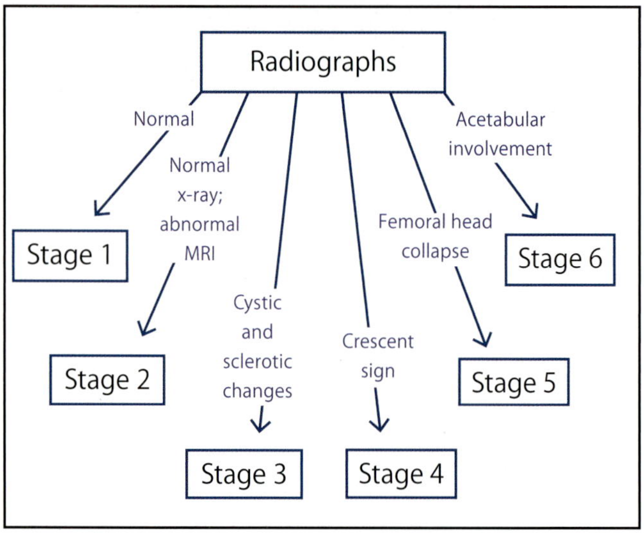

Figure 24-5. Algorithm for staging hip osteonecrosis.

Although initial studies have been positive, long-term studies are needed to determine the effect of this modality.

Pulsed electromagnetic field therapy may protect the articular cartilage from the damaging effects of inflammation while promoting osteogenic activity in the necrotic area.[53] One study demonstrated that pulsed electromagnetic field therapy in patients with Ficat II and III hip osteonecrosis was superior to core decompression.[54] However, application of this treatment needs more evidence from clinical studies. Electrical stimulation can potentially assist in fracture nonunions and encourage bone formation. However, studies have shown that used as an adjunctive therapy to core decompression and grafting, electrical stimulation does not provide any significant benefit.[55,56] Long-term and large-scale studies are needed to support the benefits of this treatment in osteonecrosis treatment.

Hyperbaric oxygen treatment has been utilized in the treatment of many other orthopedic problems with positive results, but no study specifically examined this modality in osteonecrosis.[57] The mechanism of this treatment is to increase the oxygen supply for the blood vessels and induce new vascularization. This may have potential benefits for patients with osteonecrosis. However, serious side effects can occur, including seizures, pulmonary edema, and even death.

Operative Treatments

There are many surgical options that are available to treat hip osteonecrosis when nonsurgical options fail. Furthermore, when patients present with later stages of hip osteonecrosis, surgical treatment may be the only option. In

Table 24-3

Pharmacological Agents Used in Hip Osteonecrosis

Pharmacological Agent	Author	Year	Mean Follow-Up (Range)	Level of Evidence	Clinical Outcome
Cholesterol-lowering agents	Pritchett et al[82]	2001	90 (60 to 132)	IV	Three (1%) out of the 284 patients taking statins and corticosteroids developed osteonecrosis
Anticoagulants	Glueck et al[83]	2005	161 (108 to 216)	II	Nineteen (95%) of 20 hips in Stage I and II osteonecrosis had delayed disease progression
Prostacyclin analogues	Disch et al[84]	2005	25 (11 to 37)	III	All 17 patients experienced improvement in Harris hip scores, reduction in pain and edema on MRI
Bisphosphonates	Ramachandran et al[85]	2007	38 (25 to 58)	IV	Fourteen (82%) of 17 adolescents were pain-free and there was mean improvements in Harris hip scores, Iowa Hip Rating, and Global Pediatric Outcomes Data Collection Instrument
	Nishii et al[86]	2006	12	II	Alendronate group demonstrated a decrease in bone resorption marker and hip pain compared to the control (8)
	Lai et al[87]	2005	(24 to 28)	I	Two (17%) out of 29 hips in the alendronate group required further intervention compared to 17 (68%) out of 25 hips in the control group
	Agarwala et al[88]	2005	12 (3 to 60)	II	Significant reduction in pain and disability and improvement in standing and walking times

the following section we will discuss the surgical treatments, which are categorized as joint-preserving and joint-replacing treatments.

Joint-Preserving Treatments

Prior to the collapse of the femoral head, joint-preserving surgical treatments are ideal. The major options are core decompression, nonvascularized and vascularized bone grafting with adjunctive therapies, and osteotomies (Table 24-5).

Core decompression was first used for both diagnostic and therapeutic purposes by Hungerford and Ficat and Arlet.[58,59] They believed that by reducing bone marrow pressure as well as possibly inducing neovascularization, the necrotic area could form healthy bone. Two methods of core decompression have been developed, the trephine 8 to 10 mm and the multiple small diameter techniques. Currently, the most commonly used method is an 8- to 10-mm trephine guided by fluoroscopy with either the core tract being left open or filled in with bone graft.[60] Complications associated with this technique include articular cartilage damage or subchondral fractures. Because of these complications, the multiple small diameter technique was developed by Kim et al, who reported a lower rate of collapse (14.3%) compared with the larger trephine method.[61]

Nonvascularized or vascularized bone grafting can be used with core decompression in hip osteonecrosis treatment. Nonvascularized bone grafting removes necrotic bone and replaces it with cancellous and cortical autografts to

Table 24-4

NONSURGICAL TREATMENT FOR HIP OSTEONECROSIS

TREATMENT	AUTHOR	YEAR	NUMBER OF HIPS	LEVEL OF EVIDENCE	MEAN FOLLOW-UP IN MONTHS (RANGE)	CLINICAL SUCCESS (%)
Extra corporeal shock wave therapy	Wang et al[52]	2005	29	I	25 (24 to 38)	83
	Ludwig et al[51]	2001	22	II	12	64
Pulsed electromagnetic field therapy	Massari et al[53]	2006	76	IV	28 (12 to 108)	74
Electrical stimulation	Trancik et al[56]	1990	11	IV	45 (24 to 60)	45
	Steinberg et al[55]	1990	40	III	31 (24 to 48)	19
Hyperbaric oxygen treatment	Huang et al[57]	2006	-	IV	-	-

provide mechanical support for the articular surface to prevent collapse and allow for bone healing.[62-64] Indications for nonvascularized bone grafting include femoral head collapse of less than 2 mm or unsuccessful core decompression. The 3 commonly used techniques are the core tract (also known as Phemister), trapdoor, and lightbulb techniques. Briefly, the core tract technique involves drilling a hole from the femoral head into the neck, which provides a tract in which bone grafts can be placed.[64] The trapdoor technique makes a window in the articular cartilage and then the bone grafts are placed within this window.[65] The lightbulb technique grafts bones through a window made at the neck or head-neck junction of the femur.[66] Each of these techniques has its own disadvantages and advantages.

Vascularized bone grafting is similar to nonvascularized bone grafting with an addition of the vascularization procedure. The procedure is technically challenging and time-intensive and has higher morbidity at the donor sites. The surgery requires 2 teams: one team prepares the femur while the other harvests the fibula or ilium graft. There are many studies promoting the efficacy of this procedure for early stage osteonecrosis.

Adjunctive therapies have been utilized with bone grafting to help with weight bearing, lesion heading, or growth of new bones. A variety of methods are available, including tantalum rods, bone growth factors, stem cells, gene therapy, and arthrodiastasis. Some have been well studied in clinical use while others are on the cutting edge, awaiting more evidence to support their applications.

Tantalum is a light metal that has a high yield to stress. Its features make it an ideal candidate material for use in the hips where weight bearing is necessary. Porous tantalum rods have been developed for treatment of hip osteonecrosis by introducing them into core tracks to potentially allow bone growth to occur while providing support. Although some initial short-term studies showed promise,[67,68] others have shown an implant failure rate of greater than 50% (13 out of 23 hips) at a mean 18 months after implantation.[69] Additionally, Tanzer et al recently found little bone ingrowth in 15 failed implants (of 113 hips that were followed) with these clinical failures occurring at a mean of 13 months (range, 3 to 36 months) after implantation.[70] Longer-term studies are needed to better determine the efficacy of this treatment modality.

Bone growth factors can be used to avoid donor site morbidity from vascularized bone graft surgery. These factors induce new bone formation, which may prevent femoral head collapse. Bone morphogenetic proteins have been widely studied since 1973 when Reddi and Huggins first described their roles in bone formation.[71] Currently there are more than 15 types of bone morphogenetic proteins identified. Other bone growth factors, such as fibroblast growth factors, have also been used to treat osteonecrosis of the hip.[72]

Stem cells have the potential to differentiate into bone, muscle, cartilage, tendon, and other connective tissues. Clinical studies have shown its potential in treating early osteonecrosis.[73,74] One disadvantage of utilizing stem cells

Table 24-5

Joint-Preserving Surgical Treatments for Hip Osteonecrosis

Treatment	Author	Year	Number of Hips	Level of Evidence	Mean Follow-Up in Months (Range)	Clinical Success (%)
Core decompression (multiple small drilling technique)	Radke et al[89]	2004	65	IV	- (60 to 120)	70
	Mont et al[60]	2004	45	II	24 (20 to 39)	71
	Yoon et al[90]	2001	39	IV	61 (24 to 118)	45
Core decompression (trephine 8 to 10 mm technique)	Lieberman et al[91]	2004	17	IV	53 (26 to 94)	82
	Aigner et al[92]	2002	45	IV	69 (31 to 120)	80
	Simank et al[93]	2001	94	III	72 (18 to 228)	69
	Steinberg et al[94]	2001	312	II	48 (24 to 168)	64
	Maniwa et al[95]	2000	26	II	94 (29 to 164)	66
	Chen et al[33]	2000	27	IV	28	60
	Lavernia et al[96]	2000	67	II	44	63
Nonvascular bone grafting (core tract)	Keizer et al[97]	2006	80	IV	84	46
	Wang et al[52]	2005	28	I	26 (24 to 39)	68
	Israelite et al[98]	2005	276	IV	- (24 to 145)	62
	Kim et al[99]	2005	30	III	50 (36 to 67)	78
	Lieberman et al[91]	2004	17	IV	53 (26 to 94)	82
	Rijnen et al[100]	2003	28	II	50 (24 to 119)	71
	Plakseychuk et al[101]	2003	50	III	60 (36 to 96)	36
	Mont et al[102]	2003	21	IV	48 (36 to 55)	86
Nonvascular bone grafting (trapdoor technique)	Mont et al[63]	1998	30	IV	56 (30 to 60)	73
	Ko et al[103]	1995	14	IV	53 (24 to 108)	85
Nonvascular bone grafting (lightbulb technique)	Seyler et al[104]	2007	47	IV	28 (12 to 50)	68
	Mont et al[102]	2003	21	IV	48 (36 to 55)	86
Vascularized bone grafting using the fibula	Roush et al[105]	2006	200	IV	90 (79 to 100)	76
	Yen[106]	2006	22	III	>36	82

(continued)

Table 24-5 (continued)

JOINT-PRESERVING SURGICAL TREATMENTS FOR HIP OSTEONECROSIS

TREATMENT	AUTHOR	YEAR	NUMBER OF HIPS	LEVEL OF EVIDENCE	MEAN FOLLOW-UP IN MONTHS (RANGE)	CLINICAL SUCCESS (%)
	Stubbs et al[107]	2005	7	IV	47 (36 to 75)	100
	Marciniak et al[108]	2005	102	IV	96 (60 to 180)	42
	Kim et al[99]	2005	23	III	50 (36 to 66)	43
Vascularized bone grafting using the ilium	Yen et al[106]	2006	39	III	>48	56
	Nakamura et al[109]	2005	12	IV	81 (36 to 180)	83
	Matsusaki et al[110]	2005	17	IV	51 (18 to 133)	71
Osteotomy	Yoon et al[111]	2008	43	IV	37 (24 to 52)	93
	Sugioka et al[112]	2008	51	IV	144 (14 to 252)	65
	Ikemura et al[113]	2007	42	IV	72 (24 to 150)	64
	Onodera et al[114]	2005	38	IV	48 (25 to 84)	58
	Rijnen et al[115]	2005	26	IV	104 (79 to 120)	56
	Nakamura et al[109]	2005	12	IV	81 (36 to 180)	83
	Matsusaki[110]	2005	17	IV	51 (18 to 133)	71

is donor site morbidity; therefore, gene therapy has been explored along this line. Animal models have shown promise in application in the treatment of osteonecrosis of the femoral head.[75,76] However, studies in humans need to be conducted.

Arthrodiastasis is a method to distract the joint in order to allow the osteonecrotic lesion to heal by protecting the joint from weight-bearing forces. This method was first introduced in 1979 to treat osteoarthritis, chondrolysis, and femoral head osteonecrosis.[77,78] Long-term clinical outcomes will ascertain the potential for this method in treating hip osteonecrosis.

Intertrochanteric osteotomies (varus or valgus) have been used with success but can only be generally applied to small lesions. Larger rotational osteotomies were developed to transpose the osteonecrotic region of the femoral head to the non-weight-bearing portion in order to allow for bone healing. This procedure has been largely successful in Asian countries but not elsewhere. There may be an anatomic difference in the Asian population in that the posterior capsule of the hip is more lax and allows better rotation of the anterior portion of the neck.[79] Complications are common because the procedure is technically demanding. The poor fixation with screws can cause increased varus, delayed unions, and even secondary collapse of the femoral head. The position of the lesion may also influence the outcome; a lesion at the posterior of the femoral head fares better compared to the anterior of the femoral head due to the principal weight-bearing anterolateral region. Furthermore, revision to a joint-replacing surgery may be difficult after this procedure.

Joint-Replacing Treatments

With the development of implants, hip replacements become a more optimal treatment for patients with osteonecrotic hips. Depending on the type of implants, treatment options include bipolar hemiarthroplasty, limited resurfacing, total hip arthroplasty (THA), and metal-on-metal resurfacing (Table 24-6).

In bipolar hemiarthroplasty, the femoral head is replaced but the native acetabulum is kept intact. The goal of this procedure is to decrease the shear force between the acetabulum and the femoral head with an articulating cup over the prosthetic femoral head. Clinical studies on bipolar hemiarthroplasty have typically poor outcomes. One major problem with the use of this type of implant is the tendency of developing wear of the acetabulum. In addition, complications such as osteolysis and acetabular protrusion are relatively high.

Table 24-6

Joint-Replacing Surgical Treatments for Hip Osteonecrosis

Treatment	Author	Year	Number of hips	Level of evidence	Mean follow-up in months (range)	Clinical success (%)
Bipolar hemiarthroplasty	Tsumura[116]	2005	32	IV	92 (60 to 180)	86
	Yamano[117]	2004	29	IV	144	62
	Lee[118]	2004	40-	III	96 (73 to 128)	95
	Nagai[119]	2002	12	IV	199 (144 to 216)	75
Limited resurfacing	Cuckler[120]	2004	59	IV	54	68
	Beaule[121]	2004	28	III	60 (28 to 100)	86
	Adili[122]	2003	29	IV	34 (24 to 63)	76
Total hip arthroplasty	Schneider[123]	2004	57	IV	-	82
	Kim[124]	2003	100	II	122 (96 to 120)	98
	Berend[125]	2003	89	IV	110 (60 to 180)	82
	Al-Mousawi[126]	2002	35	IV	114 (60 to 180)	80
	Fyda[127]	2002	53	IV	151	83
	Xenakis[128]	2001	36	IV	136 (120 to 180)	93
	Taylor[129]	2001	70	II	91 (60 to 156)	
	Delank[130]	2001	66	III	65 (58 to 94)	93
	Hartley[131]	2000	55	IV	117	79
	Zangger[132]	2000	26	IV	55 (21 to 124)	93
Metal-on-metal resurfacing	Mont[133]	2006	42	II	36 (24 to 48)	93
	Amstutz[134]	2004	36	IV	42 (26 to 74)	94
	Mohamad[135]	2004	12	IV	18 (17 to 46)	84
	Beaule[121]	2004	56	III	60 (28 to 100)	95
	Yoon[136]	2004	40		36 (24 to 48)	93

Another option is limited femoral resurfacing in which the femoral head prosthesis is matched with the native acetabulum. Similar to hemiarthroplasty, clinical studies on limited resurfacing have mixed results. Potential advantages with this procedure are removal of damaged cartilage, preservation of bone stock, and easy conversion to THA if needed.

THA is usually the last resort for patients with hip osteonecrosis. Both the femoral head and acetabulum are replaced. In this procedure, bone stock is often sacrificed. In addition, because of the long life expectancy of these patients, they may need a revision in their lifetime. However, it is expected that with better designs and materials, implant durability will continue to increase. Results from joint replacing treatments for hip osteonecrosis using modern-day devices are depicted in Table 24-6. Metal-on-metal resurfacing was first introduced in the 1960s. This technique was developed to reduce the sacrifice of bone stock but allow the replacement of both the femoral and acetabular sides. However, component loosening and high failure rates with the early procedures caused discontinuation of its use.[80] Recently, because of improved technology, there is a growing interest in reusing the technique to treat hip osteonecrosis. This technology may be ideal for the younger patients. Because bone stock is preserved, ease of revision to THA may be accomplished later, but recent concerns about metal wear may make this a less than ideal option.

Treatment Algorithm

When treating patients with hip osteonecrosis, several factors such as age, comorbidities, and health status are important to consider. In young patients, it is imperative to consider their age and level of activities. Often, procedures that delay joint arthroplasty may be appropriate.

In addition, treatment decisions should be based on radiographic and MRI findings. Figure 24-6 shows a proposed algorithm based on staging to determine the appropriate treatment. Future studies that elucidate the pathogenesis of osteonecrosis are likely to make more effective nonoperative and operative treatments.

References

1. Haenisch H. Arthritis dissecans der hufte. *Zentralblatt.* 1925;52:1.
2. Mont MA, Hungerford DS. Non-traumatic avascular necrosis of the femoral head. *J Bone Joint Surg Am.* 1995;77(3):459-474.
3. Nam KW, Kim YL, Yoo JJ, Koo KH, Yoon KS, Kim HJ. Fate of untreated asymptomatic osteonecrosis of the femoral head. *J Bone Joint Surg Am.* 2008;90(3):477-484.
4. Min BW, Song KS, Cho CH, Lee SM, Lee KJ. Untreated asymptomatic hips in patients with osteonecrosis of the femoral head. *Clin Orthop Relat Res.* 2008;466(5):1087-1092.
5. Hungerford DS. Osteonecrosis: avoiding total hip arthroplasty. *J Arthroplasty.* 2002;17(4 suppl 1):121-124.
6. Chryssanthou CP. Dysbaric osteonecrosis. Etiological and pathogenetic concepts. *Clin Orthop Relat Res.* 1978(130):94-106.
7. Wenstrup RJ, Roca-Espiau M, Weinreb NJ, Bembi B. Skeletal aspects of Gaucher disease: a review. *Br J Radiol.* 2002;75(suppl 1):A2-12.
8. Pietrograndi V, Mastromarino R. Osteopatia da prolunga trattamento cortisonico. *Orthop Traumatol.* 1957;25:1.
9. Mont MA, Jones LC, Hungerford DS. Nontraumatic osteonecrosis of the femoral head: ten years later. *J Bone Joint Surg Am.* 2006;88(5):1117-1132.
10. Sakamoto M, Shimizu K, Iida S, Akita T, Moriya H, Nawata Y. Osteonecrosis of the femoral head: a prospective study with MRI. *J Bone Joint Surg Br.* 1997;79(2):213-219.
11. Fink B, Degenhardt S, Paselk C, Schneider T, Modder U, Ruther W. Early detection of avascular necrosis of the femoral head following renal transplantation. *Arch Orthop Trauma Surg.* 1997;116(3):151-156.
12. Koo KH, Kim R, Kim YS, et al. Risk period for developing osteonecrosis of the femoral head in patients on steroid treatment. *Clin Rheumatol.* 2002;21(4):299-303.
13. Matsuo K, Hirohata T, Sugioka Y, Ikeda M, Fukuda A. Influence of alcohol intake, cigarette smoking, and occupational status on idiopathic osteonecrosis of the femoral head. *Clin Orthop Relat Res.* 1988(234):115-123.
14. Hirota Y, Hirohata T, Fukuda K, et al. Association of alcohol intake, cigarette smoking, and occupational status with the risk of idiopathic osteonecrosis of the femoral head. *Am J Epidemiol.* 1993;137(5):530-538.
15. Calza L, Manfredi R, Mastroianni A, Chiodo F. Osteonecrosis and highly active antiretroviral therapy during HIV infection: report of a series and literature review. *AIDS Patient Care STDS.* 2001;15(7):385-389.
16. Gutierrez F, Padilla S, Ortega E, et al. Avascular necrosis of the bone in HIV-infected patients: incidence and associated factors. *AIDS.* 2002;16(3):481-483.
17. Keruly JC, Chaisson RE, Moore RD. Increasing incidence of avascular necrosis of the hip in HIV-infected patients. *J Acquir Immune Defic Syndr.* 2001;28(1):101-102.
18. Miller KD, Masur H, Jones EC, et al. High prevalence of osteonecrosis of the femoral head in HIV-infected adults. *Ann Intern Med.* 2002;137(1):17-25.
19. Roudiere L, Viard JP. Osteonecrosis of the hip, lipodystrophy and antiretroviral treatment. *AIDS.* 2000;14(13):2056.
20. Valencia ME, Barreiro P, Soriano V, Blanco F, Moreno V, Lahoz JG. Avascular necrosis in HIV-infected patients receiving antiretroviral treatment: study of seven cases. *HIV Clin Trials.* 2003;4(2):132-136.
21. Hong N, Du XK. Avascular necrosis of bone in severe acute respiratory syndrome. *Clin Radiol.* 2004;59(7):602-608.
22. McCarthy I. The physiology of bone blood flow: a review. *J Bone Joint Surg Am.* 2006;88(suppl 3):4-9.
23. Liu YF, Chen WM, Lin YF, et al. Type II collagen gene variants and inherited osteonecrosis of the femoral head. *N Engl J Med.* 2005;352(22):2294-2301.
24. Chen WM, Liu YF, Lin MW, et al. Autosomal dominant avascular necrosis of femoral head in two Taiwanese pedigrees and linkage to chromosome 12q13. *Am J Hum Genet.* 2004;75(2):310-317.
25. Glueck CJ, Freiberg RA, Fontaine RN, Tracy T, Wang P. Hypofibrinolysis, thrombophilia, osteonecrosis. *Clin Orthop Relat Res.* 2001(386):19-33.

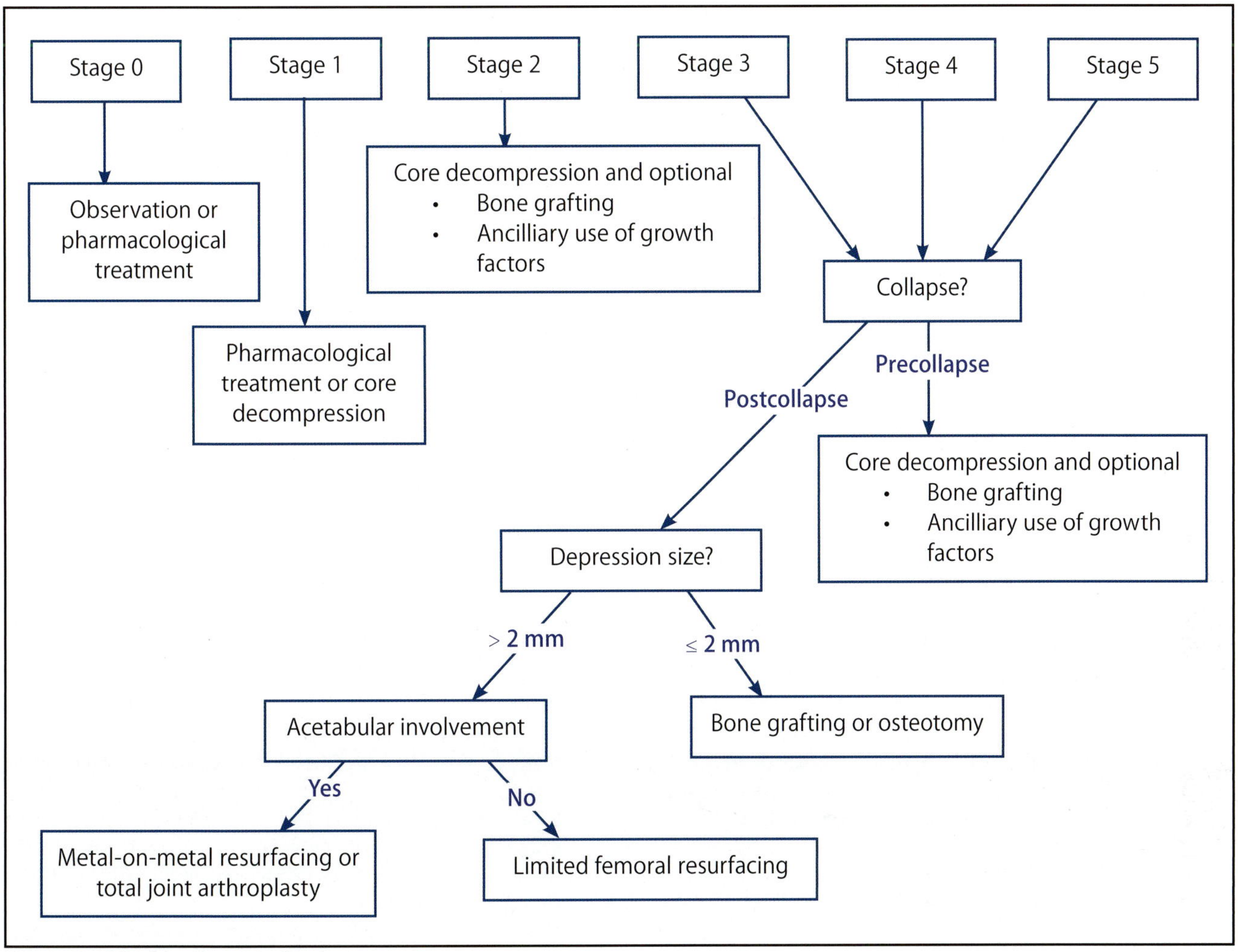

Figure 24-6. Algorithm for treating hip osteonecrosis.

26. Hirata T, Fujioka M, Takahashi KA, et al. ApoB C7623T polymorphism predicts risk for steroid-induced osteonecrosis of the femoral head after renal transplantation. *J Orthop Sci.* 2007;12(3):199-206.
27. Glueck CJ, Freiberg RA, Oghene J, Fontaine RN, Wang P. Association between the T-786C eNOS polymorphism and idiopathic osteonecrosis of the head of the femur. *J Bone Joint Surg Am.* 2007;89(11):2460-2468.
28. Kim TH, Hong JM, Oh B, et al. Genetic association study of polymorphisms in the catalase gene with the risk of osteonecrosis of the femoral head in the Korean population. *Osteoarthritis Cartilage.* 2008;16(9):1060-1066.
29. Asano T, Takahashi KA, Fujioka M, et al. ABCB1 C3435T and G2677T/A polymorphism decreased the risk for steroid-induced osteonecrosis of the femoral head after kidney transplantation. *Pharmacogenetics.* 2003;13(11):675-682.
30. Pajaczkowski JA. The stubborn hip: idiopathic avascular necrosis of the hip. *J Manipulative Physiol Ther.* 2003;26(2):107.
31. Sugano N, Kubo T, Takaoka K, et al. Diagnostic criteria for non-traumatic osteonecrosis of the femoral head. A multicentre study. *J Bone Joint Surg Br.* 1999;81(4):590-595.
32. Kerboul M, Thomine J, Postel M, Merle d'Aubigne R. The conservative surgical treatment of idiopathic aseptic necrosis of the femoral head. *J Bone Joint Surg Br.* 1974;56(2):291-296.
33. Chen CH, Chang JK, Huang KY, Hung SH, Lin GT, Lin SY. Core decompression for osteonecrosis of the femoral head at pre-collapse stage. *Kaohsiung J Med Sci.* 2000;16(2):76-82.
34. Sekiya JK, Ruch DS, Hunter DM, et al. Hip arthroscopy in staging avascular necrosis of the femoral head. *J South Orthop Assoc.* 2000;9(4):254-261.
35. Ruch DS, Sekiya J, Dickson Schaefer W, Koman LA, Pope TL, Poehling GG. The role of hip arthroscopy in the evaluation of avascular necrosis. *Orthopedics.* 2001;24(4):339-343.
36. Ficat RP. Idiopathic bone necrosis of the femoral head. Early diagnosis and treatment. *J Bone Joint Surg Br.* 1985;67(1):3-9.

37. Steinberg ME, Hayken GD, Steinberg DR. A quantitative system for staging avascular necrosis. *J Bone Joint Surg Br.* 1995;77(1):34-41.
38. Gardeniers JWM. ARCO committee on terminology and staging (report from the Nijmegen meeting). *ARCO News Letter.* 1992;4:6.
39. Gardeniers JWM. Report of the committee of staging and nomenclature. *ARCO News Letter.* 1993;5:4.
40. Ohzono K, Saito M, Sugano N, Takaoka K, Ono K. The fate of nontraumatic avascular necrosis of the femoral head. A radiologic classification to formulate prognosis. *Clin Orthop Relat Res.* 1992(277):73-78.
41. Ohzono K, Saito M, Takaoka K, et al. Natural history of nontraumatic avascular necrosis of the femoral head. *J Bone Joint Surg Br.* 1991;73(1):68-72.
42. Sugioka Y. Transtrochanteric anterior rotational osteotomy of the femoral head in the treatment of osteonecrosis affecting the hip: a new osteotomy operation. *Clin Orthop Relat Res.* 1978(130):191-201.
43. Lafforgue P, Dahan E, Chagnaud C, Schiano A, Kasbarian M, Acquaviva PC. Early-stage avascular necrosis of the femoral head: MR imaging for prognosis in 31 cases with at least 2 years of follow-up. *Radiology.* 1993;187(1):199-204.
44. Koo KH, Kim R. Quantifying the extent of osteonecrosis of the femoral head. A new method using MRI. *J Bone Joint Surg Br.* 1995;77(6):875-880.
45. Theodorou DJ, Malizos KN, Beris AE, Theodorou SJ, Soucacos PN. Multimodal imaging quantitation of the lesion size in osteonecrosis of the femoral head. *Clin Orthop Relat Res.* 2001(386):54-63.
46. Atsumi T, Kuroki Y. Modified Sugioka's osteotomy: more than 130 degrees posterior rotation for osteonecrosis of the femoral head with large lesion. *Clin Orthop Relat Res.* 1997(334):98-107.
47. Shimizu K, Moriya H, Akita T, Sakamoto M, Suguro T. Prediction of collapse with magnetic resonance imaging of avascular necrosis of the femoral head. *J Bone Joint Surg Am.* 1994;76(2):215-223.
48. Knopp RH. Drug treatment of lipid disorders. *N Engl J Med.* 1999;341(7):498-511.
49. Mont MA, Jones LC, Seyler TM, Marulanda GA, Saleh KJ, Delanois RE. New treatment approaches for osteonecrosis of the femoral head: an overview. *Instr Course Lect.* 2007;56:197-212.
50. Mont MA, Carbone JJ, Fairbank AC. Core decompression versus nonoperative management for osteonecrosis of the hip. *Clin Orthop Relat Res.* 1996(324):169-178.
51. Ludwig J, Lauber S, Lauber HJ, Dreisilker U, Raedel R, Hotzinger H. High-energy shock wave treatment of femoral head necrosis in adults. *Clin Orthop Relat Res.* 2001(387):119-126.
52. Wang CJ, Wang FS, Huang CC, Yang KD, Weng LH, Huang HY. Treatment for osteonecrosis of the femoral head: comparison of extracorporeal shock waves with core decompression and bone-grafting. *J Bone Joint Surg Am.* 2005;87(11):2380-2387.
53. Massari L, Fini M, Cadossi R, Setti S, Traina GC. Biophysical stimulation with pulsed electromagnetic fields in osteonecrosis of the femoral head. *J Bone Joint Surg Am.* 2006;88(suppl 3):56-60.
54. Aaron RK, Lennox D, Bunce GE, Ebert T. The conservative treatment of osteonecrosis of the femoral head. A comparison of core decompression and pulsing electromagnetic fields. *Clin Orthop Relat Res.* 1989(249):209-218.
55. Steinberg ME, Brighton CT, Bands RE, Hartman KM. Capacitive coupling as an adjunctive treatment for avascular necrosis. *Clin Orthop Relat Res.* 1990(261):11-18.
56. Trancik T, Lunceford E, Strum D. The effect of electrical stimulation on osteonecrosis of the femoral head. *Clin Orthop Relat Res.* 1990(256):120-124.
57. Huang KC, Hsu WH, Peng KT, Huang TJ, Hsu RW. Hyperbaric oxygen therapy in orthopedic conditions: an evaluation of safety. *J Trauma.* 2006;61(4):913-917.
58. Ficat C. [Value of the functional investigation of the bone: intramedullary pressure measurement, trans-osseus phlebography and needle biopsy]. *Acta Orthop Belg.* 1999;65(suppl 1):35-44.
59. Hungerford DS. Bone marrow pressure, venography, and core decompression in isquemic necrosis of the femoral head. Paper presented at: The Hip: Proceedings of the Seventh Open Scientific Meeting of the Hip Society. 1979; St. Louis, MO.
60. Mont MA, Ragland PS, Etienne G. Core decompression of the femoral head for osteonecrosis using percutaneous multiple small-diameter drilling. *Clin Orthop Relat Res.* 2004(429):131-138.
61. Kim SY, Kim DH, Park IH, Park BC, Kim PT, Ihn JC. Multiple drilling compared with standard core decompression for the treatment of osteonecrosis of the femoral head. *J Bone Joint Surg Br.* 2004;86B(suppl):1.
62. Ganz R, Buchler U. Overview of attempts to revitalize the dead head in aseptic necrosis of the femoral head--osteotomy and revascularization. *Hip.* 1983:296-305.
63. Mont MA, Einhorn TA, Sponseller PD, Hungerford DS. The trapdoor procedure using autogenous cortical and cancellous bone grafts for osteonecrosis of the femoral head. *J Bone Joint Surg Br.* 1998;80(1):56-62.
64. Phemister DB. Treatment of the necrotic head of the femur in adults. *J Bone Joint Surg Am.* 1949;31A(1):55-66.
65. Merle D'Aubigne R, Postel M, Mazabraud A, Massias P, Gueguen J, France P. Idiopathic necrosis of the femoral head in adults. *J Bone Joint Surg Br.* 1965;47(4):612-633.
66. Rosenwasser MP, Garino JP, Kiernan HA, Michelsen CB. Long term followup of thorough debridement and cancellous bone grafting of the femoral head for avascular necrosis. *Clin Orthop Relat Res.* 1994(306):17-27.
67. Tsao AK, Roberson JR, Christie MJ, et al. Biomechanical and clinical evaluations of a porous tantalum implant for the treatment of early-stage osteonecrosis. *J Bone Joint Surg Am.* 2005;87(suppl 2):22-27.

68. Veillette CJ, Mehdian H, Schemitsch EH, McKee MD. Survivorship analysis and radiographic outcome following tantalum rod insertion for osteonecrosis of the femoral head. *J Bone Joint Surg Am.* 2006;88(suppl 3):48-55.
69. Floerkemeier T, Thorey F, Daentzer D, et al. Clinical and radiological outcome of the treatment of osteonecrosis of the femoral head using the osteonecrosis intervention implant. *Int Orthop.* 2010;35(4):489-495.
70. Tanzer M, Bobyn JD, Krygier JJ, Karabasz D. Histopathologic retrieval analysis of clinically failed porous tantalum osteonecrosis implants. *J Bone Joint Surg Am.* 2008;90(6):1282-1289.
71. Reddi AH, Huggins CB. Influence of geometry of transplanted tooth and bone on transformation of fibroblasts. *Proc Soc Exp Biol Med.* 1973;143(3):634-637.
72. Yang C, Yang SH, Du JY, Li J, Xu WH, Xiong YF. Basic fibroblast growth factor gene transfection to enhance the repair of avascular necrosis of the femoral head. *Chin Med Sci J.* 2004;19(2):111-115.
73. Gangji V, Hauzeur JP, Matos C, De Maertelaer V, Toungouz M, Lambermont M. Treatment of osteonecrosis of the femoral head with implantation of autologous bone-marrow cells. A pilot study. *J Bone Joint Surg Am.* 2004;86-A(6):1153-1160.
74. Hernigou P, Beaujean F. Treatment of osteonecrosis with autologous bone marrow grafting. *Clin Orthop Relat Res.* 2002(405):14-23.
75. Peterson B, Zhang J, Iglesias R, et al. Healing of critically sized femoral defects, using genetically modified mesenchymal stem cells from human adipose tissue. *Tissue Eng.* 2005;11(1-2):120-129.
76. Yang C, Yang S, Du J, Li J, Xu W, Xiong Y. Vascular endothelial growth factor gene transfection to enhance the repair of avascular necrosis of the femoral head of rabbit. *Chin Med J (Engl).* 2003;116(10):1544-1548.
77. Aldegheri R. Arthodiatasi d'anca. Ortopedia E *Traumatologia Ogg.* 1981;1:1.
78. Aldegheri R, Trivella G. L'artrodiatasi nel trattamento dell'anca rigida dopo epifisiolis. *Revista Italiana di Ortopediae Traumatologia Pediatrica.* 1985;1:1.
79. Dean MT, Cabanela ME. Transtrochanteric anterior rotational osteotomy for avascular necrosis of the femoral head. Long-term results. *J Bone Joint Surg Br.* 1993;75(4):597-601.
80. Kantor SG, Huo MH, Huk OL, Salvati EA. Cemented total hip arthroplasty in patients with osteonecrosis. A 6-year minimum follow-up study of second-generation cement techniques. *J Arthroplasty.* 1996;11(3):267-271.
81. Marcus ND, Enneking WF, Massam RA. The silent hip in idiopathic aseptic necrosis. Treatment by bone-grafting. *J Bone Joint Surg Am.* 1973;55(7):1351-1366.
82. Pritchett JW. Statins and dietary fish oils improve lipid composition in bone marrow and joints. *Clin Orthop Relat Res.* 2007;456:233-237.
83. Glueck CJ, Freiberg RA, Sieve L, Wang P. Enoxaparin prevents progression of stages I and II osteonecrosis of the hip. *Clin Orthop Relat Res.* 2005(435):164-170.
84. Disch AC, Matziolis G, Perka C. The management of necrosis-associated and idiopathic bone-marrow oedema of the proximal femur by intravenous iloprost. *J Bone Joint Surg Br.* 2005;87(4):560-564.
85. Ramachandran M, Ward K, Brown RR, Munns CF, Cowell CT, Little DG. Intravenous bisphosphonate therapy for traumatic osteonecrosis of the femoral head in adolescents. *J Bone Joint Surg Am.* 2007;89(8):1727-1734.
86. Nishii T, Sugano N, Miki H, Hashimoto J, Yoshikawa H. Does alendronate prevent collapse in osteonecrosis of the femoral head? *Clin Orthop Relat Res.* 2006;443:273-279.
87. Lai KA, Shen WJ, Yang CY, Shao CJ, Hsu JT, Lin RM. The use of alendronate to prevent early collapse of the femoral head in patients with nontraumatic osteonecrosis. A randomized clinical study. *J Bone Joint Surg Am.* 2005;87(10):2155-2159.
88. Agarwala S, Jain D, Joshi VR, Sule A. Efficacy of alendronate, a bisphosphonate, in the treatment of AVN of the hip. A prospective open-label study. *Rheumatology (Oxford).* 2005;44(3):352-359.
89. Radke S, Kirschner S, Seipel V, Rader C, Eulert J. Magnetic resonance imaging criteria of successful core decompression in avascular necrosis of the hip. *Skeletal Radiol.* 2004;33(9):519-523.
90. Yoon TR, Song EK, Rowe SM, Park CH. Failure after core decompression in osteonecrosis of the femoral head. *Int Orthop.* 2001;24(6):316-318.
91. Lieberman JR, Conduah A, Urist MR. Treatment of osteonecrosis of the femoral head with core decompression and human bone morphogenetic protein. *Clin Orthop Relat Res.* 2004(429):139-145.
92. Aigner N, Schneider W, Eberl V, Knahr K. Core decompression in early stages of femoral head osteonecrosis--an MRI-controlled study. *Int Orthop.* 2002;26(1):31-35.
93. Simank HG, Brocai DR, Brill C, Lukoschek M. Comparison of results of core decompression and intertrochanteric osteotomy for nontraumatic osteonecrosis of the femoral head using Cox regression and survivorship analysis. *J Arthroplasty.* 2001;16(6):790-794.
94. Steinberg ME, Larcom PG, Strafford B, et al. Core decompression with bone grafting for osteonecrosis of the femoral head. *Clin Orthop Relat Res.* 2001(386):71-78.
95. Maniwa S, Nishikori T, Furukawa S, et al. Evaluation of core decompression for early osteonecrosis of the femoral head. *Arch Orthop Trauma Surg.* 2000;120(5-6):241-244.
96. Lavernia CJ, Sierra RJ. Core decompression in atraumatic osteonecrosis of the hip. *J Arthroplasty.* 2000;15(2):171-178.
97. Keizer SB, Kock NB, Dijkstra PD, Taminiau AH, Nelissen RG. Treatment of avascular necrosis of the hip by a non-vascularised cortical graft. *J Bone Joint Surg Br.* 2006;88(4):460-466.
98. Israelite C, Nelson CL, Ziarani CF, Abboud JA, Landa J, Steinberg ME. Bilateral core decompression for osteonecrosis of the femoral head. *Clin Orthop Relat Res.* 2005;441:285-290.

99. Kim SY, Kim YG, Kim PT, Ihn JC, Cho BC, Koo KH. Vascularized compared with nonvascularized fibular grafts for large osteonecrotic lesions of the femoral head. *J Bone Joint Surg Am.* 2005;87(9):2012-2018.
100. Rijnen WH, Gardeniers JW, Buma P, Yamano K, Slooff TJ, Schreurs BW. Treatment of femoral head osteonecrosis using bone impaction grafting. *Clin Orthop Relat Res.* 2003(417):74-83.
101. Plakseychuk AY, Kim SY, Park BC, Varitimidis SE, Rubash HE, Sotereanos DG. Vascularized compared with nonvascularized fibular grafting for the treatment of osteonecrosis of the femoral head. *J Bone Joint Surg Am.* 2003;85-A(4):589-596.
102. Mont MA, Etienne G, Ragland PS. Outcome of nonvascularized bone grafting for osteonecrosis of the femoral head. *Clin Orthop Relat Res.* 2003(417):84-92.
103. Ko JY, Meyers MH, Wenger DR. "Trapdoor" procedure for osteonecrosis with segmental collapse of the femoral head in teenagers. *J Pediatr Orthop.* 1995;15(1):7-15.
104. Seyler TM, Marker DR, Ulrich SD, Fatscher T, Mont MA. Nonvascularized Bone Grafting Defers Joint Arthroplasty in Hip Osteonecrosis. *Clin Orthop Relat Res.* 2008;466(5):1125-1132.
105. Roush TF, Olson SA, Pietrobon R, Braga L, Urbaniak JR. Influence of acetabular coverage on hip survival after free vascularized fibular grafting for femoral head osteonecrosis. *J Bone Joint Surg Am.* 2006;88(10):2152-2158.
106. Yen CY, Tu YK, Ma CH, Yu SW, Kao FC, Lee MS. Osteonecrosis of the femoral head: comparison of clinical results for vascularized iliac and fibula bone grafting. *J Reconstr Microsurg.* 2006;22(1):21-24.
107. Stubbs AJ, Gunneson EB, Urbaniak JR. Pediatric femoral avascular necrosis after pyarthrosis: use of free vascularized fibular grafting. *Clin Orthop Relat Res.* 2005;439:193-200.
108. Marciniak D, Furey C, Shaffer JW. Osteonecrosis of the femoral head. A study of 101 hips treated with vascularized fibular grafting. *J Bone Joint Surg Am.* 2005;87(4):742-747.
109. Nakamura Y, Kumazawa Y, Mitsui H, Toh S, Katano H. Combined rotational osteotomy and vascularized iliac bone graft for advanced osteonecrosis of the femoral head. *J Reconstr Microsurg.* 2005;21(2):101-105.
110. Matsusaki H, Noguchi M, Kawakami T, Tani T. Use of vascularized pedicle iliac bone graft combined with transtrochanteric rotational osteotomy in the treatment of avascular necrosis of the femoral head. *Arch Orthop Trauma Surg.* 2005;125(2):95-101.
111. Yoon TR, Abbas AA, Hur CI, Cho SG, Lee JH. Modified transtrochanteric rotational osteotomy for femoral head osteonecrosis. *Clin Orthop Relat Res.* 2008;466(5):1110-1116.
112. Sugioka Y, Yamamoto T. Transtrochanteric posterior rotational osteotomy for osteonecrosis. *Clin Orthop Relat Res.* 2008;466(5):1104-1109.
113. Ikemura S, Yamamoto T, Jingushi S, Nakashima Y, Mawatari T, Iwamoto Y. Use of a screw and plate system for a transtrochanteric anterior rotational osteotomy for osteonecrosis of the femoral head. *J Orthop Sci.* 2007;12(3):260-264.
114. Onodera S, Majima T, Abe Y, Ito H, Matsuno T, Minami A. Transtrochanteric rotational osteotomy for osteonecrosis of the femoral head: relation between radiographic features and secondary collapse. *J Orthop Sci.* 2005;10(4):367-373.
115. Rijnen WH, Gardeniers JW, Westrek BL, Buma P, Schreurs BW. Sugioka's osteotomy for femoral-head necrosis in young Caucasians. *Int Orthop.* 2005;29(3):140-144.
116. Tsumura H, Torisu T, Kaku N, Higashi T. Five- to fifteen-year clinical results and the radiographic evaluation of acetabular changes after bipolar hip arthroplasty for femoral head osteonecrosis. *J Arthroplasty.* 2005;20(7):892-897.
117. Yamano K, Atsumi T, Kajwara T. Bipolar endoprosthesis for osteonecrosis of the femoral head: a 7- to 18-year followup. *ARCO Transactions.* 2004.
118. Lee SB, Sugano N, Nakata K, Matsui M, Ohzono K. Comparison between bipolar hemiarthroplasty and THA for osteonecrosis of the femoral head. *Clin Orthop Relat Res.* 2004(424):161-165.
119. Nagai I, Takatori Y, Kuruta Y, et al. Nonself-centering Bateman bipolar endoprosthesis for nontraumatic osteonecrosis of the femoral head: a 12- to 18-year follow-up study. *J Orthop Sci.* 2002;7(1):74-78.
120. Cuckler JM, Moore KD, Estrada L. Outcome of hemiresurfacing in osteonecrosis of the femoral head. *Clin Orthop Relat Res.* 2004(429):146-150.
121. Beaule PE, Amstutz HC, Le Duff M, Dorey F. Surface arthroplasty for osteonecrosis of the hip: hemiresurfacing versus metal-on-metal hybrid resurfacing. *J Arthroplasty.* 2004;19(8 suppl 3):54-58.
122. Adili A, Trousdale RT. Femoral head resurfacing for the treatment of osteonecrosis in the young patient. *Clin Orthop Relat Res.* 2003(417):93-101.
123. Schneider W, Knahr K. Total hip replacement in younger patients: survival rate after avascular necrosis of the femoral head. *Acta Orthop Scand.* 2004;75(2):142-146.
124. Kim YH, Oh SH, Kim JS, Koo KH. Contemporary total hip arthroplasty with and without cement in patients with osteonecrosis of the femoral head. *J Bone Joint Surg Am.* 2003;85-A(4):675-681.
125. Berend KR, Gunneson E, Urbaniak JR, Vail TP. Hip arthroplasty after failed free vascularized fibular grafting for osteonecrosis in young patients. *J Arthroplasty.* 2003;18(4):411-419.
126. Al-Mousawi F, Malki A, Al-Aradi A, Al-Bagali M, Al-Sadadi A, Booz MM. Total hip replacement in sickle cell disease. *Int Orthop.* 2002;26(3):157-161.
127. Fyda TM, Callaghan JJ, Olejniczak J, Johnston RC. Minimum ten-year follow-up of cemented total hip replacement in patients with osteonecrosis of the femoral head. *Iowa Orthop J.* 2002;22:8-19.
128. Xenakis TA, Gelalis J, Koukoubis TA, Zaharis KC, Soucacos PN. Cementless hip arthroplasty in the treatment of patients with femoral head necrosis. *Clin Orthop Relat Res.* 2001(386):93-99.

129. Taylor AH, Shannon M, Whitehouse SL, Lee MB, Learmonth ID. Harris Galante cementless acetabular replacement in avascular necrosis. *J Bone Joint Surg Br.* 2001;83(2):177-182.

130. Delank KS, Drees P, Eckardt A, Heine J. [Results of the uncemented total hip arthroplasty in avascular necrosis of the femoral head]. *Z Orthop Ihre Grenzgeb.* 2001;139(6):525-530.

131. Hartley WT, McAuley JP, Culpepper WJ, Engh CA Jr, Engh CA Sr. Osteonecrosis of the femoral head treated with cementless total hip arthroplasty. *J Bone Joint Surg Am.* 2000;82-A(10):1408-1413.

132. Zangger P, Gladman DD, Urowitz MB, Bogoch ER. Outcome of total hip replacement for avascular necrosis in systemic lupus erythematosus. *J Rheumatol.* 2000;27(4):919-923.

133. Mont MA, Seyler TM, Marker DR, Marulanda GA, Delanois RE. Use of metal-on-metal total hip resurfacing for the treatment of osteonecrosis of the femoral head. *J Bone Joint Surg Am.* 2006;88(suppl 3):90-97.

134. Amstutz HC, Beaule PE, Dorey FJ, Le Duff MJ, Campbell PA, Gruen TA. Metal-on-metal hybrid surface arthroplasty: two to six-year follow-up study. *J Bone Joint Surg Am.* 2004;86-A(1):28-39.

135. Mohamad JA, Kwan MK, Merican AM, et al. Early results of metal on metal articulation total hip arthroplasty in young patients. *Med J Malaysia.* 2004;59(suppl F):3-7.

136. Yoo TC. Results of metal-on-metal resurfacing for avascular necrosis of the femoral head. *ARCO Transactions.* 2005.

25

Developmental Dysplasia of the Hip

Khalid M. Yousuf, MD, MS and Javad Parvizi, MD, FRCS

Developmental dysplasia of the hip (DDH) is one of the leading secondary causes of osteoarthritis in the young hip. Most orthopedic surgeons in training first encounter the term *DDH* in their pediatric rotations. Physicians are trained to examine the newborn hip for laxity and this is the best screening test for dysplastic hips. The term *dysplasia* implies abnormal development. In the dysplastic hip, we find that the relationship between the femoral head and acetabulum is abnormal. An abnormal relationship causes the acetabulum to be shallow and wider. The abnormal femoral head is usually smaller, the neck shaft angle is in more valgus, and the neck is more anteverted. The preferred term *developmental dysplasia* has replaced congenital dysplasia as we understand the dynamic relationship of the femoral head and acetabulum spans beyond the intrauterine period. The dysplastic hip can be associated with many congenital disorders, most commonly congenital hip dysplasia, slipped capital femoral epiphysis, and Legg-Calvé-Perthes disease.

Evaluation of the adult patient with a dysplastic hip involves appropriate imaging and a thorough history and physical. Understanding the main complaints of the patient will guide treatment. In light of the fact that most patients are young and active and want to continue this lifestyle, one must understand the options available. Nonarthroplasty options (ie, osteotomies) exist to treat the associated pain and degenerative changes yet allow for a more active lifestyle. Recognizing dysplasia early may provide the patient with this option, which could lead to additional pain-free productive years. Frequently, the surgeon encounters a patient where osteotomies are not an option and joint replacement in this young patient has to be discussed. The surgeon has to pay special consideration to the dysplastic hip when planning a total hip arthroplasty (THA). Cases with a mild deformity may be approached like most other degenerative hips. Yet the dysplastic hip complicated by leg length discrepancies, abductor dysfunction, proximal femoral deformities, and gross anatomical distortion need to be addressed meticulously. This chapter will discuss many of these considerations as well as the natural history and complications.

Etiology, Incidence, and Risk Factors

Aggressive evaluation by pediatricians, improved diagnostic imaging, and increased awareness by parents has helped decrease the catastrophic sequelae of the dislocated hip. Fortunately, most newborns found to have hip instability will require no form of treatment. This physiologic laxity resolves in a matter of weeks and the hip develops normally. Dislocated hips are seen at a rate of 1 to 1.5 of 1000 live births. The etiology of DDH is multifactorial, including genetic, intrauterine, geographic, ethnic, and cultural factors. The incidence of DDH in European countries is higher while it is rare in the Chinese and African populations. In the Native American population, swaddling of the infant has been blamed for the higher incidence of DDH.

A positive family history is found in up to one-third of the cases. The most at-risk combination is a first-born

Parvizi J, Klatt BA.
Essentials in Total Hip Arthroplasty (pp 215-222).

female in breech presentation. Cases of DDH are found in females 80% of the time; 60% involve the left hip and up to 25% of the patients presented in a breech position. DDH has been associated with intrauterine crowding and logically there is increased correlation among cases of torticollis, talipes calcaneovalgus, and metatarsus adductus.

Pathophysiology and Natural History

Development of the newborn hip revolves around the dynamic relationship between the femoral head and the acetabulum. The contact between the femoral head and the triradiate cartilage helps deepen the acetabulum. The triradiate cartilage grows by interstitial growth and concentric formation relies on the presence of a spherical femoral head. Proximal femoral growth centers and the pull of the musculature on the proximal femur help shape a spherical femoral head. The majority of the dysplasia occurs on the acetabular side. The femoral dysplasia is usually secondary to abnormal contact between the ilium and femoral head.

When considering the anatomic changes with the dysplastic hip, one must consider abductor function, bone stock on the pelvic and femoral sides, and maintenance of overall normal anatomy and version. Occasionally, in a dysplastic hip these factors are not grossly distorted and reconstruction of the hip can be straightforward. To classify the radiographs and to plan surgical options, understanding these anatomic changes becomes very important. Some common characteristics of DDH are a shallow, anteverted acetabulum. The anterior rim may be hypoplastic. The femoral head is usually smaller and the neck is anteverted. The greater trochanter may be displaced posteriorly, causing contraction of the rotator muscles. With the dislocated hip, one must consider the false acetabulum and the bone stock present to position the reconstructed acetabulum. Reconstruction of the hip should be aimed at restoring normal anatomy. As the acetabulum is reconstructed, the femur also needs to be evaluated. Leg lengths should be measured preoperatively. These measurements may change based on the planned surgical procedures, and meticulous preoperative planning will help avoid any unexpected results. These anatomic distortions can vary and every dysplastic hip has a unique presentation.

The prognosis of untreated hips depends on 2 independent factors: bilaterality and the presence of a false acetabulum. If both hips are involved, patients may actually do well from a functional standpoint and usually do not need surgical intervention until their 60s. The presence of a false acetabulum from the articulation of the dislocated head on the ilium usually results in the need for early surgical intervention secondary to the degenerative changes. The mechanical and anatomical axes may be altered in patients with a dislocated hip. This can cause multiple other problems such as back pain, scoliosis, ipsilateral knee degeneration, and limb length discrepancies. The rate of deterioration has been linked to the degree of subluxation and the age of the patient.

History and Physical Examination

Gathering relevant history is important and key points to include are birth history, neuromuscular diseases, inflammatory disorders, steroid medication usage, and trauma. Previously we discussed the epidemiological factors in DDH. Dysplastic hips have been associated with cerebral palsy. History of previous trauma and/or surgeries may influence future surgical intervention. Painful activities, the age of the patient, and expectations of the patient will play a vital role as the treatment options are discussed.

Patients with dysplastic hips will usually complain of activity-related pain. This pain may be localized laterally from abductor fatigue or in the groin from acetabular/labral pathology. A differential diagnosis should include femoroacetabular impingement syndrome, labral pathology, cartilage damage, and dysplasia.

Physical examination should begin as the patient walks into the clinic. Gait disturbances may indicate a chronic condition due to muscular atrophy, ipsilateral knee or back problems, or neuromuscular disease. The abductor function should be evaluated with the Trendelenburg sign. Quadriceps size and strength should be documented. The patient should be evaluated in the supine position and the natural lay of the extremities should be noted. The amount of internal or external rotation can indicate abnormal version at the proximal femur or development of osteoarthritis. Leg lengths should be evaluated and a discrepancy may be noted even with bilateral disease. During range of motion testing, the examiner should note if the patient has pain, mechanical symptoms, and/or limitations. Painful mechanical symptoms can indicate labral pathology. Snapping in the anteromedial thigh/hip may indicate the iliopsoas tendon is slipping over the trochanter. With internal rotation, the snapping of the psoas tendon should disappear. A snapping psoas tendon warrants a radiographic work-up since it may be caused by a proximal femoral abnormality as part of hip dysplasia. Progression of the arthritic changes will manifest as a loss of motion. Testing of abduction and adduction with the hip flexed versus extending can help isolate the pathology. With hip flexion, abduction is not limited by the greater trochanter whereas in extension, the greater trochanter can impinge on the ilium. One must evaluate the hip for the presence of impingement and instability. The impingement test involves flexing the hip to 90 degrees and adducting to 15 degrees. In this position, if the hip is internally rotated, the anterior aspect of the femoral neck impinges on the acetabular rim. Pain can indicate labral pathology. Another cause of pain with this maneuver is excessive wear of the anterior acetabulum (acetabulum rim syndrome) seen in a dysplastic acetabulum. Apprehension testing implies anterior instability. To do an apprehension test, externally rotate and hyperextend the hip. This maneuver will load the anterior rim of the acetabulum. If there is significant uncovering of the acetabulum, this should produce a sense of instability, or "apprehension." The pressure exerted by the femoral head may even be palpable in a thin patient. This patient may never complain that his or her hip is unstable, but instead may give the history of falls and giving away of the leg.

Diagnostic Imaging and Classification

Once there is a working diagnosis of acetabular dysplasia, the patient should get appropriate imaging. Despite the availability of advance imaging, the initial study should be routine radiographs. Many patients may be referred to the clinic with non-weight-bearing anteroposterior (AP) and lateral views, which are inadequate. To evaluate the dysplastic hip, the ideal views should be a standing AP, a false profile lateral, and an abduction view. One must always remember why films are ordered; these films will help the surgeon decide if the patient has a significant amount of degeneration and if the patient is a candidate for an osteotomy. On the standing AP view, the hip can be evaluated as it bears weight. Any joint narrowing can be appreciated as well as evaluating the pelvis as a whole. Shenton's line can be traced; any disruption would indicate acetabular dysplasia, hip subluxation, and therefore a poorer prognosis. This line is drawn along the superior border of the obturator foramen and the inferior aspect of the femoral neck. The acetabular index indicates the amount of acetabulum available for weight transfer. The center edge angle is formed by a line drawn from the center of the femoral head to the edge of the acetabular roof. An angle measuring less than 20 degrees indicates severe dysplasia. Similarly, the Tonnis angle, between the horizontal line from the medial edge of the weight-bearing portion of the acetabulum to the lateral edge of the acetabulum, indicates the steepness of the acetabulum. A measurement greater than 10 degrees indicates dysplasia. The femoral head extrusion index is the percentage of uncovered femoral head. The ratio is calculated by measuring the horizontal distance between the lateral femoral head and the lateral rim of the acetabulum. This value is divided by the horizontal distance between the medial and lateral femoral head. The normal value is less than 25%. Acetabular version can be inferred by looking for the crossover sign. If the anterior and posterior rims cross ("crossover sign"), the acetabulum is retroverted. To evaluate the lateral hip joint, a false profile view should be obtained. It is obtained at 60 degrees to the patient, unlike a Judet view, which is at 45 degrees. This view will provide an understanding of under coverage of the anterior femoral head. A good false profile view will show both femoral heads on the film with 4 finger breadth distance between the heads. The internal rotation abduction view is also a unique view for the evaluation of a hypoplastic acetabulum. This view is critical in preoperative planning for a periacetabular osteotomy. With the hip maximally abducted, the femoral head should be concentric within the acetabulum. This view gives the surgeon an idea of how much correction is attainable with an osteotomy.

Advanced imaging can aide with preoperative planning. Three-dimensional reconstructions using computed tomography (CT) scan can provide a better understanding of the anatomical changes. Magnetic resonance imaging (MRI) can be used with or without intra-articular contrast to evaluate the soft tissue component, including labral pathology.

Many classification systems are available to discuss the severity of the dysplastic hip. Each system has its limitations and a universally accepted system has not yet been developed. The classification system developed by Crowe classifies the degree of dysplasia. There are 4 types, I to IV, that classify the amount of proximal migration of the femoral head. The true acetabular height is defined as 20% of the total pelvic height. The vertical subluxation is calculated by measuring the vertical distance from the teardrops to the head-neck junction. In a normal hip, this should be at the same level. The degree of subluxation is calculated as a percentage of vertical subluxation over true acetabular height. This ratio represents the amount of superior migration in reference to pelvic height. Type I represents subluxation of the femoral head less than 50% out of the true acetabulum. Type II has migrated 50% to 74%, type III has migrated 75% to 100% out of the true acetabulum, and type IV hips are completely dislocated.

Table 25-1 shows the Hartofilakidis classification. As in all classification systems there is some degree of interobserver variability, and the Crowe classification system is

Table 25-1

HARTOFILAKIDIS CLASSIFICATION

Type 1	Femoral head is contained within the true acetabulum
Type 2	Femoral head articulates with false acetabulum (the false acetabulum inferior border overlaps the superior aspect of the true acetabulum)
Type 3	Femoral head has no contact with the acetabulum

used more commonly. One should be aware of these other systems since survivability data in the literature may reference these systems.

TREATMENT OPTIONS

Nonoperative

Treatment of a dysplastic hip requires patient education of the underlying pathology. Once the patient understands the pathophysiology, treatment with conservative measures will have a realistic expectation of success and effectiveness. Treatment options are similar to the options available for degenerative osteoarthritis and have a similar degree of success. Nonsteroidal anti-inflammatory medications, steroid injections, and even synthetic synovial fluid injections can be considered. The expectations of the physician and patient are to achieve pain control. The most important aspect of nonsurgical management in a young patient with a painful dysplastic hip is activity modification. Understanding what causes the pain and avoiding it may be the best modality to prolong the time until surgical intervention is necessary.

Surgical Options

Surgical options available to patients include arthroscopy, arthrodesis, osteotomy, and arthroplasty. Most patients will have to consider one of 2 options: arthroplasty or osteotomy. In a young patient with minimal degeneration, osteotomies are a good option and may allow the patient to maintain an active lifestyle. Joint replacement can provide a significant amount of pain relief but in a young patient this option may limit activities and lead to future surgery. Numerous biomechanical and clinical studies have shown us that the natural history of untreated dysplasia leads to osteoarthritis. Any surgery to delay or inhibit this progression is an option for the patient.

ARTHROSCOPY

Hip arthroscopy has an evolving list of indications as surgical techniques and instrumentation improve. Arthroscopy is used commonly to assess and treat labral pathology. McCarthy arthroscopically treated 170 dysplastic hips and found approximately 60% to have anterior labral tears, 60% to have anterior acetabular chondral injury, and 30% to have femoral chondral injury. From this group of patients, 10% with moderate dysplasia and 3% with mild dysplasia had to be converted to a THA at an average of 2.5 years.[1] Arthroscopic treatment of chondral and labral injuries can provide symptom relief. The first step in the development of osteoarthritis in the dysplastic hip is believed to be fatiguing of the labrum. The main goals of arthroscopic interventions are pain control, restoration of function, and prolonging arthroplasty.

RESECTION ARTHROPLASTY AND FUSION

Resection arthroplasty and arthrodesis are rarely indicated but in a patient who is not a candidate for other surgical intervention (arthroplasty, osteotomy) these procedures can provide pain relief. The physician and patient need to discuss the functional limitation that results from these procedures. Arthrodesis is contraindicated if bilateral disease is present. The major consequence of a fusion procedure is the limitation in motion and development of secondary osteoarthritis in the lumbar spine and knee. Similarly, with resection arthroplasty, goals are to provide pain relief in a patient who is not a candidate for the other mentioned procedures. Leg length discrepancy and weakness of the extremity is anticipated. The patient will require a walker to aide with ambulation.

OSTEOTOMIES

Restoring the rotation and anatomy of the dysplastic hip is the goal of the osteotomy whether it is a pelvic, femoral, or combination osteotomy. Restoring near normal anatomy may prolong the development of degenerative osteoarthritis for decades, leading to improved function and less pain. In a dysplastic hip the contact surface area of the acetabulum is usually decreased, and the contact area increases by rotating the acetabulum and restoring many of the radiographic angles. This is expected to decrease the pain and protect the cartilage in the hip joint. Pelvic and femoral osteotomies are indicated in patients with minimal degenerative changes.

The Tonnis system classifies osteoarthritic changes seen on radiographs. In Tonnis grade 3 or severe disease the joint is collapsed and has end-stage degenerative changes. Most studies in the literature reference this system, and have found longevity of the pelvic osteotomies in the lower Tonnis grades. Pelvic osteotomies can be either salvage or reconstructive. Salvage osteotomies are indicated in patients for pain relief; the joint congruity cannot be restored in these patients. In a reconstructive osteotomy the goal is to restore near normal acetabular anatomy and therefore improve hip biomechanics and prevent degenerative changes. Candidates for reconstructive osteotomies should have near normal range of motion, minimal degenerative changes, and be young. The Bernese periacetabular osteotomy (PAO) is preferred by most North American surgeons. Femoral osteotomies may be added to pelvic osteotomies if more correction is needed.

Bernese Periacetabular Osteotomy

The PAO, a reconstructive osteotomy popularized by Dr. Reinhold Ganz, is preferred by many surgeons for many reasons. The advantages of this procedure are that it requires a single incision and is performed with straight cuts, which are extra-articular and reproducible. Once combined, these cuts allow for a large amount of correction of the acetabulum. The posterior column is left intact and this adds to the inherent stability of the procedure, requiring minimal hardware for fixation and early mobilization. The shape of the pelvis remains unchanged and in comparison to other osteotomies, the PAO allows for a normal vaginal delivery in women. Lastly, THA after PAO has not been reported to be a problem technically.

Different surgical approaches have been described for the PAO. The exposure described here begins with a modified Smith-Petersen approach. The skin incision begins 8 to 10 cm proximal to the anterior-superior iliac spine (ASIS) and follows the iliac crest. It extends distally and laterally to end a few centimeters distal to the greater trochanter. The internervous plane is between the sartorius and tensor fascia lata. The origin of the sartorius is released off the ASIS and taken medially. The hip is then adducted and flexed to allow access to the inner table of the pelvis. The soft tissue can be stripped using a periosteal elevator. The periosteum on the inner table is usually very thick and should be elevated to help mobilize the osteotomized fragment. The rectus muscle should be cut to expose the joint capsule. The soft tissue is retracted and the pubis bone is exposed. The ischium can be palpated through the capsular incision. This incision can be extended to help with this exposure. Care should be taken not to place any retractors distal to the obturator externus to protect the medial femoral circumflex artery. Now the anterior aspect of the hip should be exposed. The ischium is osteotomized first. Fluoroscopy can be used to guide the osteotomy. This cut should be angled approximately 25 degrees posterosuperiorly. Curved retractors are placed superiorly and inferiorly around the pubic rami to protect the obturator nerve. The pubic rami cut should be angled 45 degrees toward the midline. The last osteotomy is started between the ASIS and the anterior-inferior iliac spine (AIIS). The cut is advanced up to 1 cm of the pelvic brim and then the fourth and final cut is angled toward the ischial spine. This part of the cut should be parallel to the posterior column. A Schanz pin can be inserted into the AIIS to help mobilize the osteotomized fragment. The fragment should be positioned to provide adequate coverage, and then provisionally fixed with Kirschner wires. An AP view should be obtained intraoperatively to assess the amount of correction obtained. The roof should be horizontal, the femoral head congruent, Shenton's line should be restored, and the anterior acetabular rim should cover less of the femoral head than the posterior rim for the correction to be considered a success. The acetabular fragment is stabilized using 4.5-mm cortical screws. One screw starts in the ASIS while the other in the AIIS, both stabilizing the fragment. A third screw is placed in an anterior to posterior direction to provide additional control. Closure should be done in a routine fashion over a drain.

Postoperatively, weight bearing should be limited for 8 weeks with a goal of full release by 3 months. Abduction and hip flexion exercises are started at 6 weeks. Prophylaxis for heterotopic ossification and deep vein thrombosis is usually surgeon and patient dependent.

Dr. Ganz has recently published his 20-year follow-up on his original patients. He found that 60% of the hips were preserved at 20 years and 38% had been converted to THA at a mean of 11.7 years. These data show that the PAO has good long-term survivability. They also concluded that patients that did worse were older than 30, were more symptomatic preoperatively (based on clinical scores), had preoperative osteoarthritis (Tonnis grade 2), and a radiographic extrusion index greater than 20%. Future prospective studies may help us further delineate how long the patient may have good function before needing a hip replacement.

The most common complication is lateral femoral cutaneous nerve palsy. This procedure has a steep learning curve and complications in the initial period may include intra-articular extension of the osteotomy, extension into the posterior column, and devascularization of the osteotomized fragment. As technique improves, these complications should decrease. Nonunion has been reported but most are asymptomatic and do not require additional surgery.

Chiari Osteotomy

The Chiari osteotomy is a salvage procedure and has been referred to as a capsular arthroplasty. The femoral head articulates with an interposed surface of joint capsule and underlying cancellous bone. The procedure is indicated in a hip with an incongruent joint but with minimal degenerative changes. The main goal of the procedure is to increase abduction motion and to relieve pain. Unlike other osteotomies, the Chiari osteotomy can be performed in children and in adults. The procedure has a limited lifespan and outcomes are better in younger patients. The outcome is reported to be 10 to 15 years.[2]

Femoral Osteotomies

Femoral osteotomies are indicated when the disease primarily involves the proximal femur (avascular necrosis, slipped capital femoral epiphysis, Legg-Calvé-Perthes disease) or if more correction is required after an acetabular osteotomy. Femoral osteotomies are performed in tandem with approximately 21% of periacetabular osteotomies.[3] In a dysplastic hip, an isolated femoral osteotomy may be indicated if the patient has severe coxa valga with mild acetabular deformity. In this case, a varus-producing osteotomy can increase the congruity at the joint. This osteotomy can decrease the amount of femoral head extrusion and decrease the joint reactive forces by medializing center of rotation. Pellicci followed patients with dysplastic hips who had a varus osteotomy for a mean of 9 years. He found that 13% were converted to THA in that period.[4] The results of the same cohort were presented 16 years later, with data available for 83% of the patients. Among these patients, 35% did not require additional surgeries at 21 years follow-up. The rest (65%) required total hip replacement after 9.7 years on average (range 2 to 27 years post osteotomy). The authors conclude that younger patients with minimal hip subluxation and osteoarthritis are better candidates for this procedure.[5] Other authors have described that, using a Harris hip score of less than 70 points or additional surgery as endpoint; the cumulative rates of survival for varus intertrochanteric osteotomy were 81% at 10 years, 60% at 20 years, and 50% at 25 years. They emphasized that this procedure is not indicated in grade 3 osteoarthritis or for those patients with severe acetabular dysplasia.[6]

Valgus osteotomy is indicated for disability caused by superolateral or medial sided osteoarthritis of the femoral head. Sufficient range of motion preoperatively is necessary for a good functional arc of motion after surgery. This osteotomy is preferred in the dysplastic hips with a medial femoral head osteophytes, or "capital drop," since it will rotate the medial osteophytes into a weight-bearing portion of the joint. This will increase joint congruity and decrease joint reactive forces. The entire extremity should be evaluated when planning a valgus osteotomy. The residual limb is lengthened after the osteotomy and this can have its own sequelae. Also, the mechanical axis at the knee is shifted laterally, which may lead to degeneration of the knee.

Total Hip Arthroplasty

Many surgical alternatives to arthroplasty exist but once exhausted, arthroplasty provides a good surgical option. THA in a dysplastic hip can be a standard procedure but it can also require bone grafting and osteotomies depending on the amount of anatomical variation. The Crowe classification system provides a treatment guideline as well as a systematic method of categorizing dysplastic hip.[4] Anatomical considerations in THA of the dysplastic hip include leg length discrepancies, contraction of the soft tissue, and alteration in normal anatomy. These changes can make the exposure more difficult.

The patient should be evaluated and details in regards to joint arthroplasty discussed. Indications for the procedure include pain and dysfunction. Appropriate imaging should be obtained to evaluate the degree of osteoarthritis and dysplasia. The Crowe classification can help categorize the dysplastic hip and help guide surgical treatment. In general, Crowe I and IV hips are not as degenerative as Crowe II and III hips; therefore, they do not require THA at such an early age.

Preoperative planning should be very detailed when planning a THA in a dysplastic hip. Considerations include leg length discrepancies, pre-existing deformity, previous surgical scars, planned surgical incision and approach, and pelvic bone stock. Conventional anterolateral or posterior approaches can be utilized for most dysplastic hips. Crowe IV hips may require an extensile transtrochanteric approach for adequate acetabular exposure. Current recommendations are to approach the acetabulum and femur individually. For the acetabulum, the pre-existing bone stock is of utmost importance. Special components are available for dysplastic hips. Templating preoperatively will help decide if these smaller implants need to be available. On the femoral side, plans should account for limb shortening, intramedullary canal diameter, and implant fixation.

Hips classified as Crowe I can usually be reconstructed with standard components. Occasionally, the acetabular component may need to be medialized to improve lateral coverage. Since the deformity on the acetabular side is relatively minor, leg lengths usually are stable and femoral osteotomies are rarely needed. The use of cemented versus uncemented components is surgeon dependent. Uncemented stems are preferred if the patient is young. Modular components are usually preferred in dysplastic hip surgery to allow for individualized anatomy.

Most of the THA procedures performed in dysplastic hips are classified as Crowe II or III. These hips have increasing amounts of femoral head subluxation and have developed lateral acetabular erosion. These hips also develop secondary degeneration and alteration of the femoral head. Reconstruction of the acetabulum in this case requires consideration of the pre-existing bone stock. This usually means using a small acetabular component at the site of the true acetabulum. The trend is to secure the component with screws. If there is a significant portion of the component that is uncovered, reconstruction will need to be augmented and/or placed in a nonanatomic position. Three techniques in acetabular reconstruction are superior lateral bone grafting, high hip center reconstruction, and medialization of the acetabular component.

Superior lateral bone grafting is usually performed using femoral head autograft. The graft is fixed in place and is buttressed between the pelvis and component. Femoral head autograft incorporation is usually very successful and this helps support the newly implanted component and also can improve bone stock in the case of a revision. When it is not possible to reconstruct the acetabulum in the anatomic position, the component can be placed in a superior position (high hip center) against good native bone. A concern with this technique is that the biomechanics have been altered and this can lead to early failure of the component. Medialization of the acetabulum is a third technique to help reconstruct the acetabulum. By moving the center of hip rotation medially the joint reactive forces are decreased, but the main disadvantage is that revision surgery may be more difficult.

Femoral reconstruction of Crowe II or III hips is addressed similar to Crowe I. If the reconstructed acetabulum is far removed from the false acetabulum, it results in an increased leg length and a femoral shortening osteotomy should be considered. Without shortening the femur it may be difficult to reduce the prosthetic femoral head and a significant leg length discrepancy may occur. The end result should be to lengthen the extremity as little as possible to minimize the risk of sciatic nerve palsy.

Crowe IV hips usually have good residual bone at the true acetabulum. Reconstruction with a small dysplastic acetabulum component can restore the anatomic hip center. The bone may be soft and care should be taken while reaming the socket. Femoral reconstruction principles are similar to that in Crowe II and III hips. If the leg is significantly lengthened as the acetabulum is reconstructed, a femoral osteotomy should be considered.

Long-term follow-up studies have confirmed a higher rate of complications and failures in THA for a dysplastic hip compared to a degenerative hip.[7,8] Complications that have been reported with higher rates in dysplastic hips include sciatic nerve palsy, dislocation after primary reconstruction, intraoperative femur fracture, and infection.[7,9-11]

Summary

DDH is the leading cause of secondary osteoarthritis in the adult hip. Understanding the underlying anatomic changes and performing a thorough work-up will guide the patient and surgeon down a logical treatment algorithm. In a young, active patient, performing a periacetabular osteotomy can provide years of pain relief. This procedure will also allow the patient to maintain an active lifestyle. THA is a good surgical treatment option and one that most patients will eventually require. The Crowe classification system helps categorize the dysplastic hip and guides treatment. The more severe dysplasia can require concurrent femoral osteotomies. These patients will require close follow-up, but one must remember that prevention is the key. Management in the pediatric population will dictate the severity of the disease and surgical options available to the young adult.

References

1. McCarthy JC, Lee JA. Acetabular dysplasia: a paradigm of arthroscopic examination of chondral injuries. *Clin Orthop Relat Res.* 2002;(405):122-128.
2. Lack W, Windhager R, Kutschera HP, Engel A. Chiari pelvic osteotomy for osteoarthritis secondary to hip dysplasia. Indications and long-term results. *J Bone Joint Surg Am.* 1991;73(2):229-234.
3. Steppacher SD, Tannast M, Ganz R, Siebenrock KA. Mean 20-year followup of Bernese periacetabular osteotomy. *Clin Orthop Relat Res.* 2008;466:1633–1644.
4. Pellicci PM, Hu S. Varus rotational femoral osteotomies in adults with hip dysplasia. *Clin Orthop Relat Res.* 1991;272:162-166.
5. Voos JE, Ranawat AS, Pellicci PM, Buly RL, Salvati EA. Varus rotational osteotomies for adults with hip dysplasia: a 20-year followup. *Clin Orthop Relat Res.* 2007;457:138–143.

6. Ito H, Matsuno T, Minami A. Intertrochanteric varus osteotomy for osteoarthritis in patients with hip dysplasia: 6 to 28 years followup. *Clin Orthop Relat Res.* 2005;(433):124–128.
7. Sanchez-Sotelo J, Berry DJ, Trousdale RT, Cabanela ME. Surgical treatment of developmental dysplasia of the hip in adults: II. Arthroplasty options. *J Am Acad Orthop Surg.* 2002;10(5):334-344.
8. Garvin KL, Bowen MK, Salvati EA, Ranawat CS. Long-term results of total hip arthroplasty in congenital dislocation and dysplasia of the hip. A follow-up note. *J Bone Joint Surg Am.* 1991;1348.1354.
9. Pagnano MW, Hanssen AD, Lewallen DG, Shaughnessy WJ. The effect of superior placement of the acetabular component on the rate of loosening after total hip arthroplasty. *J Bone Joint Surg Am.* 1996;78(7):1004-1014.
10. Lewallen DG. Neurovascular injury associated with hip arthroplasty. *J Bone Joint Surg Am.* 1997;79:1870-1880.
11. Gerber SD. Femroal head autografting to augment acetabular deficiency in patients requiring total hip replacement. A minimum five-year and average seven-year follow-up study. *J Bone Joint Surg Am.* 1986;68(8):1241-1248.

Suggested Readings

Chosa E, Tajima N. Anterior acetabular head index of the hip on false-profile views. New index of anterior acetabular cover. *J Bone Joint Surg Br.* 2003;85(6):826-829.

MacKenzie JR, Kelley SS, Johnston RC. Total hip replacement for coxarthrosis secondary to congenital dysplasia and dislocation of the hip. Long-term results. *J Bone Joint Surg Am.* 1996;78(1):55-61.

26

Periprosthetic Hip Fracture

CDR M.T. Newman, MD and Hari P. Bezwada, MD

The number of primary and revision arthroplasty procedures is expected to steadily increase as the population ages.[1] The incidence of periprosthetic fractures of the femur is similarly likely to increase. Therefore, the practicing orthopedic surgeon must be familiar with the management of a variety of these periprosthetic fractures.

Periprosthetic hip fractures occur in 2 distinct settings: intraoperatively and postoperatively, each with its own particular personalities and risks. Intraoperatively, the use of press fit components can lead to increased hoop stresses that may lead to fracture. Postoperatively, wear-related osteolysis and medical comorbidities are factors that can lead to altered bone stock. Risk factors exist that can help predict which patients and implants are susceptible to fracture and these factors will direct treatment of fractures that occur.

The management of these patients can be challenging and requires a combination of skill sets in both adult reconstruction and orthopedic trauma. The choice of treatment modalities depends on 4 primary factors: the condition of the patient, the location of the fracture, the stability of the implant, and the quality of underlying bone stock. Several classification systems exist[2-9]; however, most are descriptive in nature, providing only information about the location of the fracture with respect to the implant and are thus not useful for surgical decision making. The Vancouver classification of periprosthetic hip fractures, however, is comprehensive and is perhaps the most widely used and accepted system available.[2]

Recent advances have been made in the treatment of periprosthetic fractures; however, outcomes historically have only ranged from good to poor.[3,4,6,10-11] All treatment options must be considered but many are fraught with complications. Nonoperative treatment can lead to problems related to decreased functional status and longer rehabilitation. Nonoperative management can also result in nonunion or malunion. Open reduction and internal fixation may often lead to hardware breakage if not used cautiously and correctly. Instability continues to plague revision surgery in this setting as well. A comprehensive approach to these challenging patients, including identification of risks, proper surgical planning, and rehabilitation may lead to improved outcomes.

Classification

Several classification systems have been described for periprosthetic femur fractures. However, most have provided little value in guiding treatment. The Vancouver classification does both and has become the most widely used and accepted system. This classification system identifies the location of the fracture, addresses the underlying implant stability, and directs the surgeon to evaluate the underlying quality of bone stock. The classification system differs slightly between intraoperative and postoperative fractures, but we will limit the discussion and point out highlights as needed.[2,12]

Type A fractures generally occur in the setting of significant osteopenia in the intertrochanteric region of the proximal femur (Figure 26-1). They are further classified depending on the involvement of either the greater

Parvizi J, Klatt BA.
Essentials in Total Hip Arthroplasty (pp 223-232).

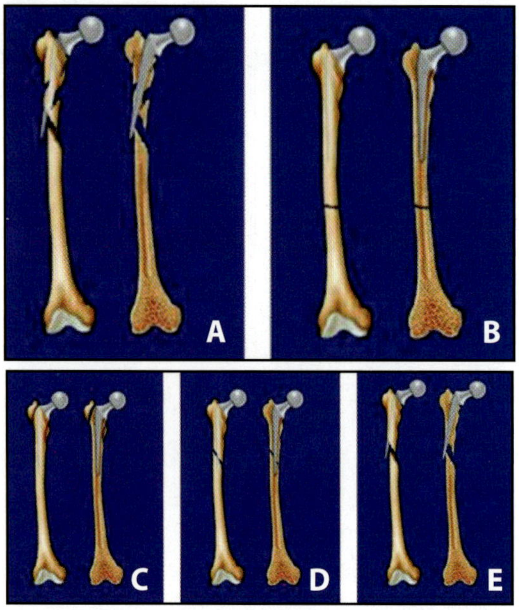

Figure 26-1. The Vancouver Classification of Periprosthetic Femoral Fractures. (A) Type A fracture with greater (g) and lesser (l) trochanteric fracture. (B) Type B1 fracture with well fixed femoral component. (C) Type B2 fracture with loose stem but good bone stock. (D) Type B3 fracture with loose stem and poor bone quality. (E) Type C fracture well distal to stem. (Reprinted with permission from Parvizi J, Rapuri VR, Purtill JJ, Sharkey PF, Rothman RH, Hozack WJ. Treatment protocol for proximal femoral periprosthetic fractures. *J Bone Joint Surg Am.* 2004;86:8-16.)

trochanter (A_{GT}) or the lesser trochanter (A_{LT}). Longitudinal fractures that occur intraoperatively can be considered a Type A fracture and are treated similarly.

Type B fractures occur around the stem or just distal to it and these are further subclassified according to implant stability and bone quality (see Figure 26-1). The B1 fracture occurs around or just distal to a well-fixed femoral stem. The B2 fracture again occurs around or just distal to a loose femoral stem. Good bone quality is evident in both B1 and B2 fractures. Type B3 fractures occur around or just distal to a loose femoral stem and have poor underlying bone due to osteopenia, osteolysis, or severe fracture comminution.

Type C fractures occur well below an intact implant and can have either adequate or poor underlying bone stock (see Figure 26-1). The implant is inherently considered stable and rarely needs to be addressed during treatment. Any fracture distal to an implant can be considered a Type C fracture, including those of the supracondylar femur, and are treated accordingly.

According to most studies, Type B fractures are the most common both intraoperatively and postoperatively and are reported to be as high as 80%[13,14] of all periprosthetic fractures. Of these, B2 fractures account for nearly 40% followed by B3 fractures at 30% of all periprosthetic fractures. B1 fractures, or those with stable implants, generally occur much less frequently and account for only 15% to 20% of periprosthetic proximal femur fractures. With this in mind, early revision of loose components for any reason could lead to decreased incidence of periprosthetic fractures. Type A and C fractures account for a much lower proportion of fractures and in most studies are reported to account for only 10% each.

Risk Factors

Several risk factors for periprosthetic fractures have been suggested and include female sex, uncemented femoral stem, age, and revision surgery. Intraoperatively certain techniques and implants have been proven to increase the risk of fracture. The use of impaction bone grafting used to augment underlying bone stock has been reported to result in fracture between 4% and 32% of cases.[15-21] In a study of 59 intraoperative fractures that occurred during revision total hip arthroplasty (THA) with impaction bone grafting, 58% were complete fractures and 42% were cortical perforations. Of these, 44% occurred during cement removal and 12% occurred during impaction bone grafting.[21] Others have looked at minimally invasive surgery as an independent risk factor and found that no fractures occurred with the use of a standard incision of >10 cm.[22] In a retrospective study of 3566 THAs where 83 fractures occurred, the only significant risk factors were use of an uncemented stem, previous surgery on the affected hip, and revision surgery.[23] In the revision setting, the presence of underlying poor bone stock due to osteopenia and osteolysis in combination with the use of longer stems and underreaming of the cortex have led to an associated increase risk of fracture[13] (Table 26-1).

Several patient factors have been associated with increased risk of fracture to include female sex, increased age, rheumatoid arthritis, and Paget's disease.[24-26] To be sure it is likely most of these risks may be confounded by osteoporosis and the surgeon should be aware that any disease associated with altered bone metabolism can increase the risk of subsequent periprosthetic fracture (Figure 26-2). This can mean early identification of implants at risk for periprosthetic fracture leading the surgeon to choose early revision, or by knowing that press fit components increase the risk of intraoperative fractures and therefore carefully sizing components.

Evaluation and Management

Diagnostic evaluation of a periprosthetic fracture begins with a thorough patient history and physical exam.

Table 26-1

RISK FACTORS ASSOCIATED WITH PERIPROSTHETIC FRACTURE

INTRAOPERATIVELY

• Revision surgery
  ◦ Impaction bone grafting
  ◦ Cement removal
• Previous surgery of affected hip
• Surgical technique
  ◦ Underreaming the femoral canal
  ◦ Large femoral stems
  ◦ Minimally invasive surgery
  ◦ Use of uncemented stems

POSTOPERATIVELY
• Paget's disease • Female sex • Increased age • Rheumatoid arthritis • Osteoporosis • Osteolysis/osteopenia

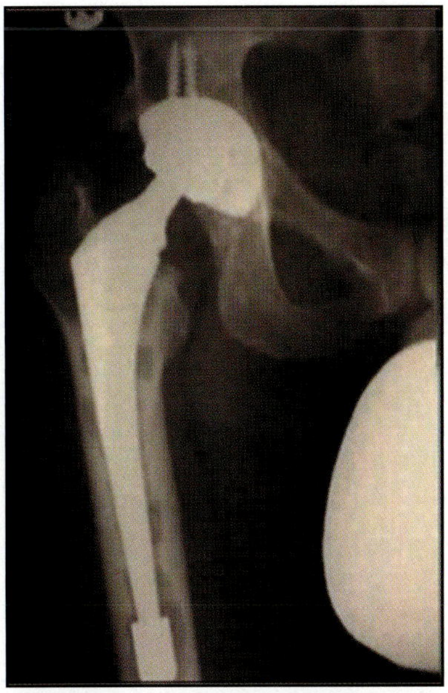

Figure 26-2. Postoperative osteolysis of THA due to polyethylene wear and cement debris, decreasing the bone quality and increasing risk of fracture.

Intraoperatively, surgeons must maintain a high index of suspicion as draping and limited exposure may lead to missed diagnosis. A close assessment of the implants and bone after insertion as well as intraoperative clues such as a sudden change in resistance while inserting components should lead the surgeon to improve exposure or order intraoperative x-rays for further assessment. For postoperative fractures, prior hip pain could indicate a loose component and an obvious deformity, including progressive leg length discrepancy, will be apparent on physical exam. Serial plain radiographic examinations will identify most cases of implant loosening and after injury is usually the only study needed to classify injury and create a plan for surgery.

Although this text is not meant to serve as an exhaustive resource for the description of operative techniques, it behooves the surgeon to know the various options available for treatment of all periprosthetic fractures. Although nonoperative treatment has been attempted in the past, most authors agree that outcomes are poor.[3] Therefore, constant reassessment of treatment options as techniques and implants evolve is likely to result in better outcomes and patient satisfaction.

Type A fractures involving the lesser trochanter are rare following total joint arthroplasty. Most commonly these occur in the setting of osteopenic bone or possibly through an osteolytic lesion. Usually no treatment is required but if the fragment is large or extends into the calcar, it may require reduction and stabilization with cerclage wiring. A treatment algorithm is outlined in Figure 26-3 for the surgeon to use in decision making for Type A fractures.

Type A fractures of the greater trochanter usually occur due to an avulsion injury and involve osteopenic bone as well (Figure 26-4). If little displacement occurs, then generally the tenodesis effect will prevent any further diastasis and no further treatment except for protected weight bearing is warranted. However, if displacement is great, then open reduction and internal fixation may be needed to prevent nonunion. A trochanteric claw may be a useful device in the treatment of these fractures (Figure 26-5). In the setting of significant osteolysis due to polyethylene wear, the underlying problem may need to be addressed, for instance, with revision surgery.

Type B fractures are by far the most common, accounting for in upwards of 80% of periprosthetic fractures in most studies. B1 fractures, or those that occur around a stable implant, are treated by open reduction and internal fixation in all but the rarest of situations. Spiral or long oblique fractures can be treated with cerclage wire or cables but short or transverse fractures should be treated with biplanar fixation with plates, cortical onlay graft, or both (Figure 26-6). Cortical onlay grafts have become an attractive option as they serve both a mechanical and biologic role by ultimately incorporating into host bone. Nonoperative

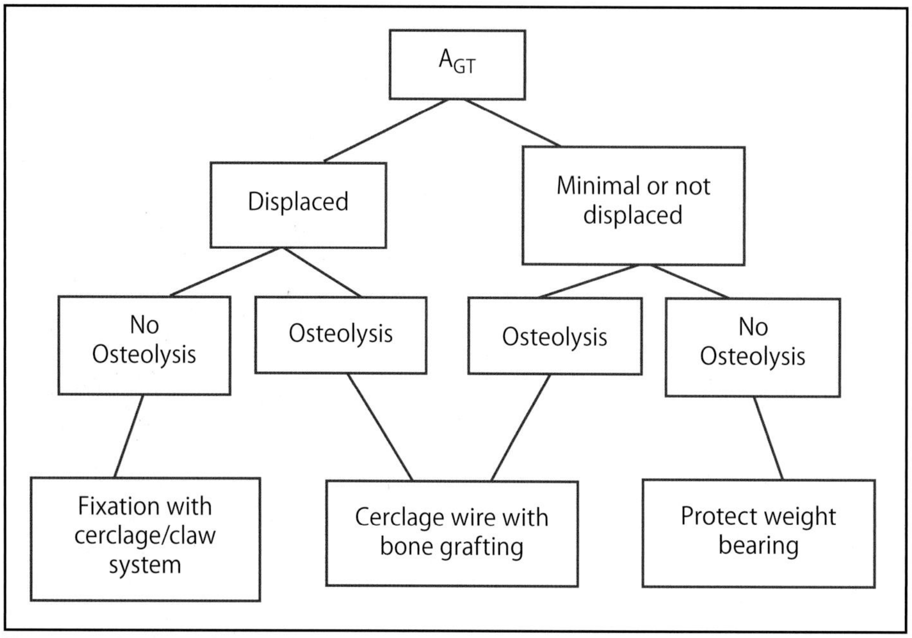

Figure 26-3. Treatment algorithm for Vancouver Type A periprosthetic fractures. (Adapted from Pike J, Davidson D, Garbuz, D, Duncan C, O'Brien PJ, Masri B. Principles of treatment for periprosthetic femoral shaft fractures around well-fixed total hip arthroplasty. *J Amer Acad Ortho Surg.* 2009;17:866-877; Parvizi J, Rapuri VR, Purtill JJ, Sharkey PF, Rothman RH, Hozack WJ. Treatment protocol for proximal femoral periprosthetic fractures. *J Bone Joint Surg Am.* 2004;86:8-16.)

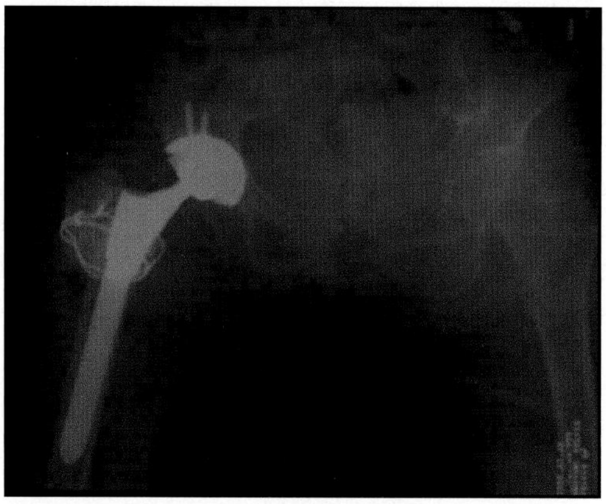

Figure 26-4. Type A_{GT} fracture prior fixation.

treatment should be avoided due to known complications of prolonged bed rest including exacerbation of pre-existing comorbidities. Nonunion or malunion can also occur with nonoperative treatment, making subsequent revisions ever more difficult. Revision of a stable implant can be deleterious to the surrounding bone and should be avoided. Again, preoperative planning is imperative and knowledge of the use of all possible constructs is necessary. Again, Figure 26-7 is useful as a guide for surgical intervention.

Vancouver B2 fractures occur in the setting of a loose component but otherwise adequate bone stock. This can become challenging as reconstruction, open reduction, and internal fixation are warranted. To make matters worse, the removal of implants can lead to further loss of underlying bone stock. The general treatment goal should be to insert long stem components that bypass the fracture site by at least 2 cortical diameters. Subsequent judicious use of plates, screws, wires and onlay bone graft allows for adequate final fixation and stability, allowing early return to weight bearing (Figure 26-8). Cemented or uncemented stems can be used and should be based on the surgeon's comfort and the underlying bone quality. Cement between fracture fragments will prevent these bones from healing, so care should be exercised in the placement of cement. Immediate weight bearing can be used with cemented stems and should be considered to allow earlier return to function. Another useful technique with poor quality bone is impaction grafting. Although challenging, this can provide greater stability to the fracture.

Vancouver B3 fractures pose the greatest challenge to the arthroplasty surgeon. These occur in a similar setting as B2 fractures, around or just distal to a loose femoral component; however, the underlying bone stock is woefully inadequate to accommodate traditional plate, screw, and wire techniques. These fractures require the revision of the femoral component and restoration of the bone stock is a necessity. Even if a proximal femoral replacement is used,

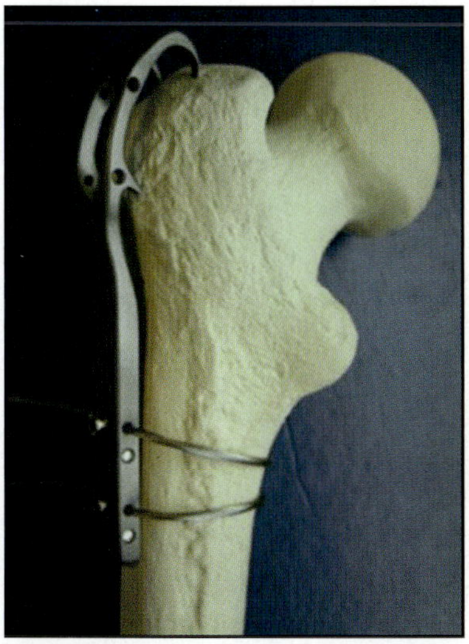

Figure 26-5. Claw plate used for greater trochanter fractures.

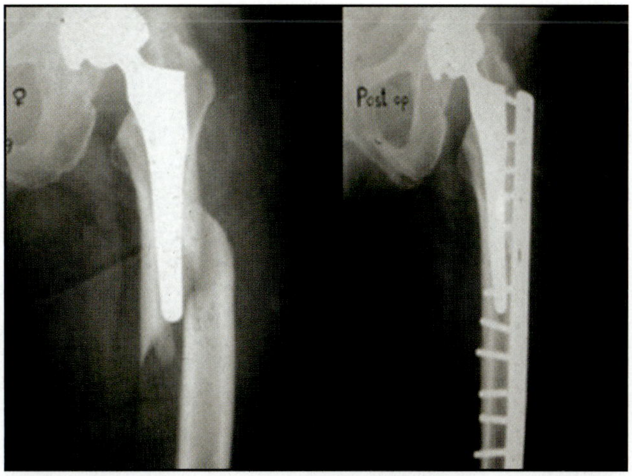

Figure 26-6. Treatment of Vancouver Type B1 fracture with long plate and cerclage wires.

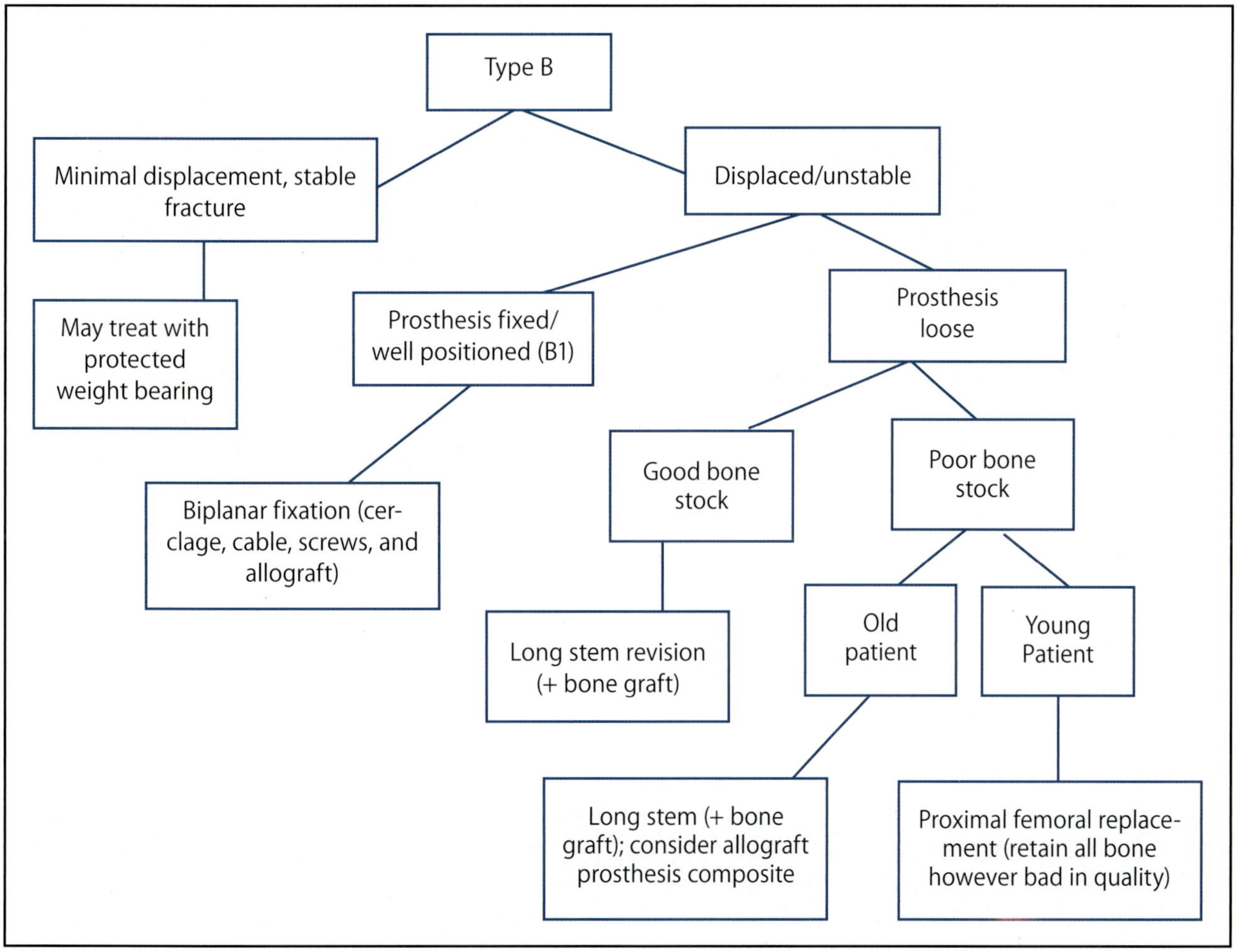

Figure 26-7. Treatment algorithm for Vancouver Type B periprosthetic fractures. (Adapted from Pike J, Davidson D, Garbuz, D, Duncan C, O'Brien PJ, Masri B. Principles of treatment for periprosthetic femoral shaft fractures around well-fixed total hip arthroplasty. *J Amer Acad Ortho Surg.* 2009;17:866-877; Parvizi J, Rapuri VR, Purtill JJ, Sharkey PF, Rothman RH, Hozack WJ. Treatment protocol for proximal femoral periprosthetic fractures. *J Bone Joint Surg Am.* 2004;86:8-16.)

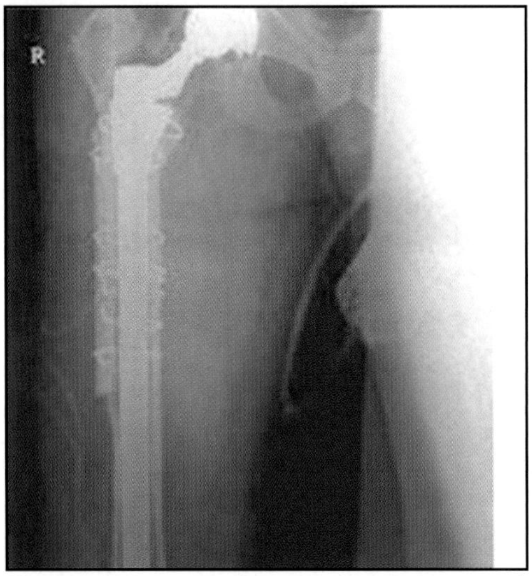

Figure 26-8. Treatment of Vancouver Type B2 fracture with revision long stemmed component and cerclage wires.

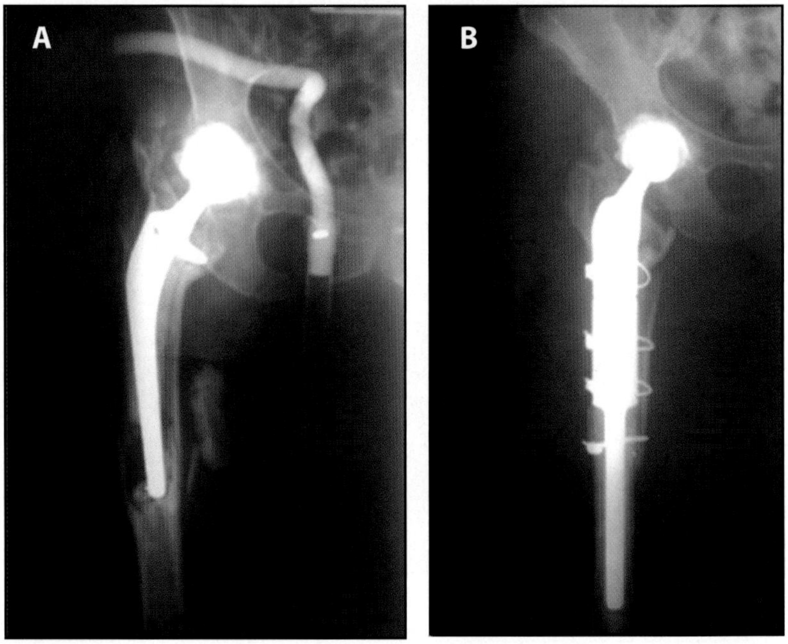

Figure 26-9. Treatment of Vancouver Type B3 fracture with proximal femoral replacement, cerclage wiring, and maintenance of underlying proximal bone stock.

retention of the native femur, regardless of quality, should be considered (Figure 26-9). Retention of the native bone can lead to impingement and instability and segments that are impinging on the acetabulum should be removed. Because of the amount of soft tissue dissection in these reconstructions, a constrained liner may also need to be considered to avoid instability. Again, by following adequate preoperative planning, revising the femoral component, restoring femoral bone stock, and accounting for soft tissue deficiency, these challenging cases can have good clinical outcomes.

Vancouver C fractures can generally be treated with standard principles of open reduction and internal fixation. However, certain pitfalls should be avoided. Primarily, avoidance of the creation of stress risers should be of utmost concern. Placement of screws should be avoided around femoral stems and, if used, retrograde nails should end at least 2 cortical diameters distal to stems. The recent emergence of newer implants requiring less soft tissue dissection (LISS, Synthes, Paoli, IN) generally are ideal for fixation of these fractures. However, a certain degree of experience in the use of these implants is a necessity. Also, less invasive plating is not possible with cerclage wiring and strut graft placement. The fixation should not be compromised. Supracondylar fractures of the femur can be treated with similar implants and blade plates can also be considered. Occasionally, strut allografts can be used to provide an improved mechanical construct. If the fracture is relatively near the femoral component, then one should consider overlapping the plate proximal to implant, but screws should still be avoided and the use of cerclage wires in this setting is encouraged (Figure 26-10). Cerclage cables should be attached to the plate for better fixation. If the cables are free to move, any movement of the cables can result in loss of reduction.

A brief discussion of periprosthetic acetabular fractures is warranted as these also can become treatment dilemmas for the operating surgery. Intraoperative fractures of the acetabulum occur much less frequently than they occur in the femur and the Mayo Clinic Total Joint Registry found only one fracture in 5400 cases.[27] Like femoral fractures, acetabular fractures occur intraoperatively and postoperatively and are broadly divided into 2 classes: those that are radiographically stable and those that are considered unstable. Intraoperatively, very little stress is delivered to the acetabulum after reaming and thus very few problems arise. Certain clues can help assist the surgeon in evaluation. For instance, a sudden change in the sound of the striking of the press-fit implant or sudden increased blood loss can indicate cancellous bleeding from the fracture. Intraoperative fractures of the acetabulum can become a problem during revision to cementless components due to use of press fit components and pre-existing osteolysis.

Acetabular fractures are treated according to fracture displacement and implant stability, similar to femoral fractures.[28,29] Treatment is straightforward intraoperatively if the fracture is nondisplaced and the component is stable;

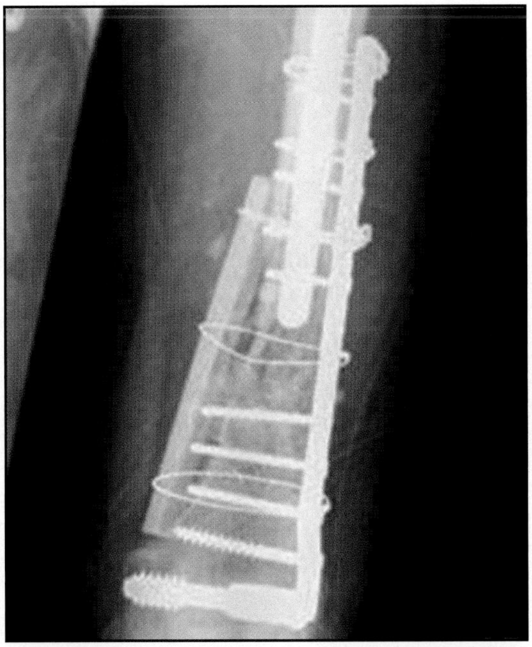

Figure 26-10. Treatment of Vancouver Type C fracture with blade plate, cortical onlay strut graft, cerclage wiring, and maintenance of underlying bone stock.

then acetabular component screw fixation can be used to stabilize. This should be followed by 8 to 12 weeks of toe-touch weight bearing. If, however, the fracture is displaced, the component should be removed and close inspection of the fracture should follow. If the posterior column is involved, then buttress plating should be performed, followed by gentle reinsertion of a press-fit component (Figure 26-11). Again, protected weight bearing should follow. If significant osteolysis exists, then cage fixation with plate augmentation may be necessary to secure the hemipelvis. Peterson and Lewallen[30] reported on 11 patients with postoperative acetabular fractures. Eight of 11 fractures were clinically and radiographically stable and 2 were unstable; one patient died of related injuries. Patients with unstable fractures were treated with revision with plate or cages, and patients with stable implants were treated nonoperatively with modified activities. Of the 10 surviving patients, 8 went on to revision due to persistent pain despite appropriate treatment. The authors concluded that initial attempts at fixation were inadequate but revision can lead to acceptable outcomes.

Outcomes and Complications

Overall, periprosthetic femur fractures are increasing in both number and complexity. In one study, an intraoperative femoral fracture was encountered during

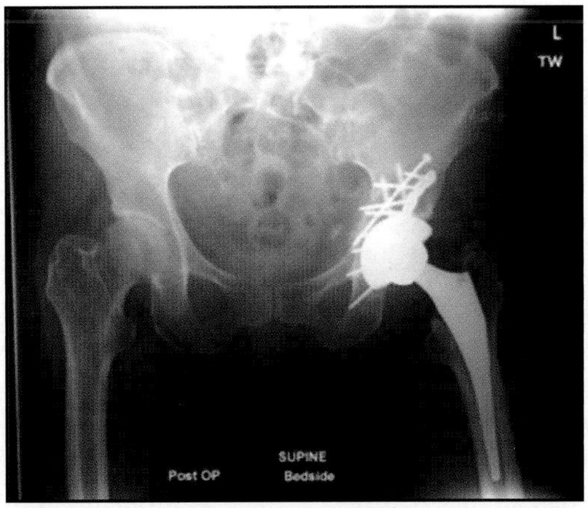

Figure 26-11. Periprosthetic acetabular fracture treated with a buttress plate column screw, and screw fixation of the acetabular component.

1% (238) of 23,980 primary THAs compared to 7.8% (497) of 6349 revisions.[31] In the same study, the rate of periprosthetic fractures was 5.4% (170 of 3121) when using a cementless stem compared with 0.3% (68 of 20,859) when a cemented stem was used. In a study by Lindahl et al[25] in 2006, they looked at 242,393 primary procedures, 28,045 reoperations, and 22,840 revision surgeries in the Swedish National Hip Arthroplasty Registry. Over a 1-year period 321 periprosthetic hip fractures were recorded, accounting for the third most common reason for reoperation (9.3%) second only to aseptic loosening and dislocation. The annual incidence of periprosthetic hip fracture was 0.13% in 1999 and 0.11% in 2000. The cumulative incidence of periprosthetic hip fracture from 1979 until 2000 was 0.4% following primary total hip replacements and 2.1% following revision total hip replacements. With these numbers likely to increase, the treatment of such fractures will require an understanding of appropriate treatment and rehabilitation.

The treatment of periprosthetic fractures after THA has been studied by several authors and has generally been associated with a high incidence of failures, complications, and poor outcomes. Difficulty arises in comparison of various results in the literature due to differences in length of follow-up, patient demographics, types of implants used, number of revision arthroplasties, differing operative techniques, and variable outcome measures utilized. In 1982, Bethea et al[3] reported the outcomes of treatment of 31 periprosthetic fractures. They found that nonoperative treatment generally yielded poor outcomes. They also reported that treatment with revision using a long-stemmed prosthesis resulted in better long-term survival. Of note, 65% of their patients had confirmed loosening or erosion of the cortex prior to fracture.

Johansson et al[4] reported the results of treatment of 37 fractures of which 23 were intraoperative and 14 were postoperative. Complications occurred in 60% of their patients. The results of treatment were satisfactory for only 43% of the intraoperative fractures and 36% of the postoperative fractures.

Mont and Maar[6] reviewed 487 periprosthetic fractures reported in 26 publications, noting great difficulty in interpreting outcomes from each treatment strategy due to the small number of patients in each study. Haddad et al[10] reported on results of a multicenter study of the treatment of Vancouver Type B1 fractures. Internal fixation was used in all 40 patients. Cortical strut grafts only were used in 19 patients, and strut graft with a lateral plate were used in 21. Union occurred in 39 of the 40 patients. Four malunions occurred during treatment but all were mild. The investigators concluded that cortical strut grafts enhanced the mechanical stability as well as the potential for healing of these challenging fractures.

Springer et al[11] recently reported the Mayo Clinic experience with 116 patients (118 hips) who had undergone revision THA to treat acute Vancouver Type B fractures. Multiple treatment modalities were used to include cemented implants, both proximally and extensively porous-coated uncemented implants, and allograft or tumor prosthesis. Mean follow-up was 5.4 years. Survival with revision or removal of femoral implant for any reason as an endpoint was 90% at 5 years and 79.2% at 10 years. Complications such as loosening, recurrent dislocation, refracture, and deep infection occurred. The authors concluded that revision THA around a femoral stem can successfully restore function for most patients and the use of uncemented, extensively porous-coated implants lead to better results.

Parvizi et al[14] in 2004 presented outcomes of surgical intervention for a variety of fractures that occurred around a total hip prosthesis in a large population. They followed the treatment algorithms initially presented by Duncan and Masri (see Figure 26-1 and Table 26-1). They reported on complications of their treatment and found that patients presenting more than 48 hours after fracture were at a high risk for deep venous thrombosis (DVT). Other complications included vascular injury, failure of fixation, nonunion, refracture, cortical perforation, loosening, instability/dislocation, and infection, accounting for a complication rate of 18.6%. The authors advocated the use of at least 10 cortices and reinforcement of fixation with biplanar strut allografts. They did not recommend screw fixation of strut allografts. They also recommended spanning the fracture with a revision stem by 5 to 8 cm.

Lindahl et al[25] noted that minor trauma, including falls from a standing height and spontaneous fractures, accounted for the majority of mechanisms of injury. A high number of patients had loose stems at the time of fracture, including 66% in the primary replacement group and 51% in the revision group. Their survival (reoperation for any reason) at 66-month follow-up was 74.8%, leading them to suggest increased scrutiny of loose implants and earlier revision to avoid fracture.

In 2007, Holley et al[32] reviewed 99 patients treated for periprosthetic fracture over a 17-year period at one institution. Sixty-six patients completed follow-up at a minimum of 12 months. Overall, 86% of patients achieved fracture union. The success rate for cemented revision in B2 and B3 fractures was 84% and 86%, respectively, for cementless revisions. Surgical complication rate was 29%. Several other findings included the increased success with the use of cortical struts and patients with rheumatoid arthritis or juvenile rheumatoid arthritis had worse outcomes regardless of fracture type or treatment. In this study, B3 fractures accounted for the highest percent of complications (66%), and with Type C fractures union was difficult regardless of treatment, thought to be due to osteopenia and stress shielding.

In a recent article by Bhattacharyya et al,[33] the association between management of periprosthetic fractures and mortality was explored. They compared 106 patients who underwent surgery for periprosthetic fracture with 309 patients who sustained either a femoral neck or intertrochanteric hip fracture and 311 patients who underwent primary hip or knee replacement as controls. They found a 1-year mortality rate of 11% (12 of 106 patients) in the periprosthetic fracture group, 16.5% mortality in the hip fracture group, and a 2.9% 1-year mortality in the arthroplasty group. They also found that a delay of greater than 2 days from admission to time of surgery was associated with an increased mortality at 1 year.

Summary

Periprosthetic fractures, which occur during and after THA, are expected to rise over the following decades. These are challenging problems that confound the surgeon with many treatment options, numerous pitfalls, complications, and historically poor outcomes. As we move forward, it behooves the arthroplasty surgeon to be cognizant of early detection of those implants that are a risk with early revision to prevent this devastating injury. However, remaining facile with the options and implants available and the current recommendations for treatment are mandatory.

REFERENCES

1. Zhan C, Kaczmarek R, Loyo-Berrios N, Sangl J, Bright RA. Incidence and short term outcomes of primary and revision hip replacement in the United States. *J Bone Joint Surg Am.* 2007;89:526-533
2. Pike J, Davidson D, Garbuz, D, Duncan C, O'Brien PJ, Masri B. Principles of treatment for periprosthetic femoral shaft fractures around well-fixed total hip arthroplasty. *J Amer Acad Ortho Surg.* 2009;17:866-877.
3. Bethea JS III, DeAndrade Jr, Fleming LL, Lindenbaum SD, Welch RB. Proximal femur fractures following total hip arthroplasty. *Clin Orthop.* 1982;170:95-106.
4. Johansson JE, McBroom R, Barrington TW, Hunter GA. Fracture of the ipsilateral femur in patients with total hip replacement. *J Bone Joint Surg Am.* 1981;63:1435-1442.
5. Kelley SS. Periprosthetic femur fractures. *J Am Acad Orthop Surg.* 1994; 2:164 -172.
6. Mont MA, Maar DC. Fractures of the ipsilateral femur after hip arthroplasty. A statistical analysis of outcome based on 487 patients. *J Arthroplasty.* 1994;9:511-519.
7. Morrey BF, Kavanagh BF. Complications with revision of the femoral component of total hip arthroplasty. Comparison between cemented and uncemented techniques. *J Arthroplasty.* 1992;7:71-79.
8. Schwartz JT Jr, Mayer JG, Engh CA. Femoral fracture during non-cemented total hip arthroplasty. *J Bone Joint Surg Am.* 1989;71:1135-1142.
9. Whittaker RP, Sotos LN, Ralston EL. Fractures of the femur about femoral endoprostheses. *J Trauma.* 1974;14:675-694.
10. Haddad FS, Duncan CP, Berry DJ, Lewallen DG, Gross AE, Chandler HP. Periprosthetic femoral fractures around well-fixed implants: use of cortical onlay allografts with or without a plate. *J Bone Joint Surg Am.* 2002;84:945-950.
11. Springer BD, Berry DJ, Lewallen DG. Treatment of periprosthetic femoral fractures following total hip arthroplasty with femoral component revision. *J Bone Joint Surg Am.* 85-A(11):2156-2162.
12. Masri BA, Meek RM, Duncan CP. Periprosthetic fractures evaluation and treatment. *Clin Orthop Relat Res.* 2004;420:80-95.
13. Meek RM, Garbuz DS, Masri BA, Greidanus NV, Duncan CP. Intraoperative fracture of the femur in revision total hip arthroplasty with a diaphyseal fitting stem. *J Bone Joint Surg Am.* 2004;86:480-485.
14. Parvizi J, Rapuri VR, Purtill JJ, Sharkey PF, Rothman RH, Hozack WJ. Treatment protocol for proximal femoral periprosthetic fractures. *J Bone Joint Surg Am.* 2004;86:8-16.
15. Gie GA, Linder L, Ling RS, Simon JP, Slooff TJ, Timperley AJ. Impacted cancellous allografts and cement for revision total hip arthroplasty. *J Bone Joint Surg Br.* 1993;75:14-21.
16. Leopold SS, Berger RA, Rosenberg AG, Jacobs JJ, Quigley LR, Galante JO. Impaction allografting with cement for revision of the femoral component. A minimum four-year follow-up study with use of a precoated femoral stem. *J Bone Joint Surg Am.* 1999;81:1080-1092.
17. Pekkarinen J, Alho A, Lepistö J, Ylikoski M, Ylinen P, Paavilainen T. Impaction bone grafting in revision hip surgery. A high incidence of complications. *J Bone Joint Surg Br.* 2000;82:103-107.
18. Piccaluga F, González Della Valle A, Encinas Fernández JC, Pusso R. Revision of the femoral prosthesis with impaction allografting and a Charnley stem. A 2- to 12-year follow-up. *J Bone Joint Surg Br.* 2002;84:544-549.
19. Ornstein E, Atroshi I, Franzén H, Johnsson R, Sandquist P, Sundberg M. Early complications after one hundred and forty-four consecutive hip revisions with impacted morselized allograft bone and cement. *J Bone Joint Surg Am.* 2002;84:1323-1328.
20. Halliday BR, English HW, Timperley AJ, Gie GA, Ling RS. Femoral impaction grafting with cement in revision total hip replacement. Evolution of the technique and results. *J Bone Joint Surg Br.* 2003;85:809-817.
21. Farfalli GL, Buttaro MA, Piccaluga F. Femoral fractures in revision hip surgeries with impacted bone allograft. *Clin Orthop Relat Res.* 2007;462:130-136.
22. Asayama I, Kinsey TL, Mahoney OM. Two-year experience using a limited-incision direct lateral approach in total hip arthroplasty. *J Arthroplasty.* 2006;21:1083-1091.
23. Moroni A, Faldini C, Piras F, Giannini S. Risk factors for intraoperative femoral fractures during total hip replacement. *Ann Chir Gynaecol.* 2000;89:113-118.
24. Lindahl H. Epidemiology of periprosthetic femur fracture around a total hip arthroplasty. *Injury.* 2007;38:651-654.
25. Lindahl H, Garellick G, Regnér H, Herberts P, Malchau H. Three hundred and twenty-one periprosthetic femoral fractures. *J Bone Joint Surg Am.* 2006;88:1215-1222.
26. Mitchell PA, Greidanus NV, Masri BA, Garbuz DS, Duncan CP. The prevention of periprosthetic fractures of the femur during and after total hip arthroplasty. *Instr Course Lect.* 2003;52:301-308.
27. McElfresh EC, Coventry MB. Femoral and pelvic fractures after total hip arthroplasty. *J Bone Joint Surg Am.* 1974;56:483-492.
28. Callaghan Y, Kim D, Pedersen T, Brown TD. Periprosthetic fractures of the acetabulum. *Orthop Clin N Am.* 30(2):221–234.
29. Callaghan JJ. Instructional Course Lectures, The American Academy of Orthopaedic Surgeons. Periprosthetic fractures of the acetabulum during and following total hip arthroplasty. *J Bone Joint Surg Am.* 1997;79:1416-21.
30. Peterson CA, Lewallen DG. Periprosthetic fracture of the acetabulum after total hip arthroplasty. *J Bone Joint Surg Am.* 1996;78:1206-1213.

31. Berry DJ. Epidemiology: hip and knee. *Orthop Clin North Am.* 1999;30:183-190.

32. Holley K, Zelken J, Padgett D, Chimento G, Yun A, Buly R. Periprosthetic fractures of the femur after hip arthroplasty: an analysis of 99 patients. *HSS J.* 2007;3(2):190-197.

33. Bhattacharyya T, Chang D, Meigs JB, Estok DM, Malchau H. Mortality after periprosthetic fracture of the femur. *J Bone Joint Surg Am.* 2007;89:2658-2662.

Suggested Readings

Callaghan JJ, Rosenberg AG, Rubash HE. *The Adult Hip.* 2nd ed. Lippincott Williams & Wilkins; 2006.

Lieberman JR, Berry DJ. *Advanced Reconstruction: Hip.* 1st ed. American Academy of Orthopaedic Surgeons; 2007.

Vail TP. *Instructional Course Lectures: Hip.* American Academy of Orthopaedic Surgeons; 2007.

27

Periprosthetic Joint Infection

Khalid Azzam, MD; James Cashman, MD; and Javad Parvizi, MD, FRCS

Periprosthetic infection (PPI) is one of the most challenging and dreaded complications in orthopedics, often resulting in repeated surgeries, patient distress and disability, increased cost and utilization of medical resources; and in rare cases even mortality.

The biggest challenge to date is to correctly diagnose PPI preoperatively or intraoperatively and implement effective treatment regimens capable of eradicating the inciting organism.

Incidence

With the introduction of laminar flow and body exhaust systems[1,2] and the administration of appropriate preoperative antibiotics, the incidence of infection after joint arthroplasty has dropped significantly from 10% after first-generation primary arthroplasty and 7% following revision to a current rate of 1%.[3,4]

Risk Factors

Some of the risk factors for PPI include[5] rheumatoid arthritis, diabetes mellitus, obesity, steroid use, malnutrition, lymphocyte count of less than 1500 cells/mm and an albumin level of less than 3.5 g/dL,[6] compromised immune status, previous surgeries on the affected limb, and excessive anticoagulation.[7] Surgical factors, such as surgeon experience, timing and dosing of antibiotic administration, long operative time (>2.5 hours), operating room (OR) traffic, and the complexity of reconstruction are all important factors influencing the incidence of PPI. Persistent postoperative wound drainage and wound healing complications are also risk factors.[8]

Etiology

The following are the 3 routes of entry of organisms into a prosthetic joint:

1. Surgical contamination: Usually manifests within the first 3 months after surgery.
2. Hematogenous spread: Can occur anytime after arthroplasty. Septic foci, dental, or other surgical procedures may result in bacteremia with settling of bacteria on the implants.
3. Local dissemination: From a contagious focus.

The mere presence of an implant reduces the number of colonies of bacteria needed to establish infection by more than 10^5. Under these circumstances, microorganisms even in small quantities are able to escape immune surveillance and attach to the implant surface. Attachment of bacteria to the implant surface and formation of biofilm accounts for the failure to isolate organisms for diagnosis and also the inability to treat PPI with antibiotics only. Bacteria in the biofilm communicate via complex molecular pathways, secrete numerous extracellular matrix products, and can develop sophisticated mechanisms to escape immune attack.[9] The virulence of bacteria such as methicillin-resistant *Staphylococcus aureus* (MRSA) is, in part, contributed to

Parvizi J, Klatt BA.
Essentials in Total Hip Arthroplasty (pp 233-240).

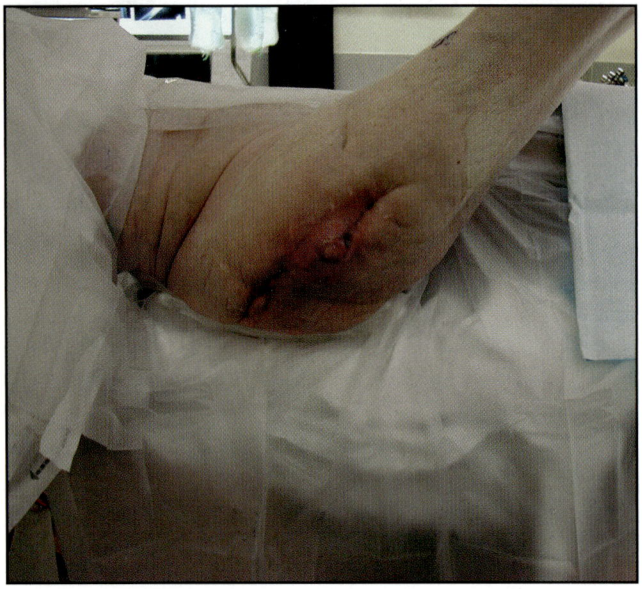

Figure 27-1. Draining sinus. A draining sinus from a hip wound is indicative of infection until proven otherwise.

by the complexity of the biofilm that they establish. Bacteria within the biofilm originally thought to maintain a low metabolic state are, in fact, more active than free-floating planktonic organisms. This high metabolism is necessary for producing extracellular polysaccharides, signaling proteins, and toxins. Biofilm is notoriously difficult to treat and common antibacterial treatment strategies effective in killing cultures extracted from biofilm have minimal effect on bacteria adherent onto implants and hidden within the biofilm.

Diagnosis

History and Physical Exam

PPI may present with nonspecific symptoms including minor hip pain. The presence of signs and symptoms such as a draining sinus tract, fever, chills, and/or a history of persistent wound drainage with concomitant painful range of motion can aid diagnosis of infection but are often absent (Figure 27-1).

Serological Tests

The erythrocyte sedimentation rate (ESR) and C-reactive protein (CRP) are traditional serological markers used as a part of diagnostic work-up for infection. ESR greater than arbitrary cut-off of 30 mm/hour and CRP greater than 1 mg/dL are considered abnormal.

The CRP begins to rise following total joint arthroplasty, reaching a peak at 48 hours postoperatively.[10] It then begins to normalize and reaches a normal level within 3 weeks.[11] On the other hand, the ESR reaches a maximum at 5 to 7 days postoperatively and may not return to normal for up to 3 months postoperatively.[12] CRP >1 mg/dL is a better prognostic indicator of infection than the ESR and has a sensitivity of 96% and a specificity of 92%.

Radiographs

Radiographs, besides providing important information about the local environment around the prosthesis, may in cases of overt infection reveal periosteal reaction, bone cysts, and focal resorption indicative of PPI. Certain changes such as focal areas of osteolysis, osteopenia, and endosteal or periosteal reaction are consistent with PPI,[13] while early loosening of the implant should alert the surgeon to the possibility of an underlying dormant infection.[14]

Radionuclide Modalities

The technetium-99m isotope bone scan, which detects areas of increased uptake, is often used by many surgeons as a part of initial work-up for PPI. Three-phase bone imaging by itself caries a sensitivity of 33% and specificity of 86% with poor predictive value.[15] This enables the bone scan to play an important role in screening and ruling out the presence of infection. It is, however, rare for the technetium bone scan to be used alone in diagnosis of PPI. Usually a dual tracer technique such as the use of an indium 111-labelled leukocyte scan is performed simultaneously with a technetium-99m diphosphonate scan.[16] The combination of technetium and indium-111 decreases the rate of false positives and improves specificity. The sulfur colloid scan combined with a leukocyte scan can result in an accuracy from 89% to 98%.[16] Both the sulfur colloid and white blood cell tracers accumulate in normal bone marrow but sulfur colloid does not accumulate in white cells present in the areas of infection. The diagnosis of infection is based, therefore, on the relative difference in the uptake of 2 tracers. Recently, positron emission tomography (PET) using fluorodeoxyglucose (FDG) imaging has been shown to have a promising role for diagnosis of PPI.[17] FDG-PET has been shown to carry 95% sensitivity and 93% specificity for diagnosis of infection around a hip prosthesis.

Joint Aspiration, Fluid Analysis, and Culture

Joint aspiration should be considered in patients with abnormal ESR and CRP.[18] Once aspirated, the joint fluid

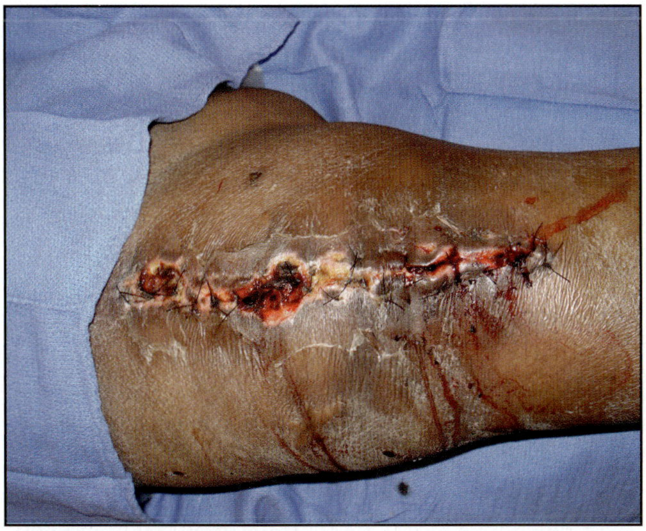

Figure 27-2. Necrotic wound. Wound necrosis requires prompt irrigation and débridement to avoid deep infection.

should be sent for cell count and neutrophil differential count as well as culture for aerobic and anaerobic bacteria and fungi. Joint aspiration does not, however, have absolute accuracy. False negative aspirations occur particularly in patients who are on antibiotics. Due to the deep location of the hip joint, aspiration under fluoroscopic guidance is recommended. Under aseptic technique, a 20-G spinal needle can be introduced under fluoroscopic control along the femoral neck and advanced until it enters the hip joint. Position can be confirmed by injecting intravenous (IV) contrast into the joint. Fluid can then be aspirated from the hip. In the absence of fluid, 5 to 10 mL of saline can be injected then aspirated and sent for culture.

Stopping Antibiotics

As per the American Academy of Orthopaedic Surgeons (AAOS) guidelines on PPI, antibiotics should be stopped for a minimum of 2 weeks prior to aspiration to avoid a false-negative aspirate. Aspiration should only be performed in patients with strong suspicion for infection as the rate of false-positive can also be unacceptably high.[19] The neutrophil percentage is more efficient in excluding infection, but a high false-positive rate could occur due to inclusion of bloody or clotted aspirates. From a practical aspect, a leukocyte count >2000 cells/µl and neutrophil percentage >70% can be used to assess for the presence of infection in patients with artificial hip or knee joints. The isolation of an organism from joint fluid, or periprosthetic tissue obtained intraoperatively, is considered the gold standard of diagnosing PPI. Although this test possesses high specificity (97% to 100%) and a near absolute positive predictive value, false positive cultures may occur in 6% of cases and an organism may not be isolated in 10% to 12% of the cases.[20,21]

Molecular Techniques

Novel molecular techniques for diagnosing PPI have previously been described.[22] During recent years, molecular techniques that are based on selective DNA amplification by the polymerase chain reaction (PCR) have been introduced.[23,24] Polymerase chain reaction analysis has been reported by some investigators to have better specificity and sensitivity than the standard culture methods.[25]

PREVENTION

Preoperative

Identification of patients who have impaired host defenses and address correctable risk factors is important[6] (steroid therapy, diabetes mellitus, decubitus ulcers, malnutrition, skin lesions, remote infection; eg, oral cavity). The Mayo group conducted an analysis of risk factors for postoperative infection. Among the univariate risk factors for infection, they found rheumatoid arthritis and steroid use along with diabetes mellitus to be significant for infection. While it may be beneficial to reduce a patient's steroid use prior to elective arthroplasty, in reality the patient's underlying medical condition may prevent this. While there is not a direct correlation with hemoglobin A1c (HbA1c) and arthroplasty outcomes, a HbA1c of <7% does correlate with a decrease in infectious complications across a wide variety of surgical procedures.[26]

Malnutrition as defined by an albumin of <34 g/L and an absolute lymphocyte count of <1.5 x 109/L was a risk factor. This was confirmed in another study that included serum transferrin less than 200 mg/dL as a marker for malnutrition.[8] Malnutrition should be reversed in the presence of a persistently draining wound (Figure 27-2). While the benefit of routine preoperative testing for malnutrition is not established, it should be considered in the revision arthroplasty setting. Psoriasis is not a risk factor for infection; however, most surgeons would advocate treatment of plaques overlying the surgical site prior to elective surgery.[6] One series of 35 patients did not identify an increased infection rate in patients with psoriasis using standard preoperative preparation.[27]

The AAOS and American Dental Association (ADA) issued a consensus statement in 2003 with regard to postoperative antibiotic prophylaxis for arthroplasty patients undergoing dental procedures.[28] While this was updated in 2009, the recommendations are largely unchanged. While there is no strong evidence to support dental clearance prior to elective arthroplasty, conventional wisdom would support removing the potentially infective burden prior to proceeding with surgery.

There are currently no widely accepted guidelines with regard to management of preoperative bladder infections in total joint arthroplasty. While there are numerous series examining the relationship between preoperative urinary tract infection and postoperative deep sepsis, no study has identified a direct relationship.[29] The patient being evaluated for surgery should be screened for symptoms of urinary obstruction and retention. In the case of patients who have immune compromise, diminished functional status, an indwelling catheter, or who have been in a nursing home for a prolonged period of time, an effort must be made to rule out a chronic asymptomatic urinary tract infection. However, the literature does not support delaying surgery simply because of the presence of bacteriuria alone in a community ambulator with no systemic risk factors. A total joint replacement may be safely performed on patients with asymptomatic bacteriuria as long as those with urine colony counts greater than 1 x 105/mL are treated with an 8- to 10-day postoperative course of an oral antibiotic appropriate to cover the organism isolated on preoperative culture.

Perioperative

A number of strategies can be employed to optimize the surgical site and minimize bacterial contamination. Shaving of the incision site should be avoided until immediately before the operative procedure or depilatory agents should be used.[30] Timing of antibiotics is critical. Antibiotics should be administered within 30 to 60 minutes of incision bearing in mind that different antibiotics have different infusion rates. Rosenberg et al found that adding confirmation of antibiotic administration to the surgical timeout for wrong-site surgery improved antibiotic administration rates.[31] Staphylococcal decolonization can be performed prior to admission using intranasal mupirocin and chlorhexidine scrubs. Rao et al have shown that decolonization for 5 days preoperatively can result in a reduction in potential infection rate.[32]

Operating Room

Prevention of infection in the OR encompasses instrument sterilization, operative site preparation, maintenance of a sterile field, and minimization of the number of personnel in the OR. When the patient is transported into the OR, ward bedding should be excluded.[33] The use of total body exhaust gowns has been advocated by some groups. Recently their use has been questioned by data from the New Zealand joint registry, which found an increased infection rate with their use.[34] However, they do provide protection to the surgeon from debris and fluids from the operative field.

Laminar flow has been advocated as a measure for preventing infection. There has been a resurgent interest in ultraviolet light technology that arose since it is considerably less expensive than laminar airflow systems.[35] However, ultraviolet light has potentially unacceptable health costs and the Centers for Disease Control and Prevention (CDC) recommends against its use. European countries have standardized laminar flow and it is used by the majority of American joint surgeons.[36] Another important factor is surgical hand washing. Chlorhexidine has been found to be more effective than alcohol hand gels.[37] The use of alcohol gels when preceded by hand washing with soap appears to be acceptable.[38] Application of a hexachlorophene foam compound provides excellent bactericidal action and is also less time consuming than traditional scrubbing methods.[39] A 3-minute scrub has been found to be more effective than lesser durations.[40] Use of double gloves and changing inner/outer gloves every 2 hours is also important. Scrub staff assisting gowning has a lower contamination rate.[41] Tips for dealing with suction include the following:

- Placement of the suction tip into the medullary canal for prolonged periods of time should be avoided.
- Changing the suction tip at 30-minute intervals and turning the suction system on only before its actual use should be done.
- Instruments that have been placed into the splash basin should not be returned to the operative wound.
- One-step water-insoluble iodophor-in-alcohol solution effectively reduces bacterial counts on the skin as does the traditional 2-step scrub-and-paint skin preparation.
- Plastic drapes impregnated with slow-release iodophor effectively eliminate any skin colonization for as long as 3 hours.[42]
- Wound irrigation with pulsatile lavage is an important factor.
- Use of antibiotic irrigating solutions results in reductions in bacterial colonization and removal of clot and tissue debris.

Surgical Technique

Several technical factors are of importance. Appropriate tissue handling is necessary to avoid devitalizing skin edges.

Tissue tension should be minimized, both with regard to the use of self-retaining retractors and overtensioning sutures in closure of the wound. Retractors should be placed carefully along fascial planes rather than in the subcutaneous tissue plane. Dissection of subcutaneous tissue from the underlying fascia can devitalize the subcutaneous tissue layer. Surgical procedures should be performed expeditiously. Longer operative durations have been associated with increased risk of infection.[43] Previous incisions should be used where possible. If this is not possible, incisions should either leave at least a 7-cm skin bridge or cross perpendicularly to older incisions.

Proper hemostasis is important to prevent hematoma formation. This can lead to persistently draining wounds and infection. Additionally, elimination of dead space by performing a multiple layered closure can aid in hematoma prevention. The use of drains is controversial. Advocates say that draining a wound prevents hematoma formation, but the use of drains is associated with increased blood loss and transfusion requirements.[44] Allogeneic blood transfusion can result in an increased infection risk due to its immunomodulatory effect.[45]

Wounds should be closed in a watertight fashion while avoiding soft tissue necrosis. Epidermal edges should be opposed and everted. After orthopedic surgery, there is a significantly higher risk of developing a wound infection when the wound is closed with staples rather than sutures. This risk is specifically greater in patients who undergo hip surgery.[16] Monofilament sutures are recommended for patients at high risk of infection. Recently, barbed sutures have been suggested as an alternative to conventional suture to distribute forces across wounds.[46]

Postoperative

Careful positioning of the patient and any padding of osseous prominences should be undertaken to prevent the development of skin ulcerations. Persistent wound drainage requires early wound irrigation and débridement. Patients should be returned to the OR promptly for hematoma evacuation. Skin necrosis calls for operative débridement. Urinary catheters should be removed as soon as the patient is ambulatory. Prophylactic antibiotics have been shown to be beneficial for 24 hours but there is no benefit to continuing beyond this time.

Treatment

Acute Infection, Irrigation, and Débridement

Although the success rate has varied in the literature depending on the patient health status, inciting organism, and duration of follow-up, the majority of investigations have reported a high failure rate. Several risk factors for failure have been identified, including the presence of a sinus tract, patient age, and prolonged duration of symptoms prior to treatment.[47,48]

The authors examined their outcomes for patients undergoing irrigation and débridement for infected arthroplasties. They found a success rate of only 44% and found that patients with staphylococcal infection, elevated American Society of Anesthesiologists score, and purulence around the prosthesis were more likely to fail. This treatment should be reserved for select healthy patients with low virulence organisms and equivocal intraoperative findings.[49]

Single-Stage Exchange Arthroplasty

Single-stage exchange arthroplasty entails resection of the components, thorough débridement of the infected tissues, reimplantation, and treatment with 6 weeks of intravenous antibiotics.[50] Despite having the advantage of being a single procedure, many current revision surgical techniques use cementless implants. Fixation without cement (no depot antibiotics) may be a contraindication to direct exchange. Furthermore, there are essentially no data on the use of bone graft in association with direct exchange. For these reasons, the indications for direct exchange are limited. The advocates of this approach are predominately European and quote excellent success rates with a single-stage approach used with a standardized protocol.[51]

Chronic Infection

Two-Stage Resection Arthroplasty With Delayed Reimplantation

Currently in the United States, resection arthroplasty with insertion of an antibiotic-laden cement spacer supplemented with 6 weeks of intravenous antibiotics is the

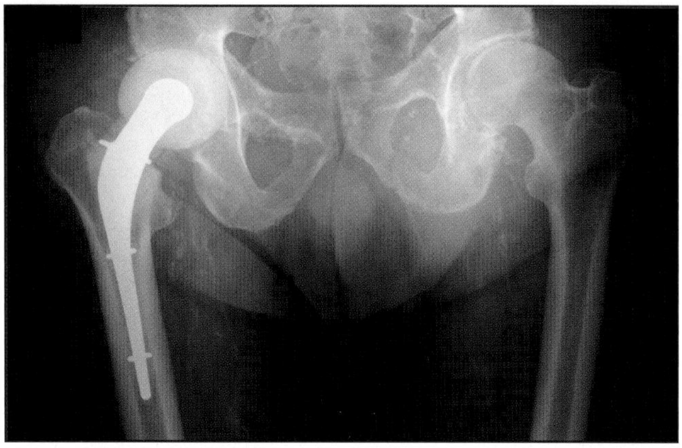

Figure 27-3. A proprietary antibiotic-impregnated spacer is used as treatment in a 2-stage revision arthroplasty.

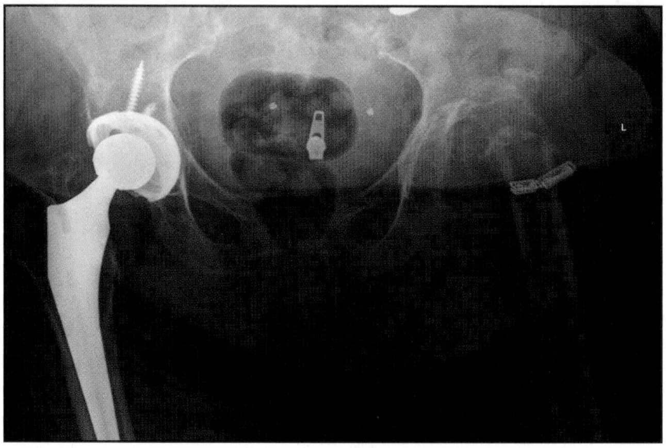

Figure 27-4. Definitive removal of all infected components and tissue with no subsequent implantation.

standard of care for infected arthroplasties. A spacer can be articulating or nonarticulating (Figure 27-3). While both help to maintain tissue plains, there are 2 schools of thought as to which is preferable. A nonarticulating spacer can be used to rest the joint and maintain the tissue planes while an articulating spacer allows for some range of motion in the treatment period. There is published literature supporting the use of both in the revision hip and knee setting. Antibiotics frequently added to bone cement include tobramycin, gentamycin, and vancomycin. The antibiotic used should reflect the sensitivities of the infecting organism. The recommended dose of antibiotics is at least 3.6 g of tobramycin and 1 to 3 g of vancomycin per packet of cement.[52] Articulating spacers have been found to abrade with time, which may aid in antibiotic elution.[53]

Antibiotics elute in greater amount and over more sustained time interval from Palacos (Zimmer, Warsaw, IN) than from Simplex-P (Stryker, Mahwah, NJ).[54] Even though a delay of 6 weeks is currently used as threshold for reimplantation time, this optimal point for spacer removal remains debatable.[47,55] With the extension of indications to perform total joint arthroplasties in patients with medical comorbidities and immune-compromised status and the emergence of multidrug-resistant organisms, there may be a substantial decrease in the success rate of 2-stage exchange arthroplasty.

Outcome rates have been variable in the literature. Most quote good results from following standardized protocols. The difficulty in interpreting this literature lies in the heterogeneity of the revision arthroplasty population.[56]

Resection (Girdlestone) Arthroplasty

A Girdlestone resection arthroplasty refers to definitive removal of all infected components and tissue with no subsequent implantation (Figure 27-4). Overall success rates for eradication of infection are between 60% and 100%. Some disadvantages are limb length discrepancy, poor function, and patient dissatisfaction. With current techniques, this procedure has few indications except those with recurrent infections, infection with multidrug-resistant organism, those with medical conditions which preclude major surgery, and failure of multiple previous exchange arthroplasties. However, those that require the procedure report satisfaction in over 80% of cases.[57]

References

1. Clohisy JC, Calvert G, Tull F, McDonald D, Maloney WJ. Reasons for revision hip surgery: a retrospective review. *Clin Orthop Relat Res.* 2004;(429):188-192.
2. Hanssen AD, Rand JA. Evaluation and treatment of infection at the site of a total hip or knee arthroplasty. *Instr Course Lect.* 1999;48:111-122.
3. Vessely MB, Whaley AL, Harmsen WS, Schleck CD, Berry DJ. The Chitranjan Ranawat Award: long-term survivorship and failure modes of 1000 cemented condylar total knee arthroplasties. *Clin Orthop Relat Res.* 2006;452:28-34.
4. Phillips JE, Crane TP, Noy M, Elliott TS, Grimer RJ. The incidence of deep prosthetic infections in a specialist orthopaedic hospital: a 15-year prospective survey. *J Bone Joint Surg Br.* 2006;88(7):943-948.
5. Salvati EA, Gonzalez Della Valle A, Masri BA, Duncan CP. The infected total hip arthroplasty. *Instr Course Lect.* 2003;52:223-245.
6. Berbari EF, Hanssen AD, Duffy MC, et al. Risk factors for prosthetic joint infection: case-control study. *Clin Infect Dis.* 1998;27(5):1247-1254.
7. Abdul-Careem MF, Hunter BD, Parvizi P, Haghighi HR, Thanthrige-Don N, Sharif S. Cytokine gene expression patterns associated with immunization against Marek's disease in chickens. *Vaccine.* 2007;25(3):424-432.

8. Jaberi FM, Parvizi J, Haytmanek CT, Joshi A, Purtill J. Procrastination of wound drainage and malnutrition affect the outcome of joint arthroplasty. *Clin Orthop Relat Res.* 2008;466(6):1368-1371.
9. Costerton W, Veeh R, Shirtliff M, Pasmore M, Post C, Ehrlich G. The application of biofilm science to the study and control of chronic bacterial infections. *J Clin Invest.* 2003;112(10):1466-1477.
10. Shih LY, Wu JJ, Yang DJ. Erythrocyte sedimentation rate and C-reactive protein values in patients with total hip arthroplasty. *Clin Orthop Relat Res.* 1987;(225):238-246.
11. White J, Kelly M, Dunsmuir R. C-reactive protein level after total hip and total knee replacement. *J Bone Joint Surg Br.* 1998;80(5):909-911.
12. Aalto K, Osterman K, Peltola H, Rasanen J. Changes in erythrocyte sedimentation rate and C-reactive protein after total hip arthroplasty. *Clin Orthop Relat Res.* 1984;(184):118-120.
13. Parvizi J, Viscusi ER, Frank HG, Sharkey PF, Hozack WJ, Rothman RR. Can epidural anesthesia and warfarin be coadministered? *Clin Orthop Relat Res.* 2007;456:133-137.
14. Della Valle CJ, Zuckerman JD, Di Cesare PE. Periprosthetic sepsis. *Clin Orthop Relat Res.* 2004;(420):26-31.
15. Mirra JM, Marder RA, Amstutz HC. The pathology of failed total joint arthroplasty. *Clin Orthop Relat Res.* 1982;(170):175-183.
16. Palestro CJ, Swyer AJ, Kim CK, Goldsmith SJ. Infected knee prosthesis: diagnosis with In-111 leukocyte, Tc-99m sulfur colloid, and Tc-99m MDP imaging. *Radiology.* 1991;179(3):645-64s8.
17. Pill SG, Parvizi J, Tang PH, et al. Comparison of fluorodeoxyglucose positron emission tomography and (111)indium-white blood cell imaging in the diagnosis of periprosthetic infection of the hip. *J Arthroplasty.* 2006;21(6 suppl 2):91-97.
18. Spangehl MJ, Masri BA, O'Connell JX, Duncan CP. Prospective analysis of preoperative and intraoperative investigations for the diagnosis of infection at the sites of two hundred and two revision total hip arthroplasties. *J Bone Joint Surg Am.* 1999;81(5):672-683.
19. Barrack ER. TGF beta in prostate cancer: a growth inhibitor that can enhance tumorigenicity. *Prostate.* 1997;31(1):61-70.
20. Pandey R, Berendt AR, Athanasou NA. Histological and microbiological findings in non-infected and infected revision arthroplasty tissues. The OSIRIS Collaborative Study Group. Oxford Skeletal Infection Research and Intervention Service. *Arch Orthop Trauma Surg.* 2000;120(10):570-574.
21. Barrack RL, Aggarwal A, Burnett RS, Clohisy JC, Ghanem E, Sharkey P, et al. The fate of the unexpected positive intraoperative cultures after revision total knee arthroplasty. *J Arthroplasty.* 2007;22(6 suppl 2):94-99.
22. Mariani BD, Levine MJ, Booth RE Jr, Tuan RS. Development of a novel, rapid processing protocol for polymerase chain reaction-based detection of bacterial infections in synovial fluids. *Mol Biotechnol.* 1995;4(3):227-237.
23. Jannes G, De Vos D. A review of current and future molecular diagnostic tests for use in the microbiology laboratory. *Methods Mol Biol.* 2006;345:1-21.
24. Tarkin IS, Dunman PM, Garvin KL. Improving the treatment of musculoskeletal infections with molecular diagnostics. *Clin Orthop Relat Res.* 2005;(437):83-88.
25. Fitzgerald RH Jr. Diagnosis and management of the infected hip prosthesis. *Orthopedics.* 1995;18(9):833-835.
26. Dronge AS, Perkal MF, Kancir S, Concato J, Aslan M, Rosenthal RA. Long-term glycemic control and postoperative infectious complications. *Arch Surg.* 2006;141(4):375-380, discussion 80.
27. Beyer CA, Hanssen AD, Lewallen DG, Pittelkow MR. Primary total knee arthroplasty in patients with psoriasis. *J Bone Joint Surg Br.* 1991;73(2):258-259.
28. Antibiotic prophylaxis for dental patients with total joint replacements. *J Am Dent Assoc.* 2003;134(7):895-899.
29. Koulouvaris P, Sculco P, Finerty E, Sculco T, Sharrock NE. Relationship between perioperative urinary tract infection and deep infection after joint arthroplasty. *Clin Orthop Relat Res.* 2009;467(7):1859-1867.
30. Seropian R, Reynolds BM. Wound infections after preoperative depilatory versus razor preparation. *Am J Surg.* 1971;121(3):251-254.
31. Rosenberg AD, Wambold D, Kraemer L, et al. Ensuring appropriate timing of antimicrobial prophylaxis. *J Bone Joint Surg Am.* 2008;90(2):226-232.
32. Rao N, Cannella B, Crossett LS, Yates AJ Jr, McGough R III. A preoperative decolonization protocol for staphylococcus aureus prevents orthopaedic infections. *Clin Orthop Relat Res.* 2008;466(6):1343-1348.
33. Nelson CL. Prevention of sepsis. *Clin Orthop Relat Res.* 1987;(222):66-72.
34. Hooper GJ, Rothwell AG, Frampton C, Wyatt MC. Does the use of laminar flow and space suits reduce early deep infection after total hip and knee replacement?: the ten-year results of the New Zealand Joint Registry. *J Bone Joint Surg Br.* 2011;93(1):85-90.
35. Berg M, Bergman BR, Hoborn J. Ultraviolet radiation compared to an ultra-clean air enclosure. Comparison of air bacteria counts in operating rooms. *J Bone Joint Surg Br.* 1991;73(5):811-815.
36. Evans RP. Current concepts for clean air and total joint arthroplasty: laminar airflow and ultraviolet radiation: a systematic review. *Clin Orthop Relat Res.* 2011;469(4):945-953.
37. Hajipour L, Longstaff L, Cleeve V, Brewster N, Bint D, Henman P. Hand washing rituals in trauma theatre: clean or dirty? *Ann R Coll Surg Engl.* 2006;88(1):13-15.
38. Carro C, Camilleri L, Traore O, Badrikian L, Legault B, Azarnoush K, et al. An in-use microbiological comparison of two surgical hand disinfection techniques in cardiothoracic surgery: hand rubbing versus hand scrubbing. *J Hosp Infect.* 2007;67(1):62-66.
39. Eitzen HE, Ritter MA, French ML, Gioe TJ. A microbiological in-use comparison of surgical hand-washing agents. *J Bone Joint Surg Am.* 1979;61(3):403-406.
40. Tanner J, Swarbrook S, Stuart J. Surgical hand antisepsis to reduce surgical site infection. *Cochrane Database Syst Rev.* 2008;23(1):CD004288.

41. Newman JB, Bullock M, Goyal R. Comparison of glove donning techniques for the likelihood of gown contamination. An infection control study. *Acta Orthop Belg.* 2007;73(6):765-771.

42. Johnston DH, Fairclough JA, Brown EM, Morris R. Rate of bacterial recolonization of the skin after preparation: four methods compared. *Br J Surg.* 1987;74(1):64.

43. Willis-Owen CA, Konyves A, Martin DK. Factors affecting the incidence of infection in hip and knee replacement: an analysis of 5277 cases. *J Bone Joint Surg Br.* 2010;92(8):1128-1133.

44. Cheung G, Carmont MR, Bing AJ, Kuiper JH, Alcock RJ, Graham NM. No drain, autologous transfusion drain or suction drain? A randomised prospective study in total hip replacement surgery of 168 patients. *Acta Orthop Belg.* 2010;76(5):619-627.

45. Shander A, Spence RK, Adams D, Shore-Lesserson L, Walawander CA. Timing and incidence of postoperative infections associated with blood transfusion: analysis of 1,489 orthopedic and cardiac surgery patients. *Surg Infect (Larchmt).* 2009;10(3):277-283.

46. Kelley BP, Heller L. A novel approach to repair of wound dehiscence in the complicated patient. *Hernia.* 2012;16(3):369-372.

47. Marculescu CE, Berbari EF, Hanssen AD, et al. Outcome of prosthetic joint infections treated with debridement and retention of components. *Clin Infect Dis.* 2006;42(4):471-478.

48. Burger RR, Basch T, Hopson CN. Implant salvage in infected total knee arthroplasty. *Clin Orthop Relat Res.* 1991;(273):105-112.

49. Azzam KA, Seeley M, Ghanem E, Austin MS, Purtill JJ, Parvizi J. Irrigation and debridement in the management of prosthetic joint infection: traditional indications revisited. *J Arthroplasty.* 2010;25(7):1022-1027.

50. Callaghan JJ, Katz RP, Johnston RC. One-stage revision surgery of the infected hip. A minimum 10-year followup study. *Clin Orthop Relat Res.* 1999;(369):139-143.

51. Oussedik SI, Dodd MB, Haddad FS. Outcomes of revision total hip replacement for infection after grading according to a standard protocol. *J Bone Joint Surg Br.* 2010;92(9):1222-1226.

52. Bloomfield MR, Klika AK, Barsoum WK. Antibiotic-coated spacers for total hip arthroplasty infection. *Orthopedics.* 2010;33(9):649.

53. Fink B, Rechtenbach A, Buchner H, Vogt S, Hahn M. Articulating spacers used in two-stage revision of infected hip and knee prostheses abrade with time. *Clin Orthop Relat Res.* 2011;469(4):1095-1102.

54. Stevens CM, Tetsworth KD, Calhoun JH, Mader JT. An articulated antibiotic spacer used for infected total knee arthroplasty: a comparative in vitro elution study of Simplex and Palacos bone cements. *J Orthop Res.* 2005;23(1):27-33.

55. Hofmann AA, Kane KR, Tkach TK, Plaster RL, Camargo MP. Treatment of infected total knee arthroplasty using an articulating spacer. *Clin Orthop Relat Res.* 1995;(321):45-54.

56. Pignatti G, Nitta S, Rani N, Dallari D, Sabbioni G, Stagni C, et al. Two stage hip revision in periprosthetic infection: results of 41 cases. *Open Orthop J.* 2010;4:193-200.

57. Sharma H, Kakar R. Outcome of Girdlestone's resection arthroplasty following complications of proximal femoral fractures. *Acta Orthop Belg.* 2006;72(5):555-559.

28

Causes of Failure of Total Hip Arthroplasty

Joshua C. Fox, MD and Michael H. Huo, MD

Total hip arthroplasty (THA) has evolved into one of the most frequently performed reconstructive operations in orthopedic surgery. Its clinical and economic efficacy has been consistently documented over the past 4 decades. There has been an evolution not just in the improvement of THA success but also in the failure mechanisms of THA. Fixation failure has traditionally been the predominant mode of primary THA failure. Innovations in the biomaterials, implant design, instrumentation, surgical techniques, perioperative protocols, and postoperative rehabilitation and surveillance have all contributed to greater durability of implant fixation. Currently, mechanisms other than loss of fixation have become major problems leading to failure.

This chapter will discuss the failure mechanisms of primary THA, including fixation failure, wear and osteolysis, infection, and instability. Emphasis is given to presenting clinical outcome data and information that is of clinical relevance. The authors will not address the failure mechanisms of revision THAs.

Fixation Failure

Aseptic fixation loosening has been the principal failure mechanism leading to revision surgery (Figure 28-1). Early reports of cemented THAs noted radiographic loosening of 20% at 5 years and upward of 30% to 40% at 10 years.[1] This was especially a problem for the younger and more active patients.[2] Many surgeons have reported improved fixation durability with newer stem designs and cementing techniques.[3,4] The emergence of cementless fixation was partially based on the failure of cement fixation 3 decades ago. There were initial challenges with stem design, surface texture, and surgical techniques that led to unpredictable clinical outcome and fixation durability of some cementless THAs. Clinical outcome has improved considerably over the past 20 years. It is estimated that cementless fixation is used in as many as two-thirds of the THAs done in the United States. In contrast, cement has remained the principal mode of implant fixation in some other countries.

The principal failure mechanism of cement fixation is debonding between cement and implant. As for cementless fixation, it is loss of bone ingrowth or bone ongrowth as a result of biological process such as osteolysis (see Figure 28-1).

Implant designs are heterogeneous as are surgical techniques and surgeon experience. Moreover, there are many patient factors that can influence the short- and long-term clinical outcome of THA. We believe it is important to understand that fixation durability is no longer an important failure mechanism based upon the clinical outcome data. The data for cement fixation are separated into 2 categories based on the surgical techniques and length of follow-up.

Parvizi J, Klatt BA.
Essentials in Total Hip Arthroplasty (pp 241-252).

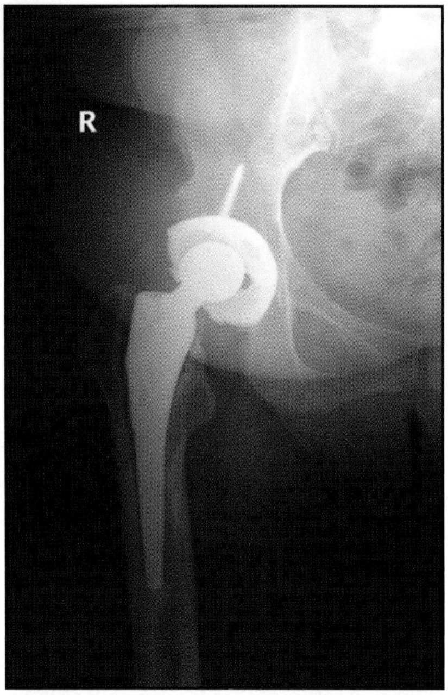

Figure 28-1. Anteroposterior radiograph of the pelvis showing aseptic loosening of the femoral stem. Please note the radiolucent line all around the stem and also subsidence of the femoral stem.

Long-Term Results of Cemented Total Hip Arthroplasty Using Techniques Earlier

Ten-Year Results

In 1973, Charnley and Cupic were the first to report the 9- to 10-year results of the low-friction arthroplasty.[5] There were 2 failed cups and 1 failed stem in 106 hips. Wroblewski reported on the 15- to 21-year result of Charnley's original series.[6] There were 32 surviving hips. No revision rate was reported. Radiographic loosening was evident in 22.5% of the cups and 29% of the stems. However, 96.5% of the patients remained relatively pain-free and were functioning well at final follow-up.

Fifteen- to 20-Year Results

McCoy et al[7] reported 4% aseptic revision rate at 15-year follow-up in 100 THAs. The 15-year fixation survival was estimated to be 98% for the cups and 93% for the stems. Kavanagh et al[8] reported on 166 Charnley THAs at a minimum 15-year follow-up. Revision for fixation failure was 12.7% overall. Loosening was 14% for the cups and 38% for the stems. Fowler et al[9] reported 5.5% aseptic failures at 13.5 years of follow-up in 426 hips done using the Exeter stem and technique. Schulte et al[10] reported the 20-year follow-up result of 330 THAs done by a single experienced surgeon. Eighty-three patients (93 hips) were alive at final follow-up. Revision was 6.3% overall and 11.1% for the surviving patients. Loosening was 23.4% for the cups and only 7.5% for the stems.

Thirty-Year Results

Berry et al[11] evaluated Charnley THAs done between 1969 and 1971 at the Mayo Clinic. Overall survival was 86.5% at 25-year follow-up. Multivariate analysis demonstrated: 1) men had 2-fold greater failure rate than women, and 2) age was a significant predictor for survival; 68.7% survival for those younger than 40 years and 100% for those older than 80 years. Callaghan et al reported the 30-year results of the patient cohort reported earlier by Schulte et al.[12] The overall revision rate was 13% for the entire group and 25% for patients who were alive 30 years after surgery. Cup revision rate was 6.4% overall and 24% for the surviving patients. The stem revision rate was only 1.2% overall and 8.8% for the surviving patients. These data should serve as a benchmark with which to evaluate the efficacy and durability of newer designs and surgical techniques.

Long-Term Results of Cemented Total Hip Arthroplasty Using Newer Techniques

Ten-Year Results

Lachiewicz and Messick[13] reported the results of 75 THAs using hybrid fixation at 10-year follow-up. The stem design was precoated. No stem was revised or determined to be loose. Meneghini et al[14] reported the results of 102 THAs done using hybrid fixation with a stem design made of cobalt-chromium alloy, collared, double-wedge geometry, and a roughened surface texture of Ra 40. Two stems were revised for loosening at 9-year follow-up. Overall fixation survival was 97.2% at 10 years.

Fifteen- to 20-Year Results

Klapach et al[15] reported the clinical results of more than 350 Charnley THAs performed using second-generation cementing technique at a minimum 20-year follow-up. Overall revision rate was 1.8%, and 5% for the surviving patients. This, however, was not significantly different from the 6.3% stem survival rate in a series of THAs done using the same stem design and the first-generation cementing technique by the same surgeon. This was perhaps partially due to the particular stem design using in both series. Callaghan et al[16] reported the results of 304 THAs done between 1984 and 1985 using a stem design with matte finish and second-generation cementing technique. Revision for any reason was 10.5% at 20-year follow-up for all patients and 25% for the surviving patients. Revision was 7.9% for the cups and 2.6% for the stems. Loosening was documented in 13.8% of the cups and 4.9% of the stems.

Durability of cement fixation has improved with newer cementing techniques even in high-risk patient groups such as those that are younger and more active. Smith et al[17] reported the results of 47 THAs done using second-generation cementing technique in patients younger than 50 years of age. Survival was 95% for the stems but only 63% for the cups at 18-year follow-up.

Stem Surface Texture in Cemented Total Hip Arthroplasty

It is important to have an understanding of stem surface texture in cemented total hip arthroplasty. There has been an intense debate over the past decade with regard to whether a matte-finished stem is at a higher risk of fixation loosening in contrast to stem designs with less cement-stem bonding. The proposed failure mechanism for a matte-finished stem is increased stress in the cement mantle leading to early cracks and debonding. Conflicting data have been reported.

Sanchez-Sotelo et al[18] reported the results of 256 hips with a matte finish and second-generation cementing techniques at mean follow-up of 15.4 years. The 15-year stem fixation survival was 92.2%. Survival was 90.1% even including radiographic loosenings. The most important predictor of fixation failure was younger age (less than 50 years) ($p < 0.0001$). Surgeons in Exeter, UK have long advocated using a polished stem with minimal cement-stem bonding. This technique has been utilized for more than 35 years. The overall rate of stem loosening was 2.8% in the initial 433 THAs performed between 1970 and 1975.[19] The stem was changed to a matte finish without changing the overall geometry in 1976. The stem revision rate increased to 10% in the next decade. Continued surveillance of patients with the more contemporary Exeter stem introduced in the 1980s demonstrated no stem revision for fixation loosening at mean follow-up of 14 years. The differences in the clinical data are most likely a function of particular stem design geometry rather than the surface texture itself. Moreover, wear at the articulation coupled with the associated osteolysis have now become the leading failure mechanism for THAs done using both cement and cementless fixation.

Long-Term Results of Cementless Total Hip Arthroplasty

Cementless fixation has undergone tremendous modifications since its introduction nearly 3 decades ago. There have been many changes in biomaterial, geometry, surface texture, extent of porous-coating, instrumentation, and surgical techniques. It is thus very difficult to make any meaningful comparison between designs or between time periods in the evolution of this technology. The North American Hip and Knee Registry[19] included over 10,000 primary THAs entered between 1995 and 2001 from participating centers. Cementless cup fixation increased from 88% in 1995 to 92% in 2001 ($p = 0.002$). Cementless stem fixation increased from 34% in 1995 to 61% in 2001 ($p < 0.0001$). This trend was attributed to improvements in design and surgical technique coupled with increasing clinical data supporting the efficacy of cementless fixation in THA.

Cementless fixation has been predictably successful and durable for the acetabular cup. Most surgeons currently use a modular cup design of hemispherical geometry with or without supplemental screw fixation. Articulation-bearing options are multiple including polyethylene, ceramic, and metal. Clinical outcome has been less predictable for the femoral stem. Fixation durability has been influenced by biomaterial, geometry, extent of porous coating, and surgical techniques.

Cementless Acetabular Cup

Clinical data on cementless cups have been consistent. Surgeons from the University of Iowa[20] have reported 15-year follow-up data of the earliest generation of cementless cup with supplemental screws and modular polyethylene bearing. The initial series included 120 THAs. It is important to note that 66 patients (72 hips) were still living at 15 years, reflecting the younger age of patients who generally received cementless fixation. It is therefore especially important to evaluate the durability of fixation and wear-related issues as these patients are expected to have longer in-situ use of their implants. No cup was revised for loosening. Pelvic osteolysis was observed in 6.9%. The linear polyethylene wear rate was on average 0.15 mm/year. Analysis was also done in a subset of patients younger than age 50 years (118 cups) from the same institution. Three cups were revised for loosening and 4 additional cup revisions were done for osteolysis. Moreover, 15 revisions were done for liner exchange for wear and osteolysis. Overall pelvic osteolysis was observed in 15%. The mean linear wear rate was higher in this more active and younger patient cohort at 0.2 mm/year. Fixation durability was significantly better

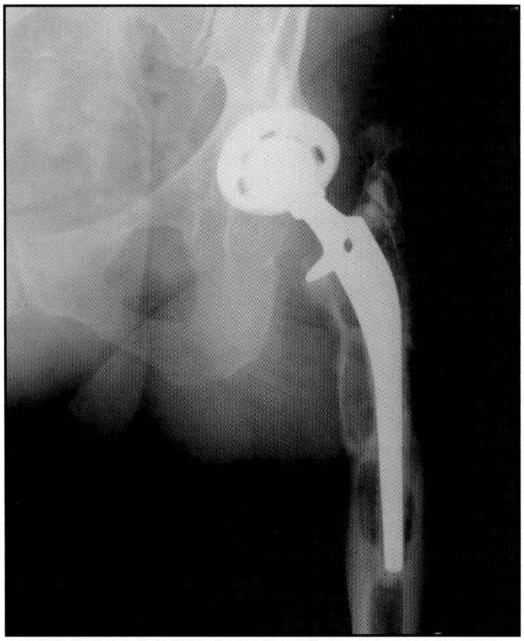

Figure 28-2. Anteroposterior radiograph of the hip showing extensive osteolysis, which was found to be due to backside wear of the polyethylene liner.

when the surgeons compared the results to their previous data with cups using cement fixation (p <0.01) at comparable follow-up interval.

Cementless Femoral Stem

Clinical efficacy of cementless stem fixation is well documented. Laupacis et al[21] conducted a prospective, randomized clinical trial including 250 patients. Patients reported no difference in outcome measures with or without cement fixation. The mean follow-up was 6.3 years. There have been numerous modifications in design and surgical technique. We will focus primarily on 2 categories of stem designs: straight cylindrical geometry with extensive-coating and tapered-wedge geometry with proximal coating.

One of the stem designs that has had the longest clinical follow-up and among the best fixation durability is the anatomical medullary lock (AML [DePuy, Warsaw, IN]). Engh et al[22] reported the 20-year follow-up data in the initial series of 223 hips. The mean age at surgery was 55 years. The mean follow-up of the 130 living (136 stems) patients was 19.2 years. Three stems were revised for loosening. Stem survival was estimated to be 97.2% at 20 years.

Durable fixation has been consistently reported with tapered wedge stems. Teloken et al[23] reported no stem revision for loosening at 15 years of follow-up in a series of 49 THAs using a tapered stem made of cobalt-chromium alloy. One important finding was that no stem progressed to loosening if it was judged to be bone-ingrown at the 2-year follow-up. This reflected that late bone remodeling due to stress transfer or bone metabolic changes did not adversely affect stem fixation durability. Garcia-Cimbrelo et al[24] reported no stem revision for loosening in 104 THAs done using a tapered stem with rectangular cross-section geometry at mean follow-up of 11 years. McLaughlin and Lee[25] followed 145 THAs done using a tapered wedge stem for 20 years. No stem was revised for loosening. Among the surviving stems 96% were judged to be bone-ingrown, 3% fibrous-stable, and 1% loose by radiographic criteria. Stem survival for all causes of failure was 91% at 22 years.

These selected citations reflect excellent mid- to long-term fixation durability for both the cup and the stem. Similar success has not been reported with other designs, many of which are no longer in clinical use. It is, however, accurate to state that fixation loosening is no longer a leading failure mechanism with cementless THAs.

Wear and Osteolysis

Wear at the articulation generates debris. The accumulation of wear debris particles in the local tissues can result in biological response, predominantly in the form of periprosthetic osteolysis (Figure 28-2). Osteolysis can lead to compromise of implant fixation. All bearing couplings regardless of hard-on-soft (metal- or ceramic-on-polyethylene), or hard-on-hard (ceramic-on-ceramic or metal-on-metal) generate wear and debris particles. The area of intense clinical and scientific focus has been with polyethylene.

Polyethylene Wear

Wear characteristics of polyethylene can be influenced by many factors including the bar stock purity, machining, sterilization, and shelf life. Gamma irradiation in air in particular has been documented to cause oxidation. Oxidation and free radicals lead to inferior wear characteristics of the material. Different wear mechanisms contribute to debris generation. These include adhesive, abrasive, and fatigue wear of the material. Not all wear debris is generated at the bearing surfaces. Particles can be produced at modular junction such as cup-shell and head-stem neck interface. Additionally, mechanisms such as impingement from component malposition can lead to accelerated wear. The quantity and size of the particles are different for different couplings and materials made from different manufacturing processes. Moreover, the threshold for osteolysis formation and progression is different for each individual patient. On average, polyethylene wear rate greater than 0.1 mm/year has been used as a predictor for osteolysis. Dowd et al[26] followed 48 hips with a single cup design and 32 mm femoral head over 10 years. All cup liners were sterilized in ethylene oxide without cross-linking. The mean linear wear rate was 0.18 mm/year. The slope of the wear rates at different time intervals was relatively linear. Osteolysis was strongly correlated with wear ($p < 0.001$). No osteolysis was observed in hips with wear of <0.1 mm/year. Another important conclusion was that future wear rates could be predicted accurately on the basis of wear rates in the early postoperative period.

Clinical wear is different from laboratory material testing data. Moreover, controversy exists with regard to the clinical correlation between wear and osteolysis generation and progression. McClung et al[27] have done extensive work correlating wear and patient activity level. They followed 37 patients whose THAs were done with conventional polyethylene sterilized with gamma radiation in air. Wear measurement demonstrated linear wear rate of 0.14 mm/year and volumetric wear rate of 73 mm^3/year. Pedometer data showed that these patients walked on average 1.9 million cycles/year. Regression analysis demonstrated the strongest correlation between male gender and increased wear. Other factors that significantly influenced wear included the patient's height ($p = 0.007$), weight ($p = 0.04$), liner thickness ($p = 0.03$), and the hip center ($p = 0.015$). Additional work from the same group demonstrated the following: 1) males walk at higher speed and for longer durations than females, 2) slower walking speed was correlated with lower wear rate, and 3) 2 million cycles of simulator testing would more accurately correspond to 1-year of in-situ usage. Thus, laboratory testing of newer polyethylene for more than 10 million cycles rather than the traditional testing limit of 6 million cycles is indicated.

Another mechanism that could contribute to wear is joint separation. Dennis et al[28] used established and validated fluoroscopic imaging techniques to evaluate patients with failing and well-functioning THAs. They found that hip separation was greater in patients with failed THA (mean 10 mm) than in those with well-functioning hips (mean 3.6 mm). The principal locus of the separation was in the superior and lateral directions that corresponded to the areas of maximal wear. Hip separation is theorized to contribute to failure by several mechanisms: 1) eccentric loading resulting in polyethylene wear, 2) impulse loading leading to loss of fixation, 3) pumping of wear debris leading to migration of particles around the pelvis and upper femoral canal resulting in periprosthetic osteolysis, and 4) instability. Impingement has been cited as a critical mechanism leading to wear and failure. Noble et al[29-31] have done much work analyzing retrieved liners. In a cohort of 120 liners made of conventional polyethylene following mean in-situ use of 18 months, they found evidence of neck-liner impingement in 32% of the liners. Subsurface cracks were found in 40%. Crack initiation from the region of impingement was observed in association with 70% of the liners with cracks. Oxidation changes were present in 90% of the liners with cracks. Noble's group also reported 31% incidence of backside wear in retrieval analysis of 113 cups. Backside wear was especially high (61%) in those cups that also demonstrated impingement. In contrast, backside wear was evident in only 16% of the liners that did not show impingement. The difference was statistically significant ($p < 0.0001$). There was also a significant difference between groups with regard to the wear rate: 0.33 mm/year with impingement versus 0.19 mm/year without impingement ($p = 0.03$). Another laboratory study was conducted to test the effect of impingement against highly cross-linked polyethylene. The liners were tested to 5 million cycles in hip simulator. Wear damage was observed in all liners after only 0.5 million cycles including pitting, delamination, and cracks at the site of impingement. The damages were most severe in the polyethylene with the highest dose of irradiation. Further improvements in implant design, component positioning, and the use of larger diameter are needed to minimize impingement in THA.

The current generation of polyethylene is manufactured using cross-linking technology in inert environment that has improved the wear characteristics of the material. Regardless of which cross-linking technology, the mechanical properties are altered. Collier et al[32] reported the results of testing of cross-linked polyethylene from 6 major orthopedic implant manufacturers. Some of the major differences among the products are as follows:

1. Gamma radiation results in uniform full-depth penetration where as electron-beam radiation results in approximately 4 cm of penetration from the surface.
2. More than 24 hours is required for gamma radiation whereas minutes to hours are required for electron-beam radiation.
3. Heating of the material after radiation facilitates further cross-linking and elimination of the free radicals generated during the cross-linking process.
4. The temperature at which heating is performed varies among the manufacturers.
5. The dose of radiation can have different effects on the mechanical properties.

Treating polyethylene with heat below melting temperature, or "annealing," will eliminate some but not all free radicals while keeping mechanical properties. Heating the material at or above the melting temperature can eliminate free radicals but the mechanical properties are substantially reduced when compared with those of conventional polyethylene. Some cases of wear and even fracture of highly cross-linked polyethylene have been reported, in particular if there was suboptimal cup position and impingement. Bradford et al[33,34] reported data from analyzing retrieved liners made of highly cross-linked polyethylene. These were compared to unused liners of the same design that served as controls. They found some evidence of wear in all liners, including scratching (96%), pitting (79%), abrasion (71%), surface cracks (67%), deformation (8%), and delamination (4%). Scanning electron microscopy demonstrated a consistent pattern of surface-crack damage parallel to and perpendicular to the machining marks. These liners were retrieved only after a very short time of in-situ service (mean 10 months). These surface cracks may progress to further subsurface cracking and fatigue wear with longer in-situ use. Second-generation of highly cross-linked polyethylene is made with modifications of the manufacturing process with the intent to improve its mechanical properties without reducing the wear resistance.

Biological Response to Wear Particles

The effects of wear debris on macrophage and monocyte cell lines have been studied extensively. Bone resorption by osteoclasts can be a result of an imbalance in the regulation of cellular activities, differentiation, proliferation, or survival. Bi et al[35] demonstrated a 30-fold increase in differentiation of cultured osteoclasts that were exposed to titanium particles. This increase led to measurably increased bone resorption. Particle phagocytosis did not affect cell survival. In contrast, Neale et al[36] demonstrated that phagocytosis of metallic particles resulted in a time and dose-dependent reduction of the osteoclast population and in bone resorption. This effect was more pronounced with cobalt-chromium and stainless steel particles than with titanium particles.

Recent studies have also shown that osteoblasts are involved in the phagocytosis of wear debris and may contribute to the development and progression of osteolysis. Vermes et al[37] demonstrated that metallic particulate debris affected osteoblast function through 2 distinct mechanisms: direct effect by the phagocytosis process itself, and an effected through down-regulation of procollagen alpha-1 gene expression along with decreased cell proliferation. Moreover, this study demonstrated that osteoblasts stimulated by particulate debris produced interleukin-6 and prostaglandin E2 leading to the activation of osteoclast function. The addition of other exogenous growth factors to the cell cultures effectively reversed the suppressive effect of wear particles on procollagen alpha-1 mRNA. This work provides possibility of pharmacological intervention for the prevention and treatment of osteolysis. Hallab et al[38] reported a decrease in H^3-thymidine incorporation into deoxyribonucleic acid in human osteoblast cell lines when exposed to synovial fluid from the hip joints of failed THAs.

One variable is the host's biological response to the wear debris. This may be a function of particle load and size. Minoda et al[39] analyzed wear particles of highly cross-linked polyethylene that were retrieved from the pseudocapsule at the time of revision surgery. They found fewer particles (5.33×10^7 particles/g) than the previously proposed critical particle load for osteolysis (1×10^{10} particles/g). The particle geometry was also smaller and rounder than those particles from conventional polyethylene. These were, however, larger than those produced from in vitro testing. These data underscore the need to develop improved models in the laboratory to test the biological effects of wear particles from newer highly cross-linked polyethylene.

Wear reduction is consistently achieved with newer material and implant designs. Questions remain whether this would result in reduction of periprosthetic osteolysis. Kitamura et al[40] examined a minimum of 6 serial radiographs for 145 THRs with identical modular cementless cup design over 10 years. The liners were made of conventional high crystalline polyethylene. Pelvic osteolysis was observed in 17.2%. The mean time to the first observation of osteolysis was 5.7 years. However, the mean x-intercept for the regression line was only 1.3 +/- 3.0 years, indicating that the onset of osteolysis was much earlier than was detectable on radiographs. In addition, progression of the 2-dimensional lesion size was on average 42.7 +/- 49.0 mm^2/year. Howie et al[41] followed 35 THAs with sequential pelvic CT scans over 1-year follow-up. They found osteolysis progression in 53%. Analysis demonstrated significant correlation with high initial wear rate ($p = 0.009$), large osteolytic lesion on the index CT scan (>10.3 cm^3, $p = 0.002$), and larger femoral head size ($p = 0.019$). These data are invaluable to guide clinical practice guidelines for surveillance of THA patients.

Metal-on-Metal Articulation

Metal-on-metal articulations provide an attractive bearing couple alternative to metal-on-polyethylene. Clinical data have demonstrated low wear rate and low incidence of osteolysis. The principal concerns are metal ion release and the biological responses to the bearing couple, in particular around some of the newer hip resurfacing implants.

Dorr et al[42] found no osteolysis in 56 THAs with a sandwich-type metal articulation after 5.2 years of follow-up. There was some initial polyethylene penetration of

0.03 mm/year from creep, and subsequent steady state of 0.03 mm/year. There was one case of metallosis due to impingement. Long's group[43] reported the midterm (6.5 years) clinical data in 161 THAs with this bearing couple. Satisfactory clinical outcome was found in 98.6%. Revision surgery was necessary in 3.7% (6 hips). Revisions specific to the bearing surface included liner dissociation (1 hip), dislocation (1 hip), unexplained pain possibly due to hypersensitivity (2 hips). There was no expansile osteolysis observed but there were radiolucencies around both the cup (21%) and the stem (9.9%).

Metal ion release is a controversial topic that has been cited as a potential failure mechanism for THA. Two centers have in particular focused on the clinical surveillance of patients with metal-on-metal bearings. MacDonald et al from University of Ontario reported on 41 patients in a prospective, randomized study comparing metal-on-metal and metal-on-polyethylene THAs.[44] There was no difference between groups in the clinical outcome at mean 2.9 years. However, there were significant differences in the urine and erythrocyte metal ion levels. The metal-on-metal group had on average 24-fold increase in the erythrocyte cobalt level ($p < 0.01$), a 2-fold increase in the chromium level ($p > 0.05$), and no difference in titanium level. With regard to urine metal levels, the metal-on-metal group had a 103-fold increase in the cobalt level ($p < 0.001$), a 29-fold increase in the chromium level ($p < 0.001$), and a 3-fold increase in the titanium level ($p < 0.02$). The levels remained elevated in 41% of the patients even after the initial bedding-in phase of in-situ wear. They followed these patients further to a mean of 7.2 years. Higher erythrocyte and urine metal levels persisted in the metal-on-metal group. Most importantly, there was no reduction over time.

Jacobs et al[45,46] from Rush-Presbyterian have done extensive work in metal ion and debris around joint implants for nearly 2 decades. They documented elevated metal ion levels even in patients with metal-on-polyethylene bearing couple. They prospectively followed serum metal levels in 58 patients. All patients had stable and well-functioning implants. All cups were made of titanium alloy with modular polyethylene bearing and inserted without cement. Different femoral stems with or without cement fixation were used. Serum and urine metal levels were measured before surgery and sequentially after surgery at defined intervals. All patients had elevated cobalt and chromium levels at 3 years in comparison to control patients without THA. The levels remained elevated in those patients with longer follow-up greater than 7 years. One source of cobalt and chromium is at the modular taper junction between the head and the stem. Potential systemic effects of disseminated metallic wear or corrosion debris are of concern. The clinical relevance has yet to be fully defined. Urban et al[47] reported dissemination of wear debris to the para-aortic lymph nodes in 78% of 28 patients. Moreover, they reported a 38% rate of metallic debris and a 14% rate of polyethylene debris in the liver and spleen. Lymphatic transport was the major mechanism of dissemination. There are reported cases of malignancy around metallic implants. Using comprehensive meta-analysis, Tharani et al[48] could not establish any link between prosthetic hip and knee implants and the development of cancer.

Metal hypersensitivity has been a subject of debate. Hallab et al[49,50] provided a comprehensive review. The prevalence of metal hypersensitivity is higher in patients with a prosthetic joint implant than it is in the general population. This issue has recently become of clinical relevance in several reports on failed THAs and hip resurfacings with metal-on-metal bearings. Korovessis et al[51] reported on the histological characteristics of tissues retrieved from the sites of 11 THAs with metal-on-metal bearing. The bearing was made of a sandwich design with polyethylene inlay. The metallurgy was a low-carbine, wrought cobalt-chromium-molybdenum alloy with a thickness of 3 mm. The investigators consistently found histiocytes and giant cells with fine intracellular metallic debris.[52] Moreover, a predominantly perivascular lymphoplasmacytic infiltrate was observed. There was no correlation of histological grading and osteolysis, however. Milosev et al[53] followed 640 THAs done using similar implant design for a mean 7.0 years. Thirty-four hips were revised. Linear or expansile femoral osteolysis was observed in 64% of the revised hips. Histology of the tissues again demonstrated perivascular lymphocyte and plasma cell infiltrates. Wear analysis demonstrated mean bearing wear of 6.3 µm/year. An abrasive wear pattern was predominant in both the cup and the femoral head. Park et al[54] reported 10 cases of osteolysis among 169 THAs done using a contemporary metal-on-metal bearing. These were observed following only 2 years of in-situ use. The patients with early osteolysis had higher prevalence of cobalt hypersensitivity than control patients did ($p = 0.03$). Histology of hip tissue from revision surgery demonstrated perivascular infiltrate of lymphocytes. Immunophenotyping demonstrated CD3-positive T cells and CD68-positive macrophages. Immunohistochemical analysis demonstrated the presence of bone-resorbing cytokines. These data suggest that delayed hypersensitivity may be the cause of early osteolysis in some patients following metal-on-metal THAs.

The surgeon should be cognizant of the propensity for systemic dissemination of the degradation products of joint arthroplasty implants through hematogenous and lymphatic routes. Expeditious revision should be considered once mechanical failure has been recognized in order to minimize the production of high concentrations of debris and metal ions. Moreover, measurement of metal ions may serve as useful clinical tools with which to identify patients who may be at the highest risk for adverse effects associated with wear debris and exposure to trace elements.

INFECTION

Infection remains to be the most feared and perhaps the most morbid complication leading to failure of a THA. There has been much reduction of its incidence with contemporary protocols of timely administration of perioperative antibiotics, surgical techniques, and improvements in the operating theater. The infection incidence based upon analysis of Medicare data is in the range of 0.5% or lower.

Patient Factors

Several risk factors have been identified to contribute to potential infection. Increasing age has been demonstrated to affect both cellular and humeral immunity in the host. Chronic diseases such as diabetes and inflammatory arthropathies are associated with a reduction of immunoresponsiveness. Malnutrition is rarely appreciated by the surgeon, particularly in patients undergoing elective THA. It can have a deleterious effect on host immunity. Pre-existing infection in the hip joint is clearly a risk. This has become much more frequent with the ever increasing volume of revision and conversion THAs. Lastly, patients with human immunodeficiency virus (HIV) infection have been reported to have higher risk of infection following THA. Lehman et al[55] reported 18% infection incidence in 29 HIV-positive patients who underwent 41 total joint arthroplasties. The infection rate was especially high (40%) in those patients who were both HIV-positive and intravenous drug abusers. Parvizi et al[56] followed 15 patients with HIV-infection who underwent 21 joint arthroplasties. All patients eventually died from their HIV infection. Infection occurred in 6 (28.6%) joints that required additional surgery.

Bacteriology

Fulkerson et al[57] reviewed positive cultures of specimens that had been obtained from 110 THAs and 84 TKAs with infection over 13 years at a tertiary medical center. Seventy percent of the infections were classified as chronic, 17% as acute postoperative, and 13% as acute hematogenous. Gram-positive organisms were isolated in 84% of the cases. *Staphylococcus aureaus* was the most common organism isolated from the site of a THA (45%), while *Staphylococcus epidermidis* was the most common organism isolated from the site of TKA (40%). With regard to antibiotic sensitivity, vancomycin 96%, gentamycin 88%, and cefazolin in only 61%. Multiple organisms were cultured in 9.3% of the cases. Based on these data, the investigators recommended the following initial antibiotic therapy: 1) chronic infections should be treated with vancomycin; 2) acute hematogenous infections should be treated with gentamycin and cefazolin; and 3) infections with multiple organisms should be treated with vancomycin and a newer-generation cephalosporin.

Management

The complex issues related to the diagnosis and treatment of infection around a THA are beyond the scope of this chapter; they will be discussed in other sections of this book. Clinically, early recognition is the most critical. Multiple laboratory tests and imaging modalities are currently used to detect infection. Diagnosis can be difficult especially if no organism is isolated from the joint fluid or tissues. Investigators from the University of Pennsylvania[58] reported distinctively different patterns of gene expression in the white blood cells retrieved from joints with implants between infected and noninfected cases. They also reported different patterns between infected cases and the cells retrieved from patients with inflammatory arthritis ($p < 0.001$). The most important finding was that abnormal gene expression was not found in noninfected cases, thus greatly improving the sensitivity and specificity of this potentially useful diagnostic methodology. Investigators from Thomas Jefferson University reported on the use of the fluorodeoxyglucose positron emission tomography (FDG-PET) imaging as a noninvasive detection test.[20] The specificity was 91.3% to identify infected cases. Even more important, infection was correctly excluded in 62 of 63 cases (specificity 98.4%). The positive and negative predictive values of this technology were 95.5% and 96.6%, respectively. These values were superior to those with using nuclear scintigraphy.

Over the past 4 decades, many treatment protocols have been proposed and shown to be clinically effective. There are, however, substantial differences in the clinical outcome from center to center. One of the problems may be that there is no standard way to quantify or qualify infections at the site of a THA. At present, treatment protocols and clinical success are both based upon some type of classification and staging system. All such systems are based on similar criteria: acute or late infection, systemic comorbidities in the host, and local comorbidities at the site of the infection.

The primary purpose of developing such staging systems is to establish some objective and reproducible criteria with the hope of influencing clinical practice and outcome.[59]

We will only briefly focus upon the most widely used treatment protocol, which is the 2-stage reimplantation. Wentworth et al[60] reported on their extensive experience of using an antibiotic-impregnated cement articulating spacer (PROSTALAC) device (DePuy) during the intervening stage in 135 patients. They compared this series to another earlier series of 134 infections treated at the same institution without PROSTALAC. The rate of persistent infection or reinfection was 17.8% for hips in the PROSTALAC groups compared to 23.1% in the patients without PROSTALAC. Complications were high: 49 complications occurred with the PROSTALAC, and 29 additional complications occurred following the second-stage reimplantation. These data clearly reflect the complexity, morbidity, and suboptimal outcome in treating THA infections.

Instability

Incidence

Recurrent dislocation is one of the most common complications leading to early revision surgery. Investigators from the Mayo Clinic have done a lot of work in the incidence of dislocation.[61] They reported that the cumulative risk for dislocation in a series of more than 6000 THAs was 1.9% at 1 month and 1.8% at 1 year. The risk rose at a constant 1% for every additional 5 years of follow-up, reaching 7% at 20 years. The risks were greater in older patients (>70 years old) (12.5% compared to 6.5% in younger patients, p = 0.018) at index surgery and in females (8.9% compared to 4.5% in males, p <0.0001). In addition, patients who underwent THA for femoral head osteonecrosis had higher dislocation than those with osteoarthritis (14.1% versus 6.4%, p <0.001).

This problem is much greater for revision THAs. Alberton et al[62] reported overall 7.4% dislocation rate in 1548 revision THAs treated at the Mayo Clinic over a 10-year period. Nonunion of the greater trochanter was associated with higher dislocation rate (p <0.001). Dislocation rate was lower in hips done using larger femoral head and an elevated rim-cup liner (p <0.05). Only 35% of the patients had one episode of dislocation without further recurrence. Reoperation was necessary in 57% of those patients who had recurrent dislocation. Most disappointing, the success rate for the revision surgeries for recurrent dislocation was only 29%. Investigators from the same institution reviewed a larger series of 4223 revision THAs done over 20 years. The overall dislocation rate was 9.2%. The cumulative risk of dislocation was 3.5% at 2 months, 6% at 1 year, 8.3% at 5 years, 10.1% at 10 years, and 13.9% at 12 years.

Mechanisms of Instability

Many factors have been identified as associated with instability in THA. One of the most frequently cited factors is surgical approach. The posterior approach has been associated with higher reported dislocation rate. Investigators from the Mayo Clinic[63] analyzed more than 22,000 THAs performed over 30 years. The cumulative risk of any dislocation was 2.2% at 1 year, 3.8% at 10 years, and 6.0% at 20 years. The 10-year cumulative risk of a dislocation was 3.2% for the anterolateral approach and 6.8% for the posterior approach (p <0.0001). The most significant factor in multivariate analysis was head size: smaller heads with higher dislocation rate. Enhanced repair of the posterior capsule and muscles has been demonstrated to reduce dislocation. This was further substantiated with cadaver study. Sioen et al[64] demonstrated significant improvement in torsional strength to failure when a transosseous repair was done compared to either soft tissue repair alone (p = 0.002) and no repair (p = 0.0002).

Investigators from the Mayo Clinic have reported different data in revision THAs in contrast to the data from analysis of dislocations following primary THAs. The risk for dislocation after revision was not correlated with age, gender, or surgical approach. There were several important findings: revision done for recurrent instability was associated with a 3.6-fold higher rate of dislocation compared with revision for aseptic loosening; multiple revisions had higher dislocation rates than those patients undergoing their first revision (p = 0.02); smaller femoral head was correlated with higher dislocation rate (p <0.0001); and revision of the stem alone was associated with a greater dislocation rate than was revision of both components or cup revision alone (p<0.001).

These data reflect the evolution in surgical techniques, implant designs, available head sizes, and rehabilitation protocols over a long time period. Regardless of the limitations of the information from these large series, the following several important points should be emphasized: 1) dislocation rate can be influenced by patient, implant, and surgical factors; 2) risk of dislocation continues to increase with longer follow-up; 3) significant improvements remain to be realized in patient selection, education, rehabilitation, surgical techniques, and implant designs to reduce the risk and incidence of dislocation following THA.

Summary

Many failure mechanisms have been reported in THA. In this short synopsis, we have emphasized in particular one of the most common mechanisms in the current clinical setting: wear and osteolysis. The volume of THA will continue to escalate as will failures. It is critical for the surgeon to appreciate the different failure mechanisms in order to identify those patients at risk and to formulate treatment plans once complications have occurred.

References

1. Stauffer RN. Ten-year follow-up study of total hip replacement. *J Bone Joint Surg Am.* 1982;64(7):983-990.
2. Chandler HP, Reineck FT, Wixson RL, McCarthy JC. Total hip replacement in patients younger than thirty years old. A five-year follow-up study. *J Bone Joint Surg Am.* 1981;63(9):1426-1434.
3. Barrack RL, Mulroy RD Jr, Harris WH. Improved cementing techniques and femoral component loosening in young patients with hip arthroplasty. A 12-year radiographic review. *J Bone Joint Surg Br.* 1992;74(3):385-389.
4. Mulroy RD Jr, Harris WH. The effect of improved cementing techniques on component loosening in total hip replacement. An 11-year radiographic review. *J Bone Joint Surg Br.* 1990;72(5):757-760.
5. Charnley J, Cupic Z. The nine and ten year results of the low-friction arthroplasty of the hip. *Clin Orthop Related Res.* 1973(95):9-25.
6. Wroblewski BM. 15-21-year results of the Charnley low-friction arthroplasty. *Clin Orthop Related Res.* 1986(211):30-35.
7. McCoy TH, Salvati EA, Ranawat CS, Wilson PD Jr. A fifteen-year follow-up study of one hundred Charnley low-friction arthroplasties. *Orthop Clin North Am.* 1988;19(3):467-476.
8. Kavanagh BF, Dewitz MA, Ilstrup DM, Stauffer RN, Coventry MB. Charnley total hip arthroplasty with cement. Fifteen-year results. *J Bone Joint Surg Am.* 1989;71(10):1496-1503.
9. Fowler JL, Gie GA, Lee AJ, Ling RS. Experience with the Exeter total hip replacement since 1970. *Orthop Clin N Am.* 1988;19(3):477-489.
10. Schulte KR, Callaghan JJ, Kelley SS, Johnston RC. The outcome of Charnley total hip arthroplasty with cement after a minimum twenty-year follow-up. The results of one surgeon. *J Bone Joint Surg Am.* 1993;75(7):961-975.
11. Berry DJ, Harmsen WS, Cabanela ME, Morrey BF. Twenty-five-year survivorship of two thousand consecutive primary Charnley total hip replacements: factors affecting survivorship of acetabular and femoral components. *J Bone Joint Surg Am.* 2002;84-A(2):171-177.
12. Callaghan JJ, Templeton JE, Liu SS, et al. Results of Charnley total hip arthroplasty at a minimum of thirty years. A concise follow-up of a previous report. *J Bone Joint Surg Am.* 2004;86-A(4):690-695.
13. Lachiewicz PF, Messick P. Precoated femoral component in primary hybrid total hip arthroplasty: results at a mean 10-year follow-up. *J Arthroplasty.* 2003;18(1):1-5.
14. Meneghini RM, Feinberg JR, Capello WN. Primary hybrid total hip arthroplasty with a roughened femoral stem: integrity of the stem-cement interface. *J Arthroplasty.* 2003;18(3):299-307.
15. Klapach AS, Callaghan JJ, Goetz DD, Olejniczak JP, Johnston RC. Charnley total hip arthroplasty with use of improved cementing techniques: a minimum twenty-year follow-up study. *J Bone Joint Surg Am.* 2001;83-A(12):1840-1848.
16. Callaghan JJ, Liu SS, Firestone DE, et al. Total hip arthroplasty with cement and use of a collared matte-finish femoral component: nineteen to twenty-year follow-up. *J Bone Joint Surg Am.* 2008;90(2):299-306.
17. Smith SE, Estok DM II, Harris WH. 20-year experience with cemented primary and conversion total hip arthroplasty using so-called second-generation cementing techniques in patients aged 50 years or younger. *J Arthroplasty.* 2000;15(3):263-273.
18. Sanchez-Sotelo J, Berry DJ, Harmsen S. Long-term results of use of a collared matte-finished femoral component fixed with second-generation cementing techniques. A fifteen-year-median follow-up study. *J Bone Joint Surg Am.* 2002;84-A(9):1636-1641.
19. Huo MH, Brown BS. What's new in hip arthroplasty. *J Bone Joint Surg Am.* 2003;85-A(9):1852-1864.
20. Huo MH, Parvizi J, Gilbert NF. What's new in hip arthroplasty. *J Bone Joint Surg Am.* 2006;88(9):2100-2113.
21. Laupacis A, Bourne R, Rorabeck C, Feeny D, Tugwell P, Wong C. Comparison of total hip arthroplasty performed with and without cement: a randomized trial. *J Bone Joint Surg Am.* 2002;84-A(10):1823-1828.
22. Engh CA Jr, Claus AM, Hopper RH Jr, Engh CA. Long-term results using the anatomic medullary locking hip prosthesis. *Clin Orthop Related Res.* 2001(393):137-146.
23. Teloken MA, Bissett G, Hozack WJ, Sharkey PF, Rothman RH. Ten to fifteen-year follow-up after total hip arthroplasty with a tapered cobalt-chromium femoral component (tri-lock) inserted without cement. *J Bone Joint Surg Am.* 2002;84-A(12):2140-2144.
24. Garcia-Cimbrelo E, Cruz-Pardos A, Madero R, Ortega-Andreu M. Total hip arthroplasty with use of the cementless Zweymuller Alloclassic system. A ten to thirteen-year follow-up study. *J Bone Joint Surg Am.* 2003;85-A(2):296-303.
25. McLaughlin JR, Lee KR. Uncemented total hip arthroplasty with a tapered femoral component: a 22- to 26-year follow-up study. *Orthopedics.* 2010;33(9):639.
26. Dowd JE, Cha CW, Trakru S, Kim SY, Yang IH, Rubash HE. Failure of total hip arthroplasty with a precoated prosthesis. 4- to 11-year results. *Clin Orthop Related Res.* 1998(355):123-136.
27. McClung CD, Zahiri CA, Higa JK, Amstutz HC, Schmalzried TP. Relationship between body mass index and activity in hip or knee arthroplasty patients. *J Orthop Res.* 2000;18(1):35-39.
28. Dennis DA, Komistek RD, Northcut EJ, Ochoa JA, Ritchie A. "In vivo" determination of hip joint separation and the forces generated due to impact loading conditions. *J Biomech.* 2001;34(5):623-629.

29. Patel AB, Wagle RR, Usrey MM, Thompson MT, Incavo SJ, Noble PC. Guidelines for implant placement to minimize impingement during activities of daily living after total hip arthroplasty. *J Arthroplasty.* 2010;25(8):1275-1281 e1271.
30. Huo MH, Gilbert NF. What's new in hip arthroplasty. *J Bone Joint Surg Am.* 2005;87(9):2133-2146.
31. Birman MV, Noble PC, Conditt MA, Li S, Mathis KB. Cracking and impingement in ultra-high-molecular-weight polyethylene acetabular liners. *J Arthroplasty.* 2005;20(7 suppl 3):87-92.
32. Collier JP, Mayor MB, Surprenant VA, Wrona M, Surprenant HP, Williams IR. The generation of wear debris from cementless hip prostheses. *Instr Course Lect.* 1994;43:257-262.
33. Bradford L, Baker DA, Graham J, Chawan A, Ries MD, Pruitt LA. Wear and surface cracking in early retrieved highly cross-linked polyethylene acetabular liners. *J Bone Joint Surg Am.* 2004;86-A(6):1271-1282.
34. Bradford L, Baker D, Ries MD, Pruitt LA. Fatigue crack propagation resistance of highly crosslinked polyethylene. *Clin Orthop Related Res.* 2004(429):68-72.
35. Bi Y, Van De Motter RR, Ragab AA, Goldberg VM, Anderson JM, Greenfield EM. Titanium particles stimulate bone resorption by inducing differentiation of murine osteoclasts. *J Bone Joint Surg Am.* 2001;83-A(4):501-508.
36. Neale SD, Haynes DR, Howie DW, Murray DW, Athanasou NA. The effect of particle phagocytosis and metallic wear particles on osteoclast formation and bone resorption in vitro. *J Arthroplasty.* 2000;15(5):654-662.
37. Vermes C, Glant TT, Hallab NJ, Fritz EA, Roebuck KA, Jacobs JJ. The potential role of the osteoblast in the development of periprosthetic osteolysis: review of in vitro osteoblast responses to wear debris, corrosion products, and cytokines and growth factors. *J Arthroplasty.* 2001;16(8 suppl 1):95-100.
38. Hallab NJ, Anderson S, Caicedo M, Brasher A, Mikecz K, Jacobs JJ. Effects of soluble metals on human peri-implant cells. *J Biomed Mater Res A.* 2005;74(1):124-140.
39. Minoda Y, Kobayashi A, Sakawa A, et al. Wear particle analysis of highly crosslinked polyethylene isolated from a failed total hip arthroplasty. *J Biomed Mater Res B Appl Biomater.* 2008;86(2):501-505.
40. Kitamura N, Sychterz-Terefenko CJ, Engh CA Sr. The temporal progression of pelvic osteolysis after uncemented total hip arthroplasty. *J Arthroplasty.* 2006;21(6):791-795.
41. Howie DW, Neale SD, Stamenkov R, McGee MA, Taylor DJ, Findlay DM. Progression of acetabular periprosthetic osteolytic lesions measured with computed tomography. *J Bone Joint Surg Am.* 2007;89(8):1818-1825.
42. Dorr LD, Wan Z, Longjohn DB, Dubois B, Murken R. Total hip arthroplasty with use of the Metasul metal-on-metal articulation. Four to seven-year results. *J Bone Joint Surg Am.* 2000;82(6):789-798.
43. Long WT. The clinical performance of metal-on-metal as an articulation surface in total hip replacement. *Iowa Orthop J.* 2005;25:10-16.
44. MacDonald SJ, McCalden RW, Chess DG, et al. Metal-on-metal versus polyethylene in hip arthroplasty: a randomized clinical trial. *Clin Orthop Related Res.* 2003(406):282-296.
45. Jacobs JJ, Campbell PA, T Konttinen Y. How has the biologic reaction to wear particles changed with newer bearing surfaces? *J Am Acad Orthop Surg.* 2008;16(suppl 1):S49-55.
46. Jacobs JJ, Urban RM, Hallab NJ, Skipor AK, Fischer A, Wimmer MA. Metal-on-metal bearing surfaces. *J Am Acad Orthop Surg.* 2009;17(2):69-76.
47. Urban RM, Jacobs JJ, Tomlinson MJ, Gavrilovic J, Black J, Peoc'h M. Dissemination of wear particles to the liver, spleen, and abdominal lymph nodes of patients with hip or knee replacement. *J Bone Joint Surg Am.* 2000;82(4):457-476.
48. Tharani R, Dorey FJ, Schmalzried TP. The risk of cancer following total hip or knee arthroplasty. *J Bone Joint Surg Am.* 2001;83-A(5):774-780.
49. Hallab N, Merritt K, Jacobs JJ. Metal sensitivity in patients with orthopaedic implants. *J Bone Joint Surg Am.* 2001;83-A(3):428-436.
50. Hallab NJ, Anderson S, Stafford T, Glant T, Jacobs JJ. Lymphocyte responses in patients with total hip arthroplasty. *J Orthop Res.* 2005;23(2):384-391.
51. Korovessis P, Petsinis G, Repanti M, Repantis T. Metallosis after contemporary metal-on-metal total hip arthroplasty. Five to nine-year follow-up. *J Bone Joint Surg Am.* 2006;88(6):1183-1191.
52. Aroukatos P, Repanti M, Repantis T, Bravou V, Korovessis P. Immunologic adverse reaction associated with low-carbide metal-on-metal bearings in total hip arthroplasty. *Clin Orthop Related Res.* 2010;468(8):2135-2142.
53. Milosev I, Trebse R, Kovac S, Cor A, Pisot V. Survivorship and retrieval analysis of Sikomet metal-on-metal total hip replacements at a mean of seven years. *J Bone Joint Surg Am.* 2006;88(6):1173-1182.
54. Park YS, Moon YW, Lim SJ, Yang JM, Ahn G, Choi YL. Early osteolysis following second-generation metal-on-metal hip replacement. *J Bone Joint Surg Am.* 2005;87(7):1515-1521.
55. Lehman CR, Ries MD, Paiement GD, Davidson AB. Infection after total joint arthroplasty in patients with human immunodeficiency virus or intravenous drug use. *J Arthroplasty.* 2001;16(3):330-335.
56. Parvizi J, Sullivan TA, Pagnano MW, Trousdale RT, Bolander ME. Total joint arthroplasty in human immunodeficiency virus-positive patients: an alarming rate of early failure. *J Arthroplasty.* 2003;18(3):259-264.
57. Fulkerson E, Valle CJ, Wise B, Walsh M, Preston C, Di Cesare PE. Antibiotic susceptibility of bacteria infecting total joint arthroplasty sites. *J Bone Joint Surg Am.* 2006;88(6):1231-1237.
58. Riggio MP, Dempsey KE, Lennon A, Allan D, Ramage G, Bagg J. Molecular detection of transcriptionally active bacteria from failed prosthetic hip joints removed during revision arthroplasty. *Eur J Clin Microbiol Infect Dis.* 2010;29(7):823-834.
59. Hanssen AD, Osmon DR. Evaluation of a staging system for infected hip arthroplasty. *Clin Orthop Related Res.* 2002(403):16-22.
60. Wentworth SJ, Masri BA, Duncan CP, Southworth CB. Hip prosthesis of antibiotic-loaded acrylic cement for the treatment of infections following total hip arthroplasty. *J Bone Joint Surg Am.* 2002;84-A (suppl 2):123-128.

61. Berry DJ, von Knoch M, Schleck CD, Harmsen WS. The cumulative long-term risk of dislocation after primary Charnley total hip arthroplasty. *J Bone Joint Surg Am.* 2004;86-A(1):9-14.
62. Alberton GM, High WA, Morrey BF. Dislocation after revision total hip arthroplasty: an analysis of risk factors and treatment options. *J Bone Joint Surg Am.* 2002;84-A(10):1788-1792.
63. Berry DJ, von Knoch M, Schleck CD, Harmsen WS. Effect of femoral head diameter and operative approach on risk of dislocation after primary total hip arthroplasty. *J Bone Joint Surg Am.* 2005;87(11):2456-2463.
64. Sioen W, Simon JP, Labey L, Van Audekercke R. Posterior transosseous capsulotendinous repair in total hip arthroplasty: a cadaver study. *J Bone Joint Surg Am.* 2002;84-A(10):1793-1798.

29

Complex Primary Total Hip Arthroplasty

Bryan D. Springer, MD

The etiology of complex primary total hip arthroplasty (THA) is multifactorial and several factors must be taken into consideration prior to performing these procedures. Dealing with the difficult primary THA involves more than dealing with just deformity/complexity that is present on radiographs. Identifying all problems preoperatively, formulating a plan to address complexity intraoperatively, and anticipating and managing problems postoperatively is paramount to achieving a successful outcome.

What makes a primary THA complex? Complexity can begin with exposure. In some patients this can be the result of soft tissue scarring from multiple operations. Exposure can also be challenging in stiff hips and in hips where there is prior hardware. Many patients have complex deformity from prior osteotomy or fracture. Childhood diseases such as Perthes disease or slipped capital femoral epiphysis can create deformity complicating the procedure. Patients with cognitive impairment from Alzheimer's disease, alcohol abuse, or with motor impairment from Parkinson's or polio create unique challenges for the arthroplasty surgeon. Patients with systemic diseases such as Gaucher's disease or sickle cell disease also require special consideration.

The purpose of this chapter is to identify those patients, diseases, and deformities that may pose potential pitfalls in hip arthroplasty.

Preoperative Planning

As has already been discussed in previous chapters, preoperative planning is critical to the success of any THA. Never is this truer than when dealing with the complex primary THA. A thorough preoperative evaluation includes a comprehensive medical evaluation, physical exam, and proper radiographs. Clinical and radiographic measures of limb lengths are an important part of this preoperative clinical exam. Preoperative templating is crucial to determine what components are necessary to complete the operation successfully. This is especially true for patients that have had prior hardware or fracture. In many cases, specialized instruments to remove prior or broken hardware may be required. In addition, custom implants may be required to deal with difficult deformity.

The Difficult Exposure

Prior Incisions and Soft Tissue Concerns

Many patients that require THA may have undergone previous hip surgery. This may result in multiple incisions and soft tissue scarring about the hip. All prior skin incisions should be considered and how they may alter the planned approach to the hip joint. Unlike the knee where blood flow to the skin is tenuous, problems with the wound around the hip with previous incisions are relatively rare. It is important, however, to follow the principles of soft tissue management when dealing with prior incisions.

Whenever possible, it is best to incorporate previous longitudinal incisions into the approach. If the patient has a single previous incision and the position is adequate for the planned approach, it should be used. In patients with

Parvizi J, Klatt BA.
Essentials in Total Hip Arthroplasty (pp 253-264).

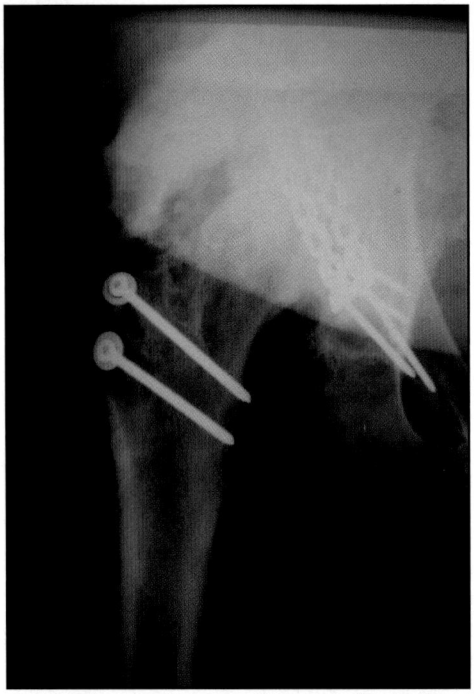

Figure 29-1. Thirty-six-year-old patient who developed massive heterotopic bone formation in his abductor muscle complex following open reduction and internal fixation of his acetabular fracture. This resulted in an essentially fused hip that required extensile exposure at the time of conversion to THA.

Table 29-1

Factors That May Influence Choice of Surgical Approach

- Prior skin incisions
- Previous surgical approach
- Retained hardware
- Need for extensile exposure
- Dislocation risk and patient compliance

Table 29-2

Common Soft Tissue Release About the Hip to Aid in Exposure of the Stiff Hip

- Anterior and superior hip capsule
- Gluteus maximus tendon
- Tendon of iliopsoas
- Adductor tendons

pliable skin, full thickness skin flaps can be created to form a mobile window that allows retraction of skin in the anterior or posterior direction to accommodate the planned approach. This is preferred to creating a parallel longitudinal incision, which may compromise circulation to the intervening skin bridge.

Old prior incisions that are not near the intended path of the procedure can generally be ignored. When prior incisions must be crossed, it is best to do so at 90-degree angles to minimize skin edge necrosis. Acute angles should be avoided. In patients with significant contracture from multiple previous scars or lack of adipose tissue resulting in noncompliant tissue, preoperative consultation with a plastic surgeon is advised. Considerations may be given to the use of "sham" incisions to ensure wound healing or the use of tissue expanders to increase the compliance of the skin.

Exposing the Stiff Hip

Many patients with prior hip surgery or trauma present with stiffness. This can be the result of soft tissue contracture, previous hardware, or bony ankylosis (Figure 29-1). These patients present a challenge during initial exposure and dislocation of the hip. Care must be taken to protect important neurovascular structures during the exposure. In addition, intraoperative fracture may occur if excessive force is required to dislocate the hip.

Preoperative planning should include evaluation of prior incisions, skin compliance, and range of motion. Musculotendinous contractures, spasticity, and bony ankylosis should be noted and compared to the normal nonoperative side. If previous surgery has been performed, the prior approach utilized and any hardware in place should be identified from the prior operative note. The approach chosen to expose the stiff hip is based on previous skin incisions (see above), prior approaches, and surgeon comfort. In addition, exposures that allow for extensile access to the hip should be utilized. Table 29-1 lists factors that should be taken into consideration when choosing surgical approach.

The initial steps in exposing the stiff hip involve release of soft tissue structures and osteophytes. Soft tissue releases are listed in Table 29-2. The gluteus maximus tendon is a thick fibrous tendon that inserts on the posterior aspect of the femur below the level of the lesser trochanter. It provides a strong restraint to anterior translation of the femur during exposure. Release of the gluteus maximus tendon and repair

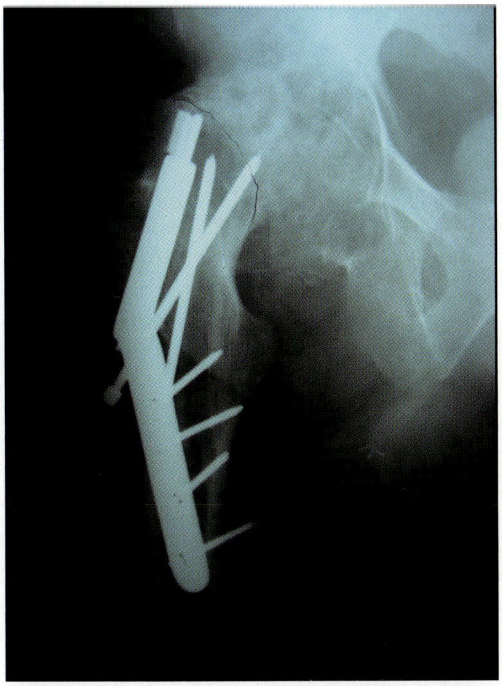

Figure 29-2. Prior hardware can lead to significant deformity and distortion of the proximal femoral anatomy.

at the conclusion of the case can be done with no functional limitations or need for added restrictions postoperatively. The tendon should be released with a 5- to 10-mm cuff of tissue to allow for reapproximation at the end of the case.

The iliopsoas tendon crosses the anterior aspect of the hip joint to insert on the lesser trochanter. In patients with significant hip flexion contracture, release of the iliopsoas tendon off the level of the lesser trochanter may aid in exposure. Patients with a neuromuscular condition often present with adduction contractures. These may be addressed at the time of surgery with direct release through the surgical site or percutaneous release/fractional lengthening though an addition medial thigh incision over the area of contracture. In addition to muscular contractures, the hip capsule itself often contributes to stiffness about the hip joint. A wide capsulectomy, particularly of the anterior and superior capsule, can substantially aid in exposure. An anterior approach releases the anterior capsule and this can help to address a flexion contracture.

Bony ankylosis secondary to osteophytes or heterotopic bone should be addressed at the time of exposure as well. All surrounding osteophytes from both the femur and acetabulum should be removed under direct visualization with an osteotome.

Osteotomy of the femoral head and neck in-situ prior to dislocation is often useful to facilitate exposure and prevent a forceful dislocation. Using a reciprocating saw with the sciatic nerve protected, the neck is osteotomized above the level of the planned resection. The head-neck segment can then be removed from the acetabulum and the femoral neck recut at the appropriate level based on preoperative templating. Occasionally extensile exposures such as classic trochanteric osteotomy, trochanteric slide osteotomy, or extended trochanteric osteotomy may be required to facilitate exposure (see Chapter 15).

Table 29-3

List of Instruments/Tools to Help Deal With Retained Hardware

- Osteotomes
- Curetts
- High-speed burr
- Metal-cutting burrs and wheels
- Broken screw removal set
- Universal extractors
- Vice-grip slap hammers

Managing Previous Hardware

Patients with prior hardware can pose a significant challenge in THA. Hardware often leads to distortion of the femoral and acetabular anatomy (Figure 29-2). This can include obliteration of the medullary canal, canal stenosis, or femoral malunion. In addition, broken hardware can be difficult to remove and prior screw holes can lead to stress risers, increasing the likelihood of intraoperatve or postoperative fracture.

Preoperative planning should include identification of hardware in place and radiographs of the entire pelvis and femur to ensure that all hardware has been identified. If extensive hardware exists, consideration may be given to a staged approach with initial removal of all hardware followed by a second surgery to perform the arthroplasty. This approach must be weighed against duration and complexity of completing the surgery in one stage.

Appropriate instruments and tools to remove hardware must be available (Table 29-3), including those needed to deal with broken hardware/screws (Figure 29-3).

At the time of surgery, hardware that is not in the way of the arthroplasty or that does not compromise the fixation of the component may be left in place. This is particularly true

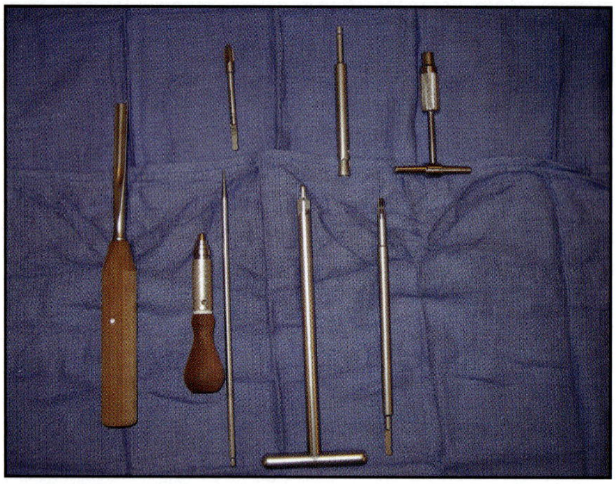

Figure 29-3. Broken screw removal set used to aid in removal of broken screws at the time of surgery.

Table 29-4 **Classification of Proximal Femoral Deformity**
Site of Deformity
• Greater trochanter • Femoral neck • Metaphysis • Diaphysis
Geometry of Deformity
• Torsional • Angular • Translational • Size abnormality
Etiology of Deformity
• Developmental (dysplasia) • Metabolic (Paget's) • Previous osteotomy • Previous fracture

in cases such as prior acetabular fractures, where a cementless socket may be placed often times with minimal or no interference from existing hardware (Figure 29-4). The rare screw that is encountered can be removed with a burr so that reaming can continue without complete hardware removal. This obviates the need for more significant dissection. Prior to removing any femoral hardware, the exposure should be completed and the hip dislocated. This limits the potential for intraoperative fracture to occur at the site of weakened

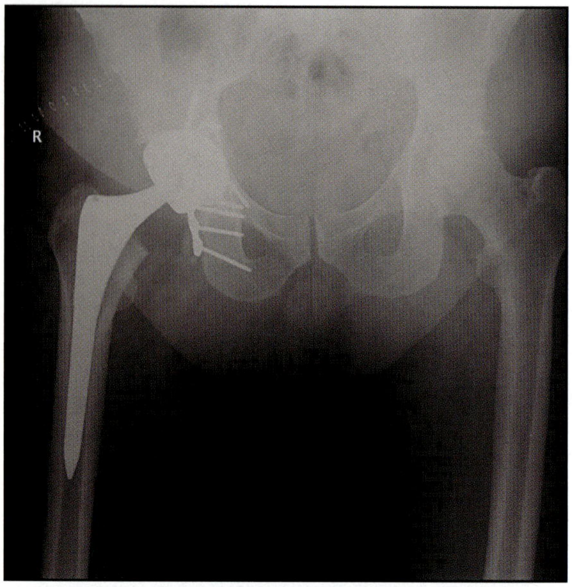

Figure 29-4. THA performed for avascular necrosis following open reduction and internal fixation of an acetabular fracture. Note that the majority of the hardware was able to be left in place at the time of surgery, obviating the need for more substantial surgical dissection to remove the hardware.

bone from prior hardware. All stress risers, such as previous screw holes, should be bypassed with the intramedullary stem by 2 cortical diameters.

Total Hip Arthroplasty in Patients With Deformity

A wide range in variation exists when dealing with deformity about the proximal femur. Most deformities can be dealt with standard or modular implants. Certain deformities, however, can be technically challenging, leading to problems such as intraoperative fracture, altered biomechanics, and failure of fixation.[1] Occasionally, such significant deformity can exist that special exposures or custom implant may be required.

Berry has described a classification of proximal femoral deformity based on the level of the deformity, geometry, and etiology of deformity (Table 29-4).[2] Deformities can be found at the greater trochanter, femoral neck, metaphysis, or diaphysis. The geometry can be torsional, angular, translational, or a size abnormality. Deformities encountered during THA are often secondary to a developmental process (dysplasia), metabolic disorders (Paget's), previous surgery that has altered the geometry of the hip (osteotomy), or fracture. Defining the deformity with this classification

Table 29-5

RESULTS OF TOTAL HIP ARTHROPLASTY AFTER PROXIMAL FEMORAL OSTEOTOMY

AUTHOR	YEAR	NUMBER OF HIPS	FOLLOW-UP	STEM TYPE	RESULTS	COMPLICATIONS
Haverkamp et al[3]	2006	121	11.9 years	Cemented	83% survivorship at 15 years	Higher rate of femoral perforation compared to controls
Breusch et al[4]	2005	48	11 years	Cementless	94% survivorship at 10 years	Complications similar to control group
Iwase et al[5]	1999	30	7 years	Both	100% survivorship with cemented stems	Better results w/ cemented stems One patient corrective osteotomy
Shinar et al[6]	1998	22	15.8 years	Cemented	10% aseptic loosening	8 patients required custom stems
Boos et al[7]	1997	74	6.9 years	Cemented	82% survival at 10 years (90% for controls)	88% required trochanteric osteotomy
Soballe et al[8]	1989	112	4.7 years	Cemented	No difference in survival compared to control	Higher rate of intraoperative femur fracture

system provides a rationale approach to plan for and deal with deformity at the time of THA.

When deformity is identified, preoperative templating is critical to determine appropriate selection and prepare for potential technical difficulties during the case. The need for modular or even custom implants should be determined. The level and degree of correction is noted should intraoperative osteotomy be required.

Prior Femoral Osteotomy

Proximal femoral osteotomy is a valuable tool to treat many conditions of the hip in the young patient. The goal is to prevent or prolong the development of end-stage arthritic disease in the hip. Ultimately, however, many of these patients will go on to develop secondary arthritis and require THA. Conversion of the failed femoral osteotomy to total hip replacement presents the challenges of not only dealing with prior hardware as mentioned above, but also the potential for complications related to distorted femoral anatomy.

Ideally, the femoral osteotomy should be performed in a way that will not significantly distort the femoral anatomy while not compromising the result of the osteotomy itself. Remodeling of the proximal femur can take place over years after an osteotomy and may not be readily apparent on radiographs secondary to distortion from the hardware. After a varus osteotomy, the trochanter tends to overhang the femoral canal, resulting in difficulty inserting the stem. A trochanteric osteotomy may be required to allow access to the femoral canal. Varus/valgus osteotomies can be combined with flexion/extension or medial/lateral displacement of the proximal segment relative to the femoral shaft. Realignment osteotomy may be required to allow for stem insertion. Rotational osteotomies may distort the anteversion and site of insertion of the stem.

The results of THA after previous femoral osteotomy are listed in Table 29-5. There are several initial reports of higher complication rates and of poorer long-term survival of THA in patients with previous femoral osteotomy.[1,9,8] More recent reports, however, show results comparable to standard primary THA.[4,3,6]

Boos et al compared a matched group of 74 patients with prior proximal femoral osteotomy with a control group of patients with standard THA.[7] All stems were cemented. No significant difference was found with regards to the rate of complications or revisions. The prior osteotomy group did have a higher rate of trochanteric osteotomy required at the time of surgery and a longer operating time owing to the

Table 29-6

RESULTS OF TOTAL HIP ARTHROPLASTY AFTER PREVIOUS ACETABULAR FRACTURE

AUTHOR	YEAR	NUMBER OF HIPS	FOLLOW-UP	CUP TYPE	RESULTS
Berry et al[10]	2002	34	10 to 16 years	Cementless	36% revision rate
Bellabarba et al[11]	2001	30	5.25 years	Cementless	97% survivorship at 10 years
Huo et al[12]	1999	21	5.4 years	Cementless	19% failure rate acetabulum
Weber et al[13]	1998	66	9.6 years	Both	78% survivorship at 10 years
Romness et al[14]	1990	55	7.5 years	Both	53% acetabular loosening

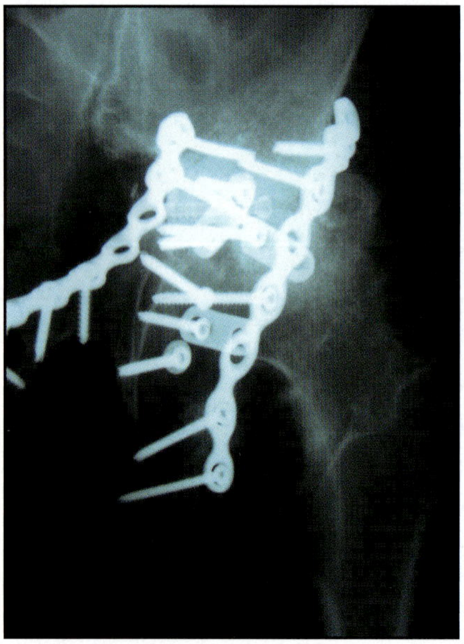

Figure 29-5. Forty-five-year-old female who developed avascular necrosis following open reduction and internal fixation of her acetabular fracture ultimately requiring conversion to THA.

complexity of the surgery. It should be noted that 55 patients in the osteotomy group had the hardware removed during a separate procedure from the arthroplasty.

Breusch et al reported on the results of uncemented hip stems in patients with failed intertrochanteric osteotomy.[4] At a mean follow-up of 10 years, the femoral survivorship using revision for any reason as an endpoint was 94%. The authors conclude that cementless fixation for the treatment of failed femoral osteotomy is comparable to those achieved in patients with regular femoral anatomy.

TOTAL HIP ARTHROPLASTY AFTER PRIOR FRACTURE

Acetabular Fracture

THA is indicated as a treatment for failed acetabular fractures in patients who develop avascular necrosis, post-traumatic osteoarthritis, or migration of hardware intra-articularly (Figure 29-5). Occasionally, THA may be indicated for the acute treatment of acetabular fractures in elderly patients or those with pre-existing arthritis.

Many of the principles used to treat patients with prior acetabular fractures have already been discussed. These include dealing with prior incisions, exposing the stiff hip, and dealing with prior hardware. In addition, patients may also have altered hip biomechanics from damaged musculature as well as heterotopic bone. Care must be taken during exposure as tethering or scarring of the sciatic nerve may have occurred. It is best to wait until fracture union has occurred prior to conversion surgery as dealing with nonunions is challenging. Hardware that is encountered at the time of surgery need not be removed unless it is in the way or compromises fixation of the acetabular component.

The results of THA following previous acetabular fracture are listed in Table 29-6.

Femoral Neck and Intertrochanteric Hip Fracture

Complications from previous hip fracture surgery of the femoral neck or intertrochanteric region may ultimately require conversion to THA. Internal fixation of femoral

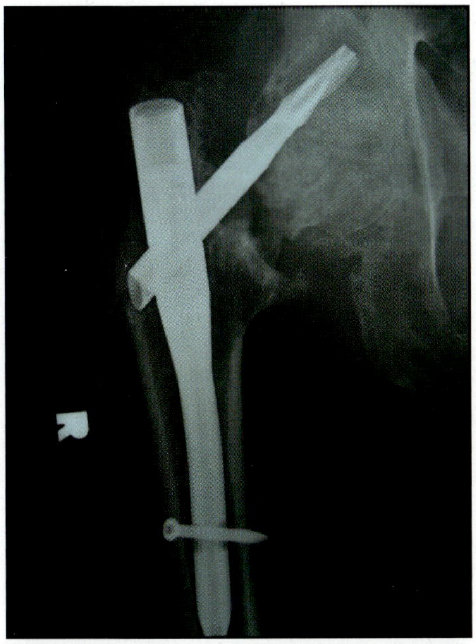

Figure 29-6. Post-traumatic arthritis and acetabular erosion secondary to failed treatment of intertrochanteric hip fracture.

neck fractures has been shown to lead to nonunion or avascular necrosis in approximately 15% to 20% of cases.[15,16] In addition, the development of post-traumatic arthritis, perforation of the acetabulum by protruding hardware, and leg length discrepancy are also indications for conversion to THA (Figure 29-6).

Preoperative considerations in dealing with the failed hip fracture include identification of prior hardware, methods of removal, and implant selection. Since many patients with previous hip fractures are elderly or debilitated, a thorough medical evaluation should be undertaken prior to proceeding with surgery. Conversion from failed hip fracture fixation to THA is associated with a higher complication rate than primary THA. Increased risk of intraoperative fracture, excessive blood loss from extensile exposures, hardware removal, leg length inequality, and risk of dislocation all must be taken into consideration and discussed preoperatively.

Patients with failed femoral neck fractures often have normal distal femoral anatomy. Once hardware is removed, stem selection can be based on surgeon comfort and patient bone quality. Both cemented and cementless implants have been shown to have predictable results. In elderly debilitated patients with minimal secondary arthritis, conversion to a hemiarthroplasty is the treatment of choice. In patients with underlying arthritis or acetabular damage secondary to hardware penetration, conversion to THA is preferred.

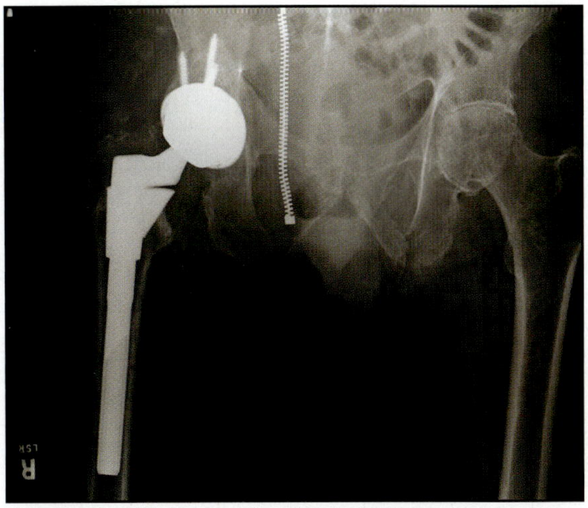

Figure 29-7. Modular stems are often helpful to deal with proximal femoral deformity following conversion of a failed intertrochanteric hip fracture.

Patients with failed intertrochanteric fractures often have distorted femoral anatomy as a result of either a malunion or nonunion. This deformity can exist in all planes and be either metaphyseal or diaphyseal. In these situations, modular stems can be useful in dealing with the deformity (Figure 29-7). Proximal femoral bone stock deficiency may require the use of calcar substituting prosthesis. In addition, defects left in the bone from prior hardware can act as stress risers and should be bypassed with the femoral stem or the addition of a cortical strut graft.

In most instances, acetabular preparation for conversion THA proceeds similarly to primary THA. Two situations often exist in these patients that should be taken into consideration. First, the acetabular bone quality is often weak and osteoporotic. This is often due to the age of the patient as well as relative disuse osteopenia secondary to inactivity. Care should be taken when reaming the acetabulum as over aggressive reaming can lead to rapid loss of bone and compromise fixation. Secondly, penetration of the acetabulum by migration of hardware can lead to both cavitary and segmental defects requiring the use of bone graft or other forms of augmentation.

Patients with prior hip fracture converted to THA have been shown to be at higher risk for development of instability postoperatively. This can be secondary to altered anatomy or biomechanics or psychological factors and poor compliance often encountered in this patient population. As such, consideration should be given to the surgical approach utilized, head size options available, and use of bipolar heads or constrained components when indicated.

Table 29-7

RESULTS OF TOTAL HIP ARTHROPLASTY AFTER FAILED TREATMENT OF HIP FRACTURE

AUTHOR	YEAR	NUMBER OF HIPS	FOLLOW-UP	FRACTURE TYPE	COMPONENTS	SURVIVORSHIP	COMPLICATIONS
Mabry et al[17]	2004	85	12.2 years	Femoral neck	Cemented	93% at 10 years, 76% at 20 years	9 dislocations
Haidukewych et al[18]	2003	60	5 months	Intertrochanteric	Mixed	87.5% at 10 years	5 reoperations 1 dislocation
Mehlhoff et al[15]	1991		2.9 years	Both	Mixed	100%	No revisions 3 dislocations

Results of conversion THA for failed femoral neck fracture or intertrochanteric fracture are listed in Table 29-7.

TOTAL HIP ARTHROPLASTY AFTER SEQUELAE OF PEDIATRIC DISEASE

Legg-Calvé-Perthes Disease

Legg-Calvé-Perthes disease is a disorder of the pediatric hip of uncertain etiology. It occurs most commonly in children 4 to 8 years of age and is more common in males than females. The disease affects the epiphyseal cartilage of the hip, leading to growth disturbance of the femoral head and often the acetabulum.

The treatment of Legg-Calvé-Perthes disease remains controversial. Little is known about the natural history of the disease and thus true comparative studies on the outcome of treatment are lacking.[19] Maintaining range of motion and containment of the femoral head during the reparative/healing process are the hallmarks of treatment. This can often be accomplished through nonoperative management with bed rest, traction, and splinting. Femoral and pelvic osteotomies can be used to achieve these goals when nonoperative management is insufficient.

The majority of patients can lead active and pain-free lives regardless of treatment and despite the fact that they often have abnormal radiographs. Clinical deterioration appears to develop with time and the majority ultimately develops degenerative disease of the hip. A series of long-term follow-up studies from the University of Iowa showed that by the fourth to fifth decade, 40% of patients required arthroplasty and an additional 10% had severe arthritis.[20] Mose demonstrated that the majority of patients followed beyond 40 years demonstrated marked reduction in function with the majority developing degenerative joint disease in their 50s and 60s.[21,22] Those with aspherical femoral heads developed degenerative changes earlier than those with a more congruent joint surface.

In patients that ultimately develop degenerative arthritis as a result of Legg-Calvé-Perthes disease, deformity often exists as a result of the disease itself or treatment. Coxa magna, an enlarged femoral head, and coxa plana, a truncated femoral head and short neck, are common sequelae of the disease.[23] In addition, femoral or pelvic osteotomy may have been performed previously not only introducing deformity but retained hardware. Physeal and epiphyseal growth arrest may lead to a shorted and deformed femoral neck. This is often complicated by trochanteric overgrowth that can make insertion of the femoral stem difficult. In these situations, a classic or extended trochanteric osteotomy may be required in order to allow for accurate insertion of the femoral stem without the risk of trochanteric fracture. In order to accommodate the misshapen femoral head, the acetabulum may also be deformed. This often results in a "shallow" socket and anterior-superior bone loss similar to that seen in the dysplastic hip.

Slipped Capital Femoral Epiphysis

Slipped capital femoral epiphysis is a disorder in which the capital femoral epiphysis displaces from the metaphysic through the physeal plate. The etiology is unknown and may be multifactorial with numerous reports citing endocrine abnormalities. It occurs most commonly between the ages of 10 to 16 years. Patients that are obese and have delayed skeletal maturation appear to be at increased risk.

Table 29-8

Commonly Found Deformity in Patients With Paget's Disease

Femoral Deformity
• Coxa vara • Trochanteric overhang • Femoral expansion (metaphyseal-diaphyseal mismatch) • Diaphyseal bowing • Sclerotic canal
Acetabular Deformity
• Acetabular protrusio • Enlarged pelvis • Cavitary/cystic degeneration

Slipped capital femoral epiphysis and its resultant deformity have been implicated as a cause of osteoarthritis.[24,25] Large numbers of hips in young patients with what was initially believed to be "primary" osteoarthritis were actually found to have subtle changes of slipped epiphysis.[26] The risk of development of osteoarthritis following slipped capital femoral epiphysis appears to be related to the degree of deformity.[27,28] Deformity predisposes patients to altered hip kinematics resulting from femoral-acetabular impingement as described by Ganz.[29] Because the slips often occur after skeletal maturity, there is little, if any, change in adaptive remolding of the acetabulum. Thus, THA in the patient population, while often of younger age than the typical arthroplasty patients with primary osteoarthritis, is relatively straightforward.

Total Hip Arthroplasty in Patients With Metabolic Bone Disease

Paget's Disease

Paget's disease is a metabolic bone disease of unknown etiology that results from increased excessive activity of both osteoclasts and osteoblasts. Histologically, Paget's results in extensive osteolysis, a large number of osteoblasts and osteoclasts, and the production of woven-type bone with wide lamella giving the bone a "mosaic" type pattern. Normal marrow spaces are replaced by highly vascularized fibrous connective tissue. The disease may involve only one bone (monostotic) or several bones (polyostotic).

The prevalence of Paget's disease in the population is approximately 4% and is the second most common metabolic bone disease after osteoporosis. Many patients are asymptomatic and the characteristic findings are noted incidentally on radiographs. For those patients that become symptomatic, they may present with joint pain, bone pain, low back pain, and have evidence of deformity. For those patients presenting with pain, it is important to differentiate the source of pain as stress fractures, lumbar compressive neuropathy, and the development of Paget's sarcoma can cause pain about the hip.

Patients who have involvement of Paget's disease near a joint often develop symptomatic arthritis. THA is the procedure of choice in patients with arthritis of the hip in conjunction with Paget's disease. Several technical considerations should be recognized prior to proceeding with THA. Table 29-8 lists the common deformities present in both the femur and acetabulum preoperatively. THA in patient with Paget's disease can be approached similarly to standard primary THA. In patients with significant coxa vara, trochanteric osteotomy and advancement may be required to facilitate stem insertion and improve hip biomechanics. The canal is often sclerotic and enlarged. Straight reamers and high speed burrs may be required to gain safe entry into the femoral canal. Acetabular protrusio is often encountered and deepening of the socket with reaming should be done with caution.

Excessive blood loss may be encountered and can be minimized with preoperative medical management. The development of heterotopic ossification can develop in up to one-half of patients with Paget's undergoing THA.[30] Consideration should be given to treatment with nonsteroidal anti-inflammatory agents or perioperative radiation.

The results of THA in patients with Paget's disease has been successful with both cemented and uncemented prosthesis.[31-35] Table 29-9 lists the results of THA in patients with Paget's disease.

Gaucher's Disease

Gaucher's disease is a lysosomal storage disease resulting in the accumulation of glucocerebrosides in the reticuloendothelial cells. It is inherited as an autosomal recessive disease. The skeletal manifestations of the disease include osteopenia, fracture, and the development of osteonecrosis.

There are a limited number of studies focusing on THA in patients with Gaucher's disease. While the majority of

Table 29-9

Results of Total Hip Arthroplasty in Patients With Paget's Disease

Author	Year	Number of Hips	Follow-Up	Implant Type	Results
McDonald et al[34]	1987	52	8.8 years	Cemented	39 good/excellent results; 9 revisions
Ludkowski et al[36]	1988	37	7.8 years	Cemented	No revisions; 27 good/excellent results
Sochart et al[37]	2000	98	10.4 years	Cemented	8 revisions; 81 good/excellent results
Hozack et al[31]	1999	5	5.8 years	Cementeless	No revisions; all good/excellent results
Kirsh et al[38]	2001	20	6 years	Cementeless	No revisions[19 good/excellent results
Parvizi et al[39]	2002	19	7 years	Cementless	No revisions; 19 good/excellent results

studies have shown improved functional outcome for this patient population there is a suggested higher incidence of aseptic loosening and infection compared to primary THA.[40-42]

Total Hip Arthroplasty in Patients With Cognitive/Motor Impairment

The indications for THA for patients with cognitive and motor impairment are no different that those of the general population. They include radiographic evidence of arthritis, pain that limits functional activities of daily living, and failure of conservative management. There are several preoperative, intraoperative, and postoperative factors that must be taken into consideration. This particular patient population, as a result of their underlying disease, is at increased risk for complications.

One of the greatest concerns in patients with underlying cognitive and motor impairment is the risk of dislocation. This is often multifactorial. Patients with motor impairment from previous stroke, cerebral palsy, or polio may demonstrate motor weakness or spasticity that places them at increased risk. Patient with cognitive impairment secondary to dementia or alcoholism are at increased risk due to noncompliance with postoperative precautions. While the operating surgeon should use the approach most familiar to him or her, consideration should be given to approaches such as the anterolateral approach to diminish the risk of dislocation. In addition, the role of larger heads and constrained liners may also need to be considered.

Parkinson's Disease

Parkinson's disease is a degenerative neurological disease of the central nervous system. Its prevalence in the general population over age 60 is approximately 1%.[43] Manifestations include tremors, rigidity, and akinesia. Patients often develop a stooped posture and "shuffling gait" as symptoms progress. Joint position sense and proprioception become impaired, often resulting in a higher incidence of hip fracture secondary to falls.[44,45]

Technically, patients with Parkinson's disease can be challenging at the time of surgery due to the presence of hip flexion and adduction contractures. Meticulous testing of stability at the time of surgery must be undertaken. Any residual tightness in the hip flexors and adductors should be released at the time of surgery. Consideration should be given to alteration in surgical approach and use of large heads.

There is a paucity of data on primary elective THA in patients with Parkinson's disease. The results are extrapolated from the literature on patients with Parkinson's treated with endoprosthetic replacement for displaced femoral neck fractures.

Weber et al reported on the results of 107 THAs performed in patient with Parkinson's disease from 1970 to 1994.[46] Complications occurred in 36% of patients and 51 patients had died at the time of latest follow-up. There were 6 dislocations, all occurring in patients with diagnosis other that osteoarthritis. The overall survivorship free of reoperation was 93% at 5 years. Pain and functional outcome improved initially but because of the progressive nature of the disease, function declines with time.

Summary

All primary total hip replacements are not routine. A variety of complex situations present unique challenges to the hip replacement surgeon, and it is possible to plan properly to improve the odds of a good outcome.

References

1. Benke GJ, Baker AS, Dounis E. Total hip replacement after upper femoral osteotomy: a clinical review. *J Bone Joint Surg Br.* 1982;64(5):570-571.
2. Berry DJ. Total hip arthroplasty in patients with proximal femoral deformity. *Clin Orthop Relat Res.* 1999;(369):262-272.
3. Haverkamp D, de Jong PT, Marti RK. Intertrochanteric osteotomies do not impair long-term outcome of subsequent cemented total hip arthroplasties. *Clin Orthop Relat Res.* 2006;444:154-160.
4. Breusch SJ, Lukoschek M, Thomsen M, Mau H, Ewerbeck V, Aldinger PR. Ten-year results of uncemented hip stems for failed intertrochanteric osteotomy. *Arch Orthop Trauma Surg.* 2005;125(5):304-309.
5. Iwase T, Hasegawa Y, Iwasada S, Kitamura S, Iwata H. Total hip arthroplasty after failed intertrochanteric valgus osteotomy for advanced osteoarthrosis. *Clin Orthop Relat Res.* 1999;(364):175-181.
6. Shinar AA, Harris WH. Cemented total hip arthroplasty following previous femoral osteotomy: an average 16-year follow-up study. *J Arthroplasty.* 1998;13(3):243-253.
7. Boos N, Krushell R, Ganz R, Muller ME. Total hip arthroplasty after previous proximal femoral osteotomy. *J Bone Joint Surg Br.* 1997;79(2):247-253.
8. Soballe K, Boll KL, Kofod S, Severinsen B, Kristensen SS. Total hip replacement after medial-displacement osteotomy of the proximal part of the femur. *J Bone Joint Surg Am.* 1989;71: 692-697.
9. Ferguson GM, Cabanela ME, Ilstrup DM. Total hip arthroplasty after failed intertrochanteric osteotomy. *J Bone Joint Surg Br.* 1994;76(2):252-257.
10. Berry DJ, Halasy M. Uncemented acetabular components for arthritis after acetabular fracture. *Clin Orthop Relat Res.* 2002;(405):164-167.
11. Bellabarba C, Berger RA, Bentley CD, et al. Cementless acetabular reconstruction after acetabular fracture. *J Bone Joint Surg Am.* 2001;83-A(6):868-876.
12. Huo MH, Solberg BD, Zatorski LE, Keggi KJ. Total hip replacements done without cement after acetabular fractures: a 4- to 8-year follow-up study. *J Arthroplasty.* 1999;14(7):827-831.
13. Weber M, Berry DJ, Harmsen WS. Total hip arthroplasty after operative treatment of an acetabular fracture. *J Bone Joint Surg Am.* 1998;80(9):1295-1305.
14. Romness DW, Lewallen DG. Total hip arthroplasty after fracture of the acetabulum. Long-term results. *J Bone Joint Surg Br.* 1990;72(5):761-764.
15. Mehlhoff T, Landon GC, Tullos HS. Total hip arthroplasty following failed internal fixation of hip fractures. *Clin Orthop Relat Res.* 1991;(269):32-37.
16. Tabsh I, Waddell JP, Morton J. Total hip arthroplasty for complications of proximal femoral fractures. *J Orthop Trauma.* 1997;11(3):166-169.
17. Mabry TM, Prpa B, Haidukewych GJ, Harmsen WS, Berry DJ. Long-term results of total hip arthroplasty for femoral neck fracture nonunion. *J Bone Joint Surg Am.* 2004;86-A(10):2263-2267.
18. Haidukewych GJ, Berry DJ. Hip arthroplasty for salvage of failed treatment of intertrochanteric hip fractures. *J Bone Joint Surg Am.* 2003;85-A(5):899-904.
19. Weinstein SL. Natural history and treatment outcomes of childhood hip disorders. *Clin Orthop Relat Res.* 1997;(344):227-242.
20. McAndrew MP, Weinstein SL. A long-term follow-up of Legg-Calve-Perthes disease. *J Bone Joint Surg Am.* 1984;66(6):860-869.
21. Mose K. Methods of measuring in Legg-Calve-Perthes disease with special regard to the prognosis. *Clin Orthop Relat Res.* 1980;(150):103-109.
22. Mose K, Hjorth L, Ulfeldt M, Christensen ER, Jensen A. Legg Calve Perthes disease. The late occurence of coxarthrosis. *Acta Orthopaedica Scandinavica.* Supplementum. 1977:169:1-39.
23. Gent E, Clarke NM. Joint replacement for sequelae of childhood hip disorders. *J Pediatr Orthop.* 2004;24(2):235-240.
24. Harris WH. Etiology of osteoarthritis of the hip. *Clin Orthop Relat Res.* 1986;(213):20-33.
25. Murray RO. The aetiology of primary osteoarthritis of the hip. *Br J Radiol.* 1965; 38(455):810-824.
26. Leunig M, Fraitzl CR, Ganz R. Early damage to the acetabular cartilage in slipped capital femoral epiphysis: therapeutic consequences. *Orthopade.* 2002;31(9):894-899.
27. Carney BT, Weinstein SL. Natural history of untreated chronic slipped capital femoral epiphysis. *Clin Orthop Relat Res.* 1996;(322):434-437.
28. Carney BT, Weinstein SL, Noble J. Long-term follow-up of slipped capital femoral epiphysis. *J Bone Joint Surg Am.* 1991;73(5):667-74.
29. Ganz R, Leunig M, Leunig-Ganz K, Harris WH. The etiology of osteoarthritis of the hip: an integrated mechanical concept. *Clin Orthop Relat Res.* 2008;466(2):264-272.
30. Ferguson DJ, Itonaga I, Maki M, McNally E, Gundle R, Athanasou NA. Heterotopic bone formation following hip arthroplasty in Paget's disease. *Bone.* 2004;34(6):1078-1083.
31. Hozack WJ, Rushton SA, Carey C, Sakalkale D, Rothman RH. Uncemented total hip arthroplasty in Paget's disease of the hip: a report of 5 cases with 5-year follow-up. *J Arthroplasty.* 1999;14(7):872-876.
32. Lewallen DG. Hip arthroplasty in patients with Paget's disease. *Clin Orthop Relat Res.* 1999;(369):243-250.
33. Lusty PJ, Walter WL, Walter WK, Zicat B. Cementless hip arthroplasty in Paget's disease at medium-term follow-up (average of 6.7 years). *J Arthroplasty.* 2007;22(5):692-696.
34. McDonald DJ, Sim FH. Total hip arthroplasty in Paget's disease. A follow-up note. *J Bone Joint Surg Am.* 1987;69(5):766-772.

35. Stauffer RN, Sim FH. Total hip arthroplasty in Paget's disease of the hip. *J Bone Joint Surg Am.* 1976;58(4):476-478.

36. Ludkowski P, Wilson-MacDonald J. Total arthroplasty in Paget's disease of the hip. A clinical review and review of the literature. *Clin Orthop Relat Res.* 1990;(255):160-167.

37. Sochart DH, Porter ML. Charnley low-friction arthroplasty for Paget's disease of the hip. *J Arthroplasty.* 2000;15(2):210-219.

38. Kirsh G, Kligman M, Roffman M. Hydroxyapatite-coated total hip replacement in Paget's disease: 20 patients followed for 4-8 years. *Acta Orthopaedica Scandinavica.* 2001;72(2):127-132.

39. Parvizi J, Schall DM, Lewallen DG, Sim FH. Outcome of uncemented hip arthroplasty components in patients with Paget's disease. *Clin Orthop Relat Res.* 2002;(403):127-134.

40. Goldblatt J, Sacks S, Dall D, Beighton P. Total hip arthroplasty in Gaucher's disease. Long-term prognosis. *Clin Orthop Relat Res.* 1988;(228):94-98.

41. Hendel D, Axer A. Total hip arthroplasty in Gaucher's disease. *Harefuah.* 1981;100(1):17-19.

42. Lebel E, Itzchaki M, Hadas-Halpern I, Zimran A, Elstein D. Outcome of total hip arthroplasty in patients with Gaucher disease. *J Arthroplasty.* 2001;16(1):7-12.

43. Frassica FJ, Wenz JF, Sim FH. *Parkinson's Disease.* In: Morrey BF, ed. *Reconstructive Surgery of the Joints.* 3rd ed. New York, NY: Churchill Livingstone; 2003:770-773.

44. Grisso JA, Kelsey JL, Strom BL, O'Brien LA, Maislin G, LaPann K, Samelson L, Hoffman S. Risk factors for hip fracture in black women. *N Engl J Med.* 1994;330(22):1555-1559.

45. Johnell O, Melton LJ III, Atkinson EJ, O'Fallon WM, Kurland LT. Fracture risk in patients with parkinsonism: a population-based study in Olmsted County, Minnesota. *Age Ageing.* 1992;21(1):32-38.

46. Weber M, Cabanela ME, Sim FH, Frassica FJ, Harmsen WS. Total hip replacement in patients with Parkinson's disease. *Int Orthop.* 2002;26(2):66-68.

30

Total Hip Arthroplasty
Wound Closure

G. Daxton Steele, MD, PharmD and Adolph J. Yates Jr, MD

It is with great peril that wound closure after total hip arthroplasty (THA) is often given minimal consideration. The act of suturing is commonly left for an assistant or the most junior resident. The conversation during closure is usually diverted from issues of technique to more casual topics. The literature concerning the avoidance of complications associated with prosthetic design or surgical approach is voluminous, whereas very few papers address issues and techniques concerning wound closure.

A cavalier attitude at the time of closing a hip arthroplasty belies the risks of prolonged wound drainage and/or dehiscence. Prolonged drainage causes longer hospital stays, and every day of late drainage has been reported as raising the risk of infection by 42%.[1] Although not as dramatic a complication as dislocation, failure of wound closure imposes a long, slow, and potentially more expensive course on the patient.

Patient Risk Factors

Preparation for successful wound closure can start as early as the day the patient is scheduled for surgery. Careful attention must be paid to potential risk factors for wound healing. Morbid obesity is clearly associated with a higher risk for drainage[1] and is rarely not appreciated. Ideally, the morbidly obese patient is asked to undergo weight loss or even bariatric surgery but this is not always feasible given the pain and immobility caused by the affected hip. Steroid use, rheumatoid arthritis, and diabetes all contribute to risk; tapering steroids, holding immunosuppressive drugs, and gaining good control of glucose levels can improve the odds for uncomplicated wound healing.

An often overlooked but more reversible risk is malnutrition. Factors that can be used to assess this include total lymphocyte counts, prealbumin, albumin, protein, transferase, and other serum levels. Nutritional supplementation, both before and after surgery can help to decrease complications.[2]

Improving Closure Through Careful Exposure

A good closure starts with attention to detail during exposure. Old incisions need to be carefully assessed to avoid tenuous flaps or consideration for wound revision/excision. Cutting at a right angle and avoidance of sharply beveled edges requires attention to the local topography of the skin. Electrocoagulation near the skin edge should be pinpointed and assisted with fine forceps to avoid burned tissue.

Deep exposure through a posterior approach should include leaving an appropriate cuff of tissue for posterior repair of the external rotators. Similar cuffs of tissue can facilitate closure of anterolateral and lateral approaches. During all layers of the approach, hemostasis should be carefully maintained.[3] Many potential postoperative bleeders are temporarily made less apparent by distraction/compression from retractors and/or lower intraoperative blood pressure.

Parvizi J, Klatt BA.
Essentials in Total Hip Arthroplasty (pp 265-268).

Incision length and wound healing requires a balanced approach. The length of the wound has been positively correlated with more postoperative drainage.[3] Mini incisions, however, have been blamed for less desirable wound healing.[4] Reducing the length of the initial incision is desirable but not to the point of jeopardizing the wound margins and the actual implantation of the prosthesis; less experienced surgeons should always be ready to widen their exposure if the skin or surgery appears to be potentially compromised.

Preparation for Closure

A routine protocol for closing after prosthetic insertion should involve several steps before the actual sutures. Hemostasis, irrigation, drains, and positioning are all to be considered in these few moments.

Even the most careful attention to hemostasis during exposure can still leave bleeders that can become apparent after removal of retractors and final reduction of the hip. Special attention should be given to the lateral circumflex as well as potential bleeding in the gluteal muscles. There are also early reports on various fibrin sealants as adjuvants for bone and wound hemostasis that show promise in reducing bleeding and thus hematoma formation.[5-7]

Copious irrigation is important, especially after longer or more difficult cases where the risk of contamination rises. Antibiotics are often used in the irrigation fluid, but their risk/benefit ratio in orthopedics,[8] let alone hip arthroplasty,[9] has yet to be fully demonstrated. It is common practice in our operating room to use pulse lavage as the method of delivery of the irrigation. One study involving hemiarthroplasty for femoral neck fractures showed a significant reduction in deep infection rates when more than 2 L of pulse lavage was used in comparison to bulb syringe irrigation.[10]

Placement of a drain remains controversial with guardedly more support for not using drains than there is for their use.[11] Studies have shown variably: no difference except the need to reinforce the wounds of the undrained hips[12]; no differences[13,14]; no differences except for more blood loss in the drained hips[15]; and more infections and transfusions in the drained hips.[16] In one meta-analysis of 18 investigations, there was no overall difference in outcomes other than a trend toward more bruising and a higher incidence of needing to reinforce wounds for drainage in the undrained hips. The authors felt that there were too few patients in any or all of the studies to show a lack of benefit from the use of a drain, especially in terms of the low-incidence complication of infection.[11] One of the authors (AJY) has had a positive anecdotal experience using a drain but leaving it over the fascia. This helps to diminish the postoperative drainage and reduces hematoma formation in the fat layer without the more significant loss of blood from leaving the drain subfascial. It is also felt to have a positive effect in helping to seal the fat layer to the fascial closure helping to obtain an earlier seal than if the drain was left in the more cavernous subfascial space.

Positioning of the leg can improve both the efficacy and the efficiency of the deep and fascial closures. A padded Mayo stand can be used to support the knee and lower leg in a more abducted position helping to close the fascia as well as diminishing the tension on the abductors when an anterolateral or lateral approach is used. The use of towels under the foot can help in the repair of the muscle cuffs with internal rotation assisting the reattachment of the gluteus medius for an anterolateral approach and external rotation assisting the reattachment of the external rotators for a posterior approach.

Deep Wound Closure

The closure of hip wounds involves a deep muscle layer of closure for both the posterior and anterolateral/lateral approaches, each carrying technical challenges.

The historical higher incidence of dislocation through the posterior approach has led to more attention to the deep closure with some form of deep posterior repair having become the norm when possible. The posterior capsular repair coupled with reattachment of the external rotators and the piriformis has been demonstrated in more than one study to lower the incidence of posterior dislocation.[17,18]

The actual success rate of such closure has been called into doubt. One study used radiopaque tantalum balls to mark the intervals of the repair of the short external rotators with heavy nonabsorbable suture through drill holes in bone; 70% of the repairs were demonstrated to fail, with half of the repairs having shown failure within the first day.[19] Enhanced repairs using a Krackow locking loop stitch[20] and another utilizing FiberWire (Arthrex, Inc, Naples, FL) have been reported,[21] but without any methodology to demonstrate survival of the repairs. Despite the question of the muscular repair failing to remain anatomic, the overall success rate of posterior repair in reducing dislocations has been replicated enough times to warrant continued use.

The lateral and anterolateral approaches require careful attention to retrieval and repair of the gluteus medius and vastus lateralis sleeves, both of which will retract anteriorly under the often thickened bursal layer of the hip. With a lateral approach, the true cuff of the gluteus medius needs to be repaired to bone with heavy nonabsorbable sutures through bone. The more proximal reapproximation of the split in the medius can be accomplished with a number 2-0 absorbable suture such as Vicryl (Ethicon, Johnson & Johnson, Somerville, NJ). An anterolateral approach needs interrupted suture repair with absorbable suture through the cuff portion of the exposure and subsequent running repair of the muscle-to-muscle intervals of the gluteus medius and vastus lateralis. An incompetent or avulsed greater trochanter has been described as being salvaged through an interpositional gluteus maximus flap transfer.[22]

The fascia lata is a critical layer in the defense of the prosthetic hip from the external environment, but it is frequently a layer put into more tension from the reconstruction due to the restoration of offset and length. Heavy nonabsorbable sutures in this plane can be irritable to very thin patients and the already relatively high rate of trochanteric bursitis after hip arthroplasty can be worsened by heavier suture retained on the other side. As such, multiple figures of 8 absorbable number 2-0 sutures are used with an emphasis on good, consistent approximation of the edges. Early in the repair, especially if there is not an assistant, a towel clamp can be used to approximate the edges, making the locking down of the suture easier. As already discussed, raising the leg into greater abduction can also help to approximate the layers with less tension. If a split was performed for exposure, a horizontal, or "u," stitch will be most efficient because of the direction of the fascia's fibers.

Superficial Wound Closure

After closure, the subcutaneous fat and skin closures remain. Careful attention must be given to both; even if the deep layer is sealed, a draining wound from failure of the superficial layers can lead to longer hospitalizations and infection, ultimately jeopardizing the reconstruction.

Repair of at least one layer of the subcutaneous fat is advisable in the obese, especially if a drain is not going to be used. A prospective study of patients treated with hemiarthroplasty after hip fracture looked at the use of a fat stitch (2-0 Vicryl) when a drain was not used. The group that did not have a fat stitch had a significantly higher rate of complications (33%) compared to the fat stitch group (6.8%).[23] Even with the use of a drain, a fat plane closure is recommended in the obese patient.

The deep dermal layer is routinely approximated using interrupted 2-0 absorbable sutures such as Vicryl or an equivalent. Care at this point must be given to wound edge handling with the use of fine skin forceps being mandatory. Once a few sutures are in place to take advantage of any preoperative markings to assist closure, adhesive occlusive dressings should be peeled back to better watch for external skin penetration or "buttonholes." Good approximation does not mean strangulation with simple sutures being the norm. Poorly approximated edges and "dog ears" should not be accepted at this level since they are not adequately addressed with the final subcuticular or transcutaneous layer of closure, whatever the technique used.

The final layer of closure can consist of staples, subcuticular sutures, or octyl cyanoacrylate (OCA). Evidence can be quoted to support any of the 3. One blinded, prospective, randomized trial looked at these 3 techniques and found no overall difference in hip arthroplasty wounds except for the speed of closure with staples.[24] Another study, however, reported a higher complication rate using skin staples in comparison to subcutaneous Vicryl.[25] Our routine is the use of a subcuticular running 4-0 monofilament absorbable suture (Monocryl [Ethicon]) supplemented with Steri-Strips (3M, St. Paul, MN). We make exceptions when the skin is very thin, such as in rheumatoid or steroid-dependent patients; staples, if not interrupted nylons, are more appropriate.

The final layer of closure often revolves around the different needs of a practice. The speed of closure with staples is advantageous in terms of length of case and duration of anesthetic. There is, however, a tendency for low-grade erythema to become apparent around retained staples in more fair-skinned patients, which can lead to undue concerns for family, visiting nurses, and outside physicians unfamiliar with surgical wounds. This can lead to inappropriate starting of antibiotics and unnecessary anxiety. Staples in a wound with local swelling can act as small stents for serous drainage; removal of staples at around day 7 can paradoxically cause a decrease in superficial drainage. Ideally, the patient returns within the first 2 weeks for staple removal.

A subcuticular closure does add time to the operative procedure but it carries some advantages. In a practice with a wide geographic distribution, the patient's first return can be at a later date such as 3 weeks. Time lost in the operating room is gained in the office where time is not needed for staple removal. Suture line care is also simplified at home. Staples can also be removed by home nursing at 2 weeks with follow-up only required when the nursing staff is uncertain of the wound's integrity.

The use of OCA is the least validated in terms of specifically hip arthroplasty. The limited literature does not allow firm recommendations. Interrupted nylons remain an acceptable alternative repair, especially in complicated incisions or wound revisions.

Summary

Safe closure of the wound after hip arthroplasty requires forethought and more than skill with suture. Minimizing preoperative risks, preparing for closure during exposure, maximization of the local environment at the time of closure, and careful selection of techniques all play into minimizing wound complications. A dry wound that heals uneventfully greatly diminishes the risks of more profound complications.

References

1. Patel VP, Walsh M, Bantoo S, Preston C, Hargovind DW, Di Cesare Pe. Factors associated with prolonged wound drainage after primary total hip and knee arthroplasty. *J Bone and Joint Surg Am.* 2007;89(1):33-38.
2. Lavernia CJ, Sierra RJ, Baerga MS. Nutritional parameters and short term outcome in arthroplasty. *J Am Coll Nutr.* 1999;18(3):274-278.
3. Wood JJ, Bevis PM, Bannister GC. Wound oozing after total hip arthroplasty. *Ann R Coll Surg Engl.* 2007;89:140-142.
4. Mow CS, Woolson ST, Ngarmukos SG, Park EH, Lorenz HP. Comparison of scars from total hip replacements done with a standard or a mini-incision. *Clin Orthop Relat Res.* 2005;441:80-85.
5. Lassen MR, Solgaard S, Kjersgaard AG, Olsen C, Lind B, Mittet, K, Ganes HC. A pilot study of the effects of Vivostat patient-derived fibrin sealant in reducing blood loss in primary hip arthroplasty. *Clin Appl Thromb Hemos.* 2006;12(3):352-357.
6. Mawatari M, Higo T, Tsutsumi Y, Shigematsu M, Hotokebuchi T. Effectiveness of autologous fibrin tissue adhesive in reducing postoperative blood loss during total hip arthroplasty: a prospective randomized study of 100 cases. *J Orthop Surg (Hong Kong).* 2006;14(2):117-121.
7. Wang GJ, Goldthwaite CA Jr, Burks S, Crawford R, Spotnitz WD; Orthopaedic Investigators Group. Fibrin sealant reduces perioperative blood loss in total hip replacement. *J Long Term Eff Med Implants.* 2003;3(5):399-411.
8. Anglen JO. Wound irrigation in musculoskeletal injury. *J Am Acad Orthop Surg.* 2001;9(4):219-226.
9. Hanssen AD, Osmon DR. The use of prophylactic antimicrobial agents during and after total hip arthroplasty. *Clin Orthop Relat Res.* 1999;369:124-138.
10. Hargrove R, Ridgeway S, Russell R, Norris M, Packham I, Levy B. Does pulse lavage reduce hip hemiarthroplasty infection rates? *J Hosp Infect.* 2006:62(4):446-449.
11. Parker MJ, Roberts CP, Hay D. Closed suction drainage for hip and knee arthroplasty. *J Bone and Joint Surg Am.* 2004;86(6):1146-1152.
12. Niskanen RO, Korkala OL, Haapala J, Kuokkanen HO, Kaukonen JP, Salo SA. Drainage is of no use in primary uncomplicated cemented hip and knee arthroplasty for osteoarthritis: a prospective randomized study. *J Arthroplasty.* 2000;15(5):567-569.
13. Crevoisier XM, Reber P, Noesberger B. Is suction drainage necessary after total joint arthroplasty? *Arch Orthop Trauma Surg.* 1998;117:121-124.
14. Kumar S, Penematsa S, Parekh S. Are drains required following a routine primary total joint arthroplasty? *Int Orthop.* 2007;31:593-596.
15. Gonzalez Della Valle A, Slullitel G, Vestri R, Comba F, Buttaro M, Piccaluga F. No need for routine closed suction drainage in elective arthroplasty of the hip: a prospective randomized trial in 104 operations. *Acta Orthop Scand.* 2004;75(1):30-33.
16. Walmsley PJ, Kell MB, Hill RMF, Brenkel I. A prospective, randomized, controlled trial of the use of drains in total hip arthroplasty. *J Bone and Joint Surg Br.* 2005;87-B:1397-1401.
17. Chiu FY, Chen CM, Chung TY, Lo WH, Chen TH. The effect of posterior capsulorrhaphy in primary total hip arthroplasty. *J Arthroplasty.* 2000;15(2):194-199.
18. Weeden SH, Paprosky WG, Bowling JW. The early dislocation rate in primary total hip arthroplasty following the posterior approach with posterior soft-tissue repair. *J Arthroplasty.* 2003;18(6):709-713.
19. Stahelin T, Vienne P, Hersche O. Failure of reinserted short external rotator muscles after total hip arthroplasty. *J Arthroplasty.* 2002;17(5):604-607.
20. Ko CK, Law SW, Chiu KH. Enhanced soft tissue repair using locking loop stitch after posterior approach for hip hemiarthroplasty. *J Arthroplasty.* 2001;16(2):207-211.
21. Osmani O, Malkani A. Posterior capsular repair following total hip arthroplasty: a modified technique. *Orthopedics.* 2004;27(6):553-555.
22. Whiteside LA, Nayfeh T, Katerberg BJ. Gluteus maximus flap transfer for greater trochanter reconstruction in revision THA. *Clin Orthop Relat Res.* 2006;453:203-210.
23. Lemon M, Bali SL, Ibery N, Elliott DS, Khaleel A. Is a fat stitch required when closing a hip hemiarthroplasty wound without a drain? *Injury.* 2006;37:190-193.
24. Khan RJK, Fick D, Yao F, Tang K, Hurworth M, Nivbrant B, Wood D. A comparison of three methods of wound closure following arthroplasty; A prospective, randomized, controlled trial. *J Bone and Joint Surg Br.* 2006;88B(2):238-242.
25. Shetty AA, Kumar VS, Morgan-Hough C, Georgeu GA, James KD, Nicholl JE. Comparing wound complication rates following closure of hip wounds with metallic skin staples or subcuticular vicryl suture: a prospective randomized trial. *J Orthop Surg.* 2004;12(2):191-193.

31

Rehabilitation After Total Hip Arthroplasty

Kristen Hines, PT; Erika Davis, MD; Katie O'Shea, PT, DPT, MBA; and Kristen Vogl, PT, DPT

The Initial Evaluation of the Presurgical Patient

Rehabilitation for total hip arthroplasty (THA) may begin with the presurgical patient. The initial evaluation by a physical therapist should address the following:

- Strength and range of motion in the affected and contralateral hip
- Knee and ankle joints bilaterally; strength, range of motion (ROM), previous injuries
- Assessment of gait pattern; is an assistive device used at baseline? Are there any gait deviations noted?
- Upper extremity strength potential and ROM; carpal tunnel syndrome?
- Neurological status
- Vital signs
- Endurance functional level; patient's baseline activity level? Has pain significantly affected quality of life or was patient less active at baseline?
- Leg lengths should be measured prior to surgery; did the patient use shoe orthotics?
- Contractures and deformities; scoliosis? Pelvic/sacroiliac joint laxity? Does the patient use bracing to accommodate?

The therapist must keep in mind that patients with degenerative joint disease typically develop joint stiffness after rest and this may limit assessment of ROM in extension, internal rotation, and extreme flexion. Spasms of the adductor, flexor, and external rotator muscles can lead to contractures and joint deformity. Finally, the muscles surrounding the hip, namely gluteus maximus and the adductor muscles, may be atrophied due to decreased activity. Joint crepitus and grating is common prior to surgery and a moderate effusion may be present within the joint preoperatively. Secondary to the above musculoskeletal deficits, the therapist should anticipate gait deviations, assistive device use, and decreased participation in community activities.

Preoperative Training

The preoperative training session can be extremely beneficial by reducing the length of hospital stay and improving cooperation during the postoperative period secondary to decreased anxiety. Some institutions may even supply patients with educational videos on postoperative exercises and transfers prior to surgery. The therapist may consider performing the preoperative training in the patient's home so safety adaptations can be made for the postsurgical period. If the patient is to be placed on hip precautions after surgery, they should be taught and understood at this time. Hip precautions are measures that are aimed at reducing the incidence of dislocation of the hip. They avoid placing the hip in the position where it is most likely to dislocate during the acute postoperative period. The therapist must be aware of the approach to the hip to apply these properly. Some surgeons are no longer using hip precautions after surgery,

Parvizi J, Klatt BA.
Essentials in Total Hip Arthroplasty (pp 269-275).

so this issue may require clarification from the surgeon. For patients without precautions, the patients are instructed to use the hip as comfort dictates.

Hip Precautions (Posterolateral Approach)

These precautions are intended to avoid overstressing the posterior capsular and short rotator muscle repair during the early stages of healing. It is a combination of flexion, internal rotation, and adduction that will maximally stress the posterolateral approach.

- Avoid flexion past 90 degrees
- Avoid adduction past the body's midline
- Avoid internal rotation of the hip

Hip Precautions (Anterolateral Approach)

These measures intend to minimize stressing the anterior musculature. It is a combination of extension, adduction, and external rotation that will stress the anterolateral approach.

- Avoid extension
- Avoid adduction past the body's midline
- Avoid external rotation

The proper use of assistive devices following surgery should be addressed also at this time. The patient will aim for twice daily physical therapy sessions following surgery, although it is important to progress the patient based on his or her comfort level and musculoskeletal ability. Sessions range from 30 to 45 min in length.

Exercises that can be taught during the preoperative training session include the following:

- Ankle pumps
- Quadriceps sets
- Gluteal sets
- Heel slides (supine and sitting)
- Short arc quads
- Long arc quads
- Isometric hip abduction*
- Active hip abduction*

*The usefulness of hip abduction exercises in THA patients is debatable and largely institution-dependent. Surgeons who perform the anterolateral approach usually prefer not to stress the abductor repair in the acute postoperative period. Resistive abduction in these patients is avoided for at least the first 8 weeks postoperatively.

The patient should be made aware that it is possible to dislocate the new prosthesis if inappropriate activities are attempted after surgery. The best way to prevent this complication is strong adherence to musculoskeletal recovery and respect of pain limitations.

Recently there has been some controversy over the traditional rehabilitation exercises following total hip replacement surgery. The contact pressures on the hip joint during straight leg raises, isometric hip extension, and active hip flexion were shown to produce the greatest stress on the joint. It is feared that these exercises may cause dislocation in the postoperative patient.[1,2] Therapy should be focused on neuromuscular re-education of the hip, knee, and ankle joints. Overall, emphasis should be placed on mobility over strength and no resistance training or weight training should be used in these patients.

Postoperative Day 0

Goal: Sitting Upright

Rehabilitation can begin the same day of surgery once the patient has recovered from anesthesia. The physical therapist should contact the nurse to perform a screen for presence of residual spinal block and symptoms of orthostatic hypotension secondary to anesthesia. If the spinal block is still causing sensory and/or motor deficits, physical therapy (PT) evaluation will be initiated in the morning of postoperative day 1 (POD 1). If there is no presence of spinal block, nursing staff may proceed to mobilize the patient to the edge of the bed or sitting upright in bed with the head of bed elevated 90 degrees for 5 min with stable vital signs. Stable vital signs include blood pressure change > or <20 mm from baseline and/or symptoms of orthostatic hypotension, nausea, vomiting, and dizziness. After screening, nursing may address the patient's symptoms with appropriate intervention (ie, fluid bolus, nausea, pain medication) to facilitate the patient's tolerance of the upcoming PT evaluation. Also, patients should be instructed on the use of an incentive spirometer at this time.

In order to initiate PT/occupational therapy (OT) evaluations, the following must be clearly documented in physician orders:

- Activity orders (ie, activity as tolerated, out of bed [OOB] with assist)
- PT/OT orders
- Weight bearing status orders (ie, toe touch weight bearing [TTWB], partial weight bearing [PWB], weight bearing as tolerated [WBAT])

- Total hip precautions (THP) orders as needed
- ROM restriction orders, as needed
- Hip abduction brace orders, as needed
- Oxygen titration/wean orders and parameters

The physical therapist should find the postoperative patient resting supine perhaps with an adductor pillow between the legs to prevent adduction. Ankle pumps, quadriceps sets, and gluteal sets can be initiated at this time. Ankle circles should be avoided at this time as the patient may inadvertently rotate the whole limb. The therapist should include foot and ankle ROM exercises in addition to strengthening exercises for the upper body and nonoperated lower limb. Isometric exercises of the major muscle groups on the operated side should be initiated also. Patient education should include proper transfer techniques for moving in bed. Traditionally, the patient should be moved toward the nonoperated side during bed activities and transfers at this stage. The therapist may assist the patient in moving from supine to sitting and from sitting to standing. The therapist can transfer the patient to an elevated chair cautiously while avoiding positions of hip instability. The patient should be able to sit upright for 30 to 60 min. The patient should be repositioned with the abductor pillow every few hours to prevent pressure ulcers and thromboembolic disease. Placing a knee immobilizer on the affected leg at this time may be helpful if the patient is groggy or prone to forgetting ROM precautions. Submaximal contraction of muscles is recommended in order to place the least amount of stress on the hip joint. One study recommends repeating lower extremity exercises 10 times per hour.[3]

Adequate pain control is essential to a good recovery. This can be accomplished in a variety of ways, which are described in further detail in Chapter 20. Additionally, ice is used as a vasoconstrictor throughout the first few postoperative days to decrease swelling and slow mechanisms of pain production.

Patients who have been advised by the treating physician to follow traditional hip precautions will need the following activities modified accordingly:

- Transfers: getting OOB, a chair, a car, etc; elevated surfaces will be more mechanically efficient
- Bed mobility/sleeping: patient positions during sleep are often awkward, involving some degree of flexion, adduction, and rotation of the hips
- Dressing and washing of the involved extremity: patients will need to be retrained with a temporary modified approach to activities of daily living (ADLs)
- Elevated toilet seat
- Place a pillow between legs when sleeping on side for about 3 months when muscle tone has increased

The role of OT is to evaluate and treat patients who are targeted for home discharge. OT will teach ADLs until patients reach their discharge goals. Patients who are going to rehab facilities will receive OT services at the rehab facility, unless social work or case management alerts OT that a precertification is needed to obtain insurance authorization for transfer. PT and OT will make an immediate assessment of the approximate number of PT and OT treatment sessions that are recommended to achieve goals set at the initial evaluation and to enable timely discharge planning by the interdisciplinary team. OT does not typically evaluate patients until POD 2.

Postoperative Day 1

Goals: Gait Training, Ambulation With Walker, Out of Bed to Chair

Patients who were unable to get up on day 0 or had a later surgery are evaluated by the physical therapist on POD 1 in the morning. The evaluation includes general ROM assessment of upper and lower extremities with specific ROM and manual muscle test of the operated extremity: pain, cognitive screening, sensation, balance, vital sign response, bed mobility, transfers, and ambulation. The goal is OOB to chair on POD 1 using a bilateral upper extremity assistive device such as a walker. If the patient is unable to stand up during the initial evaluation, the physical therapist may see the patient again in the afternoon to try to accomplish this. Of note, patients can get in or out of bed on either side of the bed, although it is usually less painful to transfer towards the operated side.

Gait training can be started in the parallel bars as soon as the patient is able to sit upright comfortably without getting dizzy or nauseous. The stance phase can be practiced as TTWB, PWB, or WBAT depending on the surgeon's orders. Adherence to weight bearing status established by the surgeon is imperative for proper recovery. WBAT allows patients to return to their normal and highest level of functioning in the timeliest fashion; however, the orthopedic surgeon may initially assign obese patients to a restricted weight-bearing status. This is because of the risk of dislocation secondary to increased loading forces if a larger patient were to fall. There are also concerns that the stem may not grow into the bone properly if the forces through the stem are too great. The patient may also begin heel slides and isometric or active assistive hip abduction with submaximal force while continuing to avoid internal rotation.

The physical therapist can begin active ROM at this time doing the following:

- Avoiding adduction
- Limiting flexion to 30 degrees
- Avoiding extension if anterior surgical approach is taken
- Avoiding resisted abduction for 8 weeks if trochanteric osteotomy is done

The majority of patients will be ready for ambulation with a bilateral upper extremity assistive device on POD 1. A front-wheeled rolling walker is useful in gait training for older patients whereas younger patients may use crutches or a cane if capable. Patients who have undergone a bilateral total hip replacement can be instructed in the 4-point crutch pattern in addition to a rolling walker. However, the therapist must be mindful of the patient's weight-bearing status as assistive device selection relates to it. The patient should be able to walk on a level surface for 100 ft before being discharged home. Emphasis of gait training includes heel strike and toe off as to promote recovery of natural gait cycle.

It is important to note that the physical therapist should document blood pressure and heart rate response to all initial position changes in the medical record. If a hypotensive episode necessitates holding a patient's treatment session, the therapist should plan to revisit the patient in the afternoon and inform the nurse and doctor.

Postoperative Days 2 to 4

Goals: Transfers and Gait Normalization/Independence

During this time period, patients are discharged home or to a rehabilitation facility. Patients should be reminded of home instructions related to commode transfers and automobile transfers at this time if for discharge home. Physical therapists can continue all previous exercises twice daily until transfer or discharge. Hip flexion generally can be progressed to 60 degrees on day 6 and to 90 degrees on day 10 pending the surgeon's protocol. However, the patient is not to exceed 90 degrees of flexion. A step-to-gait pattern may be encouraged starting day 3. The patient should be taught to negotiate stair ascent with the unaffected leg and descent with the affected (operated) leg.

If possible, patients will come to the therapy gym areas starting on POD 2. The evaluating physical therapist will determine which patients are allowed to travel to the gym. Typical requirements include the ability to tolerate at least 1 hour OOB with appropriate vital sign responses to activity. These patients should receive one PT session in the gym and the second session either in the gym or bedside as appropriate. If the evaluating therapist deems that the patient is unable to tolerate therapy in the gym, the patient can be seen bedside for both sessions. Treatment should continue at the bedside until gym tolerance is established.

Importantly, hip precaution instruction (if ordered) continues until the patient can either demonstrate independence, has appropriate assistance/supervision at home, or rehab transfer occurs. Stair-climbing instruction can occur as the patient tolerates, keeping in mind that patients must have at least unilateral upper extremity support for all functional activities including stair climbing. Ultimately, the intensity and content of each patient's treatment sessions should vary to meet the needs of each individual.

Most hospitals have developed pathways. Patients on a pathway should be seen once daily until discharge. A patient is considered off-pathway if orthopedics is no longer their primary service or there was a medical change in status that caused a hold in treatment.

Return to Home

If a patient is returning directly home from the hospital, OT will perform an evaluation on POD 2. The evaluation is to assesses cognitive status, upper extremity strength and ROM, general ROM and strength screening of lower extremities, and ADLs (ie, toileting, upper and lower body washing, dressing using adaptive equipment as necessary [see below], and home management tasks [preparing meals, light laundry, etc]).

Commonly used adaptive equipment includes the following:

- Leg lifter
- Reacher
- Long-handled shoe horn
- Long-handled sponge
- Walker basket
- Elastic shoelaces

Patients arrive to surgery with an established discharge plan; however, it is important to confirm this plan by POD 2 to prevent confusion on discharge day. If the initial discharge plan is changed due to patient performance in therapy or medical complication, the therapist should notify case management, social work, and the orthopedic surgeon. PT or OT will continue to assess the patient's progress on a daily basis and modify discharge plans as needed.

Discharge criteria include the following:

- Home discharge
    - Independent ambulation with the appropriate assistive device on a level surface at least 100 feet
    - Independent transfers from bed, toilet, and chair
    - Independent ADL and appropriate home activities
    - Independent with total hip replacement precautions (as appropriate)
    - Supervision on stairs if required, otherwise independent
    - Independent with home exercise program
    - Independent with a car transfer
    - Appropriate assistance and supervision at home if not fully independent and family member has completed training
- Inpatient rehabilitation discharge
    - Minimum to maximum assistance with mobility (transfers, ambulation, stairs)
    - OOB tolerance >1 hour
    - Ambulation at least 5 feet with an assistive device

Patients who return home routinely receive a home PT referral with transition to outpatient PT after their staples are removed and incision well approximated. Staple removal will usually occur on the 12th to 14th day after surgery. PT will also issue the appropriate assistive device to patient prior to discharge. Commonly, case management will order commodes and set up home care referrals and OT will arrange for and issue appropriate adaptive materials.

Patients can travel home via car provided they are able to safely perform a car transfer. If the physical therapist or physician determines the patient is unsafe to travel via car, alternative transportation should be arranged by case management. Instructing the patient to move the seat as far back from the dashboard as possible and recline the seat to approximately a 70-degree angle will make this position more comfortable.

In summary, the patient with precautions should be instructed to avoid specific activities and positions. The patient should not sit in low chairs, sleep on their sides, cross legs, flex his or her hips more than 90 degrees, force his or her hips to bend, drive, sit in the bottom of a bath tub, squat, or do any exercises not given by the physical therapist. Three to 4 weeks after surgery the patient may progress from a walker or crutches to a single-point cane. The patient will be seen for a follow-up appointment with his or her orthopedic surgeon in 4 to 6 weeks. At that time, some of these restrictions may be lifted. Complications that warrant a referral back to the orthopedic surgeon include symptoms of intermittent claudication (pain with walking that improves with rest), a positive Trendelenburg sign, wound infection, signs of thromboembolic disease, systemic symptoms indicating allergy or infection, or persistent severe pain.

Patients should be instructed to do the following:

- Use a pain medication prior to initiating exercise
- Use ice to assist with swelling 20 to 30 minutes at a time once an hour
- Perform home exercise program 3 times per day in 10-repetition sets
- Increase activity daily

The following includes common patient concerns prior to discharge:

- Sports: Running, jumping, football, basketball, karate, soccer, and heavy lifting should be avoided. Sports that the total hip replacement patient can look forward to include walking, swimming, bowling, golf, and cycling. Further investigation is being conducted as to what constitutes a safe sport after THA.
- New shoes should be worn after surgery so as not to continue previous abnormal gait.
- Stairs: Step-over-step stair climbing may be achieved during the home therapy phase.
- Driving: Patients can drive approximately 3 to 4 weeks after right total hip replacement. For a left hip replacement, driving can start earlier. The issues that determine the ability to drive are 1) patient must be off narcotics as driving while on narcotics could impair function, and 2) patient must have full control and reaction to stop vehicle in an emergency. Although some surgeons may want to release patients to drive at their discretion, others prefer this judgment to be made by the patient with an understanding of those 2 criteria. It is impossible for the surgeon to conduct a safety test and to evaluate each patient's ability to drive.
- Return to work: Most patients can return to work within the month as long as their jobs do not require heavy manual labor. Lifting should be limited to less than 10 lbs until 8 to 12 weeks after surgery.
- Sexual activity: It is acceptable to resume sexual activity in the supine position after an uncomplicated total hip replacement within 1 to 2 months. The

prone position may be assumed within 2 to 3 months following an uncomplicated total hip replacement. Handouts are available with suggestions for safe sexual positions.

Rapid Recovery Protocols

This chapter focuses on the most common rehabilitation path used after THA. There are newer, rapid recovery protocols that allow for a quicker recovery and an earlier discharge. Patients begin immediate weight bearing and transition to a cane on POD 1. Many centers are discharging THA patients on POD 1, and a select few centers are doing discharge on POD 0. The rapid recovery protocols compress what is done in the longer admissions into a day. They are dependent on healthy patients, good pain control, weight bearing as tolerated, and no hip precautions. These protocols will not work for all patients but have shown dramatic, rapid results when applied to the right patients.

References

1. Givens-Heiss DL, Krebs DE, Riley PO, et al. In vivo acetabular contact pressures during rehabilitation, part II: postacute phase. *Phys Ther.* 1992;72:700-705.
2. Foran, JRH. Joint replacement. American Academy of Orthopaedic Surgeons. URL: http://orthoinfo.aaos.org/menus/arthroplasty.cfm. Accessed August 2011.
3. Enloe LJ, Shields RK, Smith K, Leo K, Miller B. Total hip and knee replacement treatment programs: a report using consensus. *J Orthop Sports Phys Ther.* 1996;23:3-11.

Suggested Readings

Biring GS, Masri BA, Greidanus NV, Duncan CP, Garbuz DS. Predictors of quality of life outcomes after revision total hip replacement. *J Bone Joint Surg Br.* 2007;89:1446-1451.

Brander V, Stulberg SD. Rehabilitation after hip- and knee-joint replacement. An experience- and evidence-based approach to care. *Am J Phys Med Rehabil.* 2006;85:S98-118.

Brotzman SB, Wilk KE. *Clinical Orthopaedic Rehabilitation.* 2nd ed. Philadelphia, PA: Mosby, Inc; 2003.

Forrest G, Roque J, Dawodu S. Decreasing length of stay after total joint arthroplasty: effect on referrals to rehabilitation units. *Arch Phys Med Rehabil.* 1999;80(2):192-194.

Frost KL, Bertocci GE, Wassinger CA, Munin MC, Burdett RG, Fitzgerald SG. Isometric performance following total hip arthroplasty and rehabilitation. *J Rehabil Res Dev.* 2006;43:435-444.

Giaquinto S, Ciotola E, Margutti F, Valentini F. Gait during hydrokinesitherapy following total hip arthroplasty. *Disabil Rehabil.* 2007;29:743-749.

Hurkmans HL, Bussmann JB, Selles RW, Benda E, Stam HJ, Verhaar JA. The difference between actual and prescribed weight bearing of total hip patients with a trochanteric osteotomy: long-term vertical force measurements inside and outside the hospital. *Arch Phys Med Rehabil.* 2007;88:200-206.

Iyengar KP, Nadkarni JB, Ivanovic N, Mahale A. Targeted early rehabilitation at home after total hip and knee joint replacement: does it work? *Disabil Rehabil.* 2007;29:495-502.

Katz JN, Wright EA, Guadagnoli E, Liang MH, Karlson EW, Cleary PD. Differences between men and women undergoing major orthopaedic surgery for degenerative arthritis. *Arthritis Rheum.* 1994;37:687-694.

Klein GR, Levine BR, Hozack WJ, et al. Return to athletic activity after total hip arthroplasty. Consensus guidelines based on a survey of the hip society and american association of hip and knee surgeons. *J Arthroplasty.* 2007;22:171-175.

Kottke FJ, Lehmann JF. *Krusen's Handbook of Physical Medicine and Rehabilitation.* 4th ed. Philadelphia, PA: WB Saunders Company; 1990.

Krebs DE, Elbaum L, Riley PO, Hodge WA, Mann RW. Exercise and gait effects on in vivo hip contact pressures. *Phys Ther.* 1991;71:301-309.

Laupacis A, Bourne R, Rorabeck C, et al. The effect of elective total hip replacement on health-related quality of life. *J Bone Joint Surg Am.* 1993;75:1619-1626.

Levine B, Kaplanek B, Scafura D, Jaffe WL. Rehabilitation after total hip and knee arthroplasty: a new regimen using pilates training. *Bull NYU Hosp Jt Dis.* 2007;65:120-125.

Magee DJ. *Orthopedic Physical Assessment.* 4th ed. Philadelphia, PA: WB Saunders Company; 2002.

Maire J, Dugue B, Faillenet-Maire AF, et al. Influence of a 6-week arm exercise program on walking ability and health status after hip arthroplasty: a 1-year follow-up pilot study. *J Rehabil Res Dev.* 2006;43:445-450.

Maxey L, Magnusson J. *Rehabilitation for the Postsurgical Orthopedic Patient.* St. Louis, MO: Mosby, Inc; 2001.

McGrory BJ, Stuart MJ, Sim FH. Participation in sports after hip and knee arthroplasty: review of literature and survey of surgeon preferences. *Mayo Clin Proc.* 1995;70:342-348.

Michlovitz S, Nolan T. *Modalities for Therapeutic Intervention (Contemporary Perspectives in Rehabilitation).* 4th ed. Philadelphia, PA: FA Davis Company; 2005.

Munin MC, Kwoh CK, Glynn N, Crossett L, Rubash HE. Predicting discharge outcome after elective hip and knee arthroplasty. *Am J Phys Med Rehabil.* 1995;74:294-301.

Ng CY, Ballantyne JA, Brenkel IJ. Quality of life and functional outcome after primary total hip replacement. A five-year follow-up. *J Bone Joint Surg Br.* 2007;89:868-873.

O'Donnell S, Kennedy D, MacLeod AM, Kilroy C, Gollish J. Achieving team consensus on best practice rehabilitation guidelines following primary total hip replacement (THR) surgery. *Healthc Q.* 2006;9:60-64.

Ranawat AS, Ranawat CS. Pain management and accelerated rehabilitation for total hip and total knee arthroplasty. *J Arthroplasty.* 2007;22:12-15.

Richardson JK, Iglarsh ZA. *Clinical Orthopaedic Physical Therapy.* Philadelphia, PA: WB Saunders Company; 1994.

Santavirta N, Lillqvist G, Sarvimaki A, Honkanen V, Konttinen YT, Santavirta S. Teaching of patients undergoing total hip replacement surgery. *Int J Nurs Stud.* 1994;31:135-142.

Stern SH, Fuchs MD, Ganz SB, Classi P, Sculco TP, Salvati EA. Sexual function after total hip arthroplasty. *Clin Orthop Relat Res.* 1991:228-235.

Stevens M, Wagenmakers R, Groothoff JW, Bulstra SK, van den Akker-Scheek I, Zijlstra W. Physical activity behavior after total hip arthroplasty (THA): a prediction based on patient characteristics. *Patient Educ Couns.* 2007;69:196-199.

Strickland EM, Fares M, Krebs DE, et al. In vivo acetabular contact pressures during rehabilitation, part I: acute phase. *Phys Ther.* 1992;72:691-699.

Strom H, Nilsson O, Milbrink J, Mallmin H, Larsson S. The effect of early weight bearing on migration pattern of the uncemented CLS stem in total hip arthroplasty. *J Arthroplasty.* 2007;22:1122-1129.

Unlu E, Eksioglu E, Aydog E, Aydog ST, Atay G. The effect of exercise on hip muscle strength, gait speed and cadence in patients with total hip arthroplasty: a randomized controlled study. *Clin Rehabil.* 2007;21:706-711.

van den Akker-Scheek I, Stevens M, Groothoff JW, Bulstra SK, Zijlstra W. Preoperative or postoperative self-efficacy: which is a better predictor of outcome after total hip or knee arthroplasty? *Patient Educ Couns.* 2007;66:92-99.

Vincent HK, Weng JP, Vincent KR. Effect of obesity on inpatient rehabilitation outcomes after total hip arthroplasty. *Obesity (Silver Spring).* 2007;15:522-530.

Vincent KR, Vincent HK, Lee LW, Weng J, Alfano AP. Outcomes after inpatient rehabilitation of primary and revision total hip arthroplasty. *Arch Phys Med Rehabil.* 2006;87:1026-1032.

Wiklund I, Romanus B. A comparison of quality of life before and after arthroplasty in patients who had arthrosis of the hip joint. *J Bone Joint Surg Am.* 1991;73:765-769.

Zavadak KH, Gibson KR, Whitley DM, Britz P, Kwoh CK. Variability in the attainment of functional milestones during the acute care admission after total joint replacement. *J Rheumatol.* 1995;22:482-487.

Financial Disclosures

Dr. Christopher S. Adams has no financial or proprietary interest in the materials presented herein.

Dr. Matt Austin has not disclosed any relevant financial relationships.

Dr. Khalid Azzam has no financial or proprietary interest in the materials presented herein.

Dr. Robert L. Barrack has not disclosed any relevant financial relationships.

Dr. Ravi K. Bashyal has no financial or proprietary interest in the materials presented herein.

Dr. Benjamin Bender has not disclosed any relevant financial relationships.

Dr. Hari P. Bezwada receives research support from the Genzyme speaker's bureau and is a consultant for Zimmer.

Dr. Orhan Bican has not disclosed any relevant financial relationships.

Dr. James Cashman has no financial or proprietary interest in the materials presented herein.

Dr. Michael E. Ciminiello has not disclosed any relevant financial relationships.

Dr. Erika Davis has no financial or proprietary interest in the materials presented herein.

Dr. Craig J. Della Valle has not disclosed any relevant financial relationships.

Dr. Joshua C. Fox has no financial or proprietary interest in the materials presented herein.

Dr. Mitchell K. Freedman has no financial or proprietary interest in the materials presented herein.

Dr. Kishor Gandhi is a consultant for B. Braun Medical, Inc.

Dr. Elie Ghanem has no financial or proprietary interest in the materials presented herein.

Dr. Ashok Gowda has no financial or proprietary interest in the materials presented herein.

Dr. Eric L. Grossman has no financial or proprietary interest in the materials presented herein.

Dr. Sanaz Hariri has not disclosed any relevant financial relationships.

Dr. Kristen Huber has no financial or proprietary interest in the materials presented herein.

Dr. Pooya Hosseinzadeh has no financial or proprietary interest in the materials presented herein.

Dr. William J. Hozack is a consultant for and receives royalties from Stryker and is Editor in Chief of the *Journal of Arthroplasty.*

Dr. Ronald Huang has no financial or proprietary interest in the materials presented herein.

Dr. Michael H. Huo has not disclosed any relevant financial relationships.

Dr. S. Mehdi Jafari has no financial or proprietary interest in the materials presented herein.

Dr. Thomas K. John has no financial or proprietary interest in the materials presented herein.

Dr. Lauren K. Kahl has no financial or proprietary interest in the materials presented herein.

Dr. Brian A. Klatt has no financial or proprietary interest in the materials presented herein.

Dr. Steven Kurtz has not disclosed any relevant financial relationships.

Dr. Lawrence P. Lai has no financial or proprietary interest in the materials presented herein.

Dr. Eric Levicoff has not disclosed any relevant financial relationships.

Dr. Junaid Makda has not disclosed any relevant financial relationships.

Dr. Henrik Malchau has not disclosed any relevant financial relationships.

Dr. Michael Manley has not disclosed any relevant financial relationships.

Dr. Richard L. McGough III receives research support from DePuy/Johnson & Johnson.

Dr. Michael A. Mont has not disclosed any relevant financial relationships.

Dr. S.M. Javad Mortazavi has no financial or proprietary interest in the materials presented herein.

Dr. M.T. Newman has no financial or proprietary interest in the materials presented herein.

Dr. Ali Oliashirazi has not disclosed any relevant financial relationships.

Dr. Katie O'Shea has no financial or proprietary interest in the materials presented herein.

Dr. Javad Parvizi has nothing personally to disclose but as part of the Rothman Research Group, they disclose the following: research support from NIH, OREF, Stryker Orthopedics, DePuy, Zimmer, Baxter, 3M, Biomemetics, Ceramtec, and Smith and Nephew; consultants for Zimmer, Smith and Nephew, Convatech, TissueGene, Ceramtec, OsteoMEM, 3M, and Cadence; board members/advisers for the *Journal of Arthroplasty*, the Philadelphia Orthopaedic Society, the Eastern Orthopedic Association, United Healthcare, Magnifi Group (Publishers), 3M, and JBJS-A; and intellectual property/royalty/ownership from SmarTech, Elsevier, Wolters Kluwer, SLACK Incorporated, Hip Innovation Technology, CD Diagnostics, Jaypee Publishers, and Datatrace.

Dr. Brett Perricelli has not disclosed any relevant financial relationships.

Dr. Manny Porat has no financial or proprietary interest in the materials presented herein.

Dr. Luis Pulido has not disclosed any relevant financial relationships.

Dr. James J. Purtill has no financial or proprietary interest in the materials presented herein.

Dr. Aaron G. Rosenberg is a consultant for Medtronics and Zimmer and has royalty arrangements for intellectual property with Zimmer.

Dr. Adam J. Schwartz has no financial or proprietary interest in the materials presented herein.

Dr. Eric Schwenk has no financial or proprietary interest in the materials presented herein.

Dr. Thorsten M. Seyler has not disclosed any relevant financial relationships.

Dr. Peter F. Sharkey receives royalties from Knee Creations, Stryker Orthopedics, and StelKast, Inc; is on the speaker's bureau for Stryker and Knee Creations; is a paid consultant for Stryker, Knee Creations, and Arthrex; has stock or stock options in Physican Recommended Nutriceuticals and Knee Creations; receives research support as a PI from Convatec; is on the editorial/governing board of the *Journal of Arthropalsty*, the *American Journal of Orthopaedics*, and *Clinical Orthopaedics & Related Research;* and is a board member of the American Association of Hip and Knee Surgeons.

Dr. Eric B. Smith has not disclosed any relevant financial relationships.

Dr. Bryan D. Springer has not disclosed any relevant financial relationships.

Dr. G. Daxton Steele has not disclosed any relevant financial relationships.

Dr. Eugene R. Viscusi is a consultant and on advisory boards for AcelRx, Cadence, Incline, Pacira, Salix, Cubist, Purdue, and Merck, and is a speaker for Cadence. Thomas Jefferson University receives grants from Adolor, Cadence, and AcelRx.

Dr. Kristen Vogl has no financial or proprietary interest in the materials presented herein.

Dr. Adolf J. Yates Jr has no financial or proprietary interest in the materials presented herein.

Dr. Khalid M. Yousuf has not disclosed any relevant financial relationships.

Index